Dermatology

Editor

ROY M. COLVEN

MEDICAL CLINICS OF NORTH AMERICA

www.medical.theclinics.com

Consulting Editors
DOUGLAS S. PAAUW
EDWARD R. BOLLARD

November 2015 • Volume 99 • Number 6

ELSEVIER

1600 John F. Kennedy Boulevard • Suite 1800 • Philadelphia, Pennsylvania, 19103-2899

http://www.theclinics.com

MEDICAL CLINICS OF NORTH AMERICA Volume 99, Number 6
November 2015 ISSN 0025-7125, ISBN-13: 978-0-323-41456-2

Editor: Jessica McCool
Developmental Editor: Alison Swety

Medical Clinics of North America (ISSN 0025-7125) is published bimonthly by Elsevier Inc., 360 Park Avenue South, New York, NY 10010-1710. Months of publication are January, March, May, July, September, and November. Business and editorial offices: 1600 John F. Kennedy Boulevard, Suite 1800, Philadelphia, PA 19103-2899. Periodicals postage paid at New York, NY, and additional mailing offices. Subscription prices are USD $255.00 per year (US individuals), $471.00 per year (US institutions), $125.00 per year (US Students), $320.00 per year (Canadian individuals), $612.00 per year (Canadian institutions), $200.00 per year (Canadian and foreign students), $390.00 per year (foreign individuals), and $612.00 per year (foreign institutions). To receive student/resident rate, orders must be accompanied by name of affiliated institution, date of term, and the signature of program/residency coordinator on institution letterhead. Orders will be billed at individual rate until proof of status is received. Foreign air speed delivery is included in all Clinics' subscription prices. All prices are subject to change without notice. **POSTMASTER:** Send address changes to *Medical Clinics of North America*, Elsevier Health Sciences Division, Subscription Customer Service, 3251 Riverport Lane, Maryland Heights, MO 63043. **Customer Service: Telephone: 1-800-654-2452** (U.S. and Canada); **1-314-447-8871** (outside U.S. and Canada). **Fax: 314-447-8029. E-mail: journalscustomerserviceusa@elsevier.com** (for print support); **journalsonlinesupport-usa@elsevier.com** (for online support).

Reprints. For copies of 100 or more of articles in this publication, please contact the Commercial Reprints Department, Elsevier Inc., 360 Park Avenue South, New York, NY 10010-1710. Tel.: 212-633-3874; Fax: 212-633-3820; E-mail: reprints@elsevier.com.

Medical Clinics of North America is also published in Spanish by McGraw-Hill Interamericana Editores S. A., P.O. Box 5-237, 06500 Mexico, D.F., Mexico.

Medical Clinics of North America is covered in *MEDLINE/PubMed (Index Medicus), Current Contents, ASCA, Excerpta Medica, Science Citation Index,* and *ISI/BIOMED.*

PROGRAM OBJECTIVE

The goal of the *Medical Clinics of North America* is to keep practicing physicians up to date with current clinical practice by providing timely articles reviewing the state of the art in patient care.

TARGET AUDIENCE

All practicing physicians and other healthcare professionals.

LEARNING OBJECTIVES

Upon completion of this activity, participants will be able to:
1. Review common dermatologic conditions and procedures.
2. Discuss treatments for acute dermatologic conditions such as nail disease and blisters.
3. Recognize management strategies in long term conditions such as psoriasis and skin cancer.

ACCREDITATION

The Elsevier Office of Continuing Medical Education (EOCME) is accredited by the Accreditation Council for Continuing Medical Education (ACCME) to provide continuing medical education for physicians.

The EOCME designates this enduring material for a maximum of 15 *AMA PRA Category 1 Credit*(s)™. Physicians should claim only the credit commensurate with the extent of their participation in the activity.

All other healthcare professionals requesting continuing education credit for this enduring material will be issued a certificate of participation.

DISCLOSURE OF CONFLICTS OF INTEREST

The EOCME assesses conflict of interest with its instructors, faculty, planners, and other individuals who are in a position to control the content of CME activities. All relevant conflicts of interest that are identified are thoroughly vetted by EOCME for fair balance, scientific objectivity, and patient care recommendations. EOCME is committed to providing its learners with CME activities that promote improvements or quality in healthcare and not a specific proprietary business or a commercial interest.

The planning committee, staff, authors and editors listed below have identified no financial relationships or relationships to products or devices they or their spouse/life partner have with commercial interest related to the content of this CME activity:
Lauren K. Biesbroeck, MD; Roy M. Colven, MD; Ramin Fathi, MD; Philip Fleckman, MD; Anjali Fortna; Sumul Ashok Gandhi, MD; Deepti Gupta, MD; Tarannum Jaleel, MD; Jolene R. Jewell, MD; Andrea Kalus, MD; Jeremy Kampp, MD; Young Kwak, MD; Jessica McCool; Sarah A. Myers, MD; Douglas S. Paauw, MD, MACP; Santha Priya; Naveed Sami, MD; Michi M. Shinohara, MD; Megan Suermann; Laura Swanson, MD; Alison Swety; Jay C. Vary Jr, MD, PhD; Shelley Yang, MD.

The planning committee, staff, authors and editors listed below have identified financial relationships or relationships to products or devices they or their spouse/life partner have with commercial interest related to the content of this CME activity:
April Wang Armstrong, MD, MPH is a consultant/advisor for AbbVie Inc.; Janssen Global Services; Eli Lilly and Company; Amgen Inc.; Celgene Corporation; Merck & Co., Inc.; Novartis AG; and Pfizer Inc.; and has research support from AbbVie Inc.; Janssen Global Services; and Eli Lilly and Company.
Alexa B. Kimball, MD, MPH is a consultant/advisor for, with research support from, Amgen Inc.; AbbVie Inc.; Janssen Global Services; Novartis AG; Celgene Corporation; and Pfizer Inc., and is a consultant/advisor for Eli Lilly and Company.
Kathryn T. Shahwan, MD has research support from Janssen Global Services, LLC.
John D. Whited, MD, MHS receives royalties/patents from Cambridge University Press.

UNAPPROVED/OFF-LABEL USE DISCLOSURE

The EOCME requires CME faculty to disclose to the participants:
1. When products or procedures being discussed are off-label, unlabelled, experimental, and/or investigational (not US Food and Drug Administration [FDA] approved); and
2. Any limitations on the information presented, such as data that are preliminary or that represent ongoing research, interim analyses, and/or unsupported opinions. Faculty may discuss information about pharmaceutical agents that is outside of FDA-approved labelling. This information is intended solely for CME and is not intended to promote off-label use of these medications. If you have any questions, contact the medical affairs department of the manufacturer for the most recent prescribing information.

TO ENROLL

To enroll in the *Medical Clinics of North America* Continuing Medical Education program, call customer service at 1-800-654-2452 or sign up online at http://www.theclinics.com/home/cme. The CME program is available to subscribers for an additional annual fee of USD $295.

METHOD OF PARTICIPATION

In order to claim credit, participants must complete the following:

1. Complete enrolment as indicated above.
2. Read the activity.
3. Complete the CME Test and Evaluation. Participants must achieve a score of 70% on the test. All CME Tests and Evaluations must be completed online.

CME INQUIRIES/SPECIAL NEEDS

For all CME inquiries or special needs, please contact elsevierCME@elsevier.com.

MEDICAL CLINICS OF NORTH AMERICA

FORTHCOMING ISSUES

January 2016
Managing Chronic Pain
Charles E. Argoff, *Editor*

March 2016
Travel and Adventure Medicine
Paul S. Pottinger and
Christopher A. Sanford, *Editors*

May 2016
Medical Care for Kidney and Liver
Transplant Recipients
David A. Sass and
Alden M. Doyle, *Editors*

RECENT ISSUES

September 2015
Comprehensive Care of the Patient with
Chronic Illness
Douglas S. Paauw, *Editor*

July 2015
Management of Cardiovascular Disease
Deborah L. Wolbrette, *Editor*

May 2015
Women's Health
Joyce E. Wipf, *Editor*

RELATED INTEREST

Primary Care: Clinics in Office Practice
December 2015 (Vol. 42, Issue 4)
Primary Care Dermatology
George G.A. Pujalte, *Editor*
http://www.primarycare.theclinics.com/

Contributors

CONSULTING EDITORS

DOUGLAS S. PAAUW, MD, MACP
Professor of Medicine, Division of General Internal Medicine, Rathmann Family
Foundation Endowed Chair for Patient-Centered Clinical Education; Medicine Student
Programs, Professor of Medicine, University of Washington School of Medicine, Seattle,
Washington

EDWARD R. BOLLARD, MD, DDS, FACP
Professor of Medicine, Associate Dean of Graduate Medical Education, Designated
Institutional Official, Department of Medicine, Penn State-Hershey Medical Center/Penn
State University College of Medicine, Hershey, Pennsylvania

EDITOR

ROY M. COLVEN, MD
Professor of Medicine, Division of Dermatology, University of Washington School of
Medicine, Seattle, Washington

AUTHORS

APRIL WANG ARMSTRONG, MD, MPH
Vice Chair of Clinical Research, Associate Professor, Department of Dermatology,
Director of Clinical Trials and Outcomes Research, Director of the Psoriasis Program,
University of Colorado Denver, Aurora, Colorado

LAUREN K. BIESBROECK, MD
Acting Instructor, Division of Dermatology, University of Washington School of
Medicine, Seattle, Washington

ROY M. COLVEN, MD
Professor of Medicine, Division of Dermatology, University of Washington School
of Medicine, Seattle, Washington

RAMIN FATHI, MD
Resident Physician, Department of Dermatology, University of Colorado Denver,
Aurora, Colorado

PHILIP FLECKMAN, MD
Professor, Division of Dermatology, University of Washington School of Medicine,
Seattle, Washington

SUMUL ASHOK GANDHI, MD
Division of Dermatology, University of Washington School of Medicine, Seattle,
Washington

DEEPTI GUPTA, MD
Pediatric Dermatologist, Assistant Professor, Division of Dermatology, Department of Pediatrics, Seattle Children's Hospital; Adjunct Assistant Professor, Division of Dermatology, Department of Medicine, University of Washington, Seattle, Washington

TARANNUM JALEEL, MD
Department of Dermatology, University of Alabama at Birmingham, Birmingham, Alabama

JOLENE R. JEWELL, MD
Chief Resident, Department of Dermatology, Duke University Medical Center, Durham, North Carolina

ANDREA KALUS, MD
Dermatology Division, Associate Professor, Department of Medicine, University of Washington School of Medicine, Seattle, Washington

JEREMY KAMPP, MD
Assistant Clinical Professor, Director of Dermatologic Surgery, Division of Dermatology, University of Washington School of Medicine, Seattle, Washington

ALEXA B. KIMBALL, MD, MPH
Director, Clinical Unit for Research Trials and Outcomes in Skin (CURTIS), Professor, Department of Dermatology, Massachusetts General Hospital, Harvard Medical School, Boston, Massachusetts

YOUNG KWAK, MD
Department of Dermatology, University of Alabama at Birmingham, Birmingham, Alabama

SARAH A. MYERS, MD
Associate Professor, Department of Dermatology, Duke University Medical Center, Durham, North Carolina

NAVEED SAMI, MD
Associate Professor, Director, Autoimmune Bullous Disease Clinic, Department of Dermatology, University of Alabama at Birmingham, Birmingham, Alabama

KATHRYN T. SHAHWAN, MD
Fellow, Clinical Unit for Research Trials and Outcomes in Skin (CURTIS), Department of Dermatology, Massachusetts General Hospital, Harvard Medical School, Boston, Massachusetts

MICHI M. SHINOHARA, MD
Clinical Assistant Professor, Division of Dermatology, University of Washington School of Medicine, Seattle, Washington

LAURA SWANSON, MD
Division of Dermatology, University of Washington, Seattle, Washington

JAY C. VARY Jr, MD, PhD
Assistant Professor, Division of Dermatology, Department of Medicine, University of Washington, Seattle, Washington

JOHN D. WHITED, MD, MHS
Associate Chief of Staff, Research and Development, Durham Veterans Affairs Medical Center; Associate Professor of Medicine, Division of General Internal Medicine, Duke University School of Medicine, Durham, North Carolina

SHELLEY YANG, MD
Division of Dermatology, University of Washington School of Medicine, Seattle, Washington

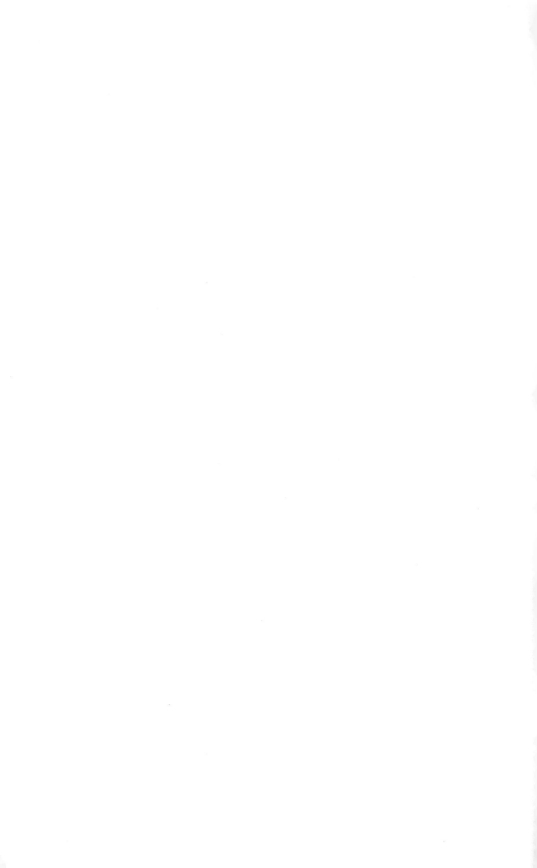

Contents

Foreword: Dermatology   xv

Douglas S. Paauw

Preface: Dermatology   xvii

Roy M. Colven

Topical Therapy Primer for Nondermatologists   1167

Jolene R. Jewell and Sarah A. Myers

> Topical medications are the foundation upon which dermatologic care is built. The proper use of topical therapeutics requires consideration of the active ingredient, potency, vehicle, and medication quantity. This article provides a concise but non-comprehensive list of topical medications used for acne, rosacea, psoriasis, actinic keratoses, and non-melanoma skin cancers. Common treatment regimens and pitfalls in prescribing topicals are discussed via clinical vignettes.

The Role of Biologic Therapies in Dermatology   1183

Ramin Fathi and April Wang Armstrong

> Primary care physicians frequently encounter patients on biologic therapies, and it is valuable to understand the how biologics are used in dermatology. This article provides a practical and clinically relevant discussion on the dermatologic use of biologic medications, their dermatologic indications, mechanisms of actions, and adverse effects.

Selected Disorders of Skin Appendages—Acne, Alopecia, Hyperhidrosis   1195

Jay C. Vary Jr

> This article reviews some of the more common diseases of the skin appendages that are encountered in medicine: hyperhidrosis, acne, alopecia areata, female pattern hair loss, androgenetic alopecia, and telogen effluvium. The pathophysiology behind the conditions and their treatments are discussed so that clinicians can make logical therapeutic choices for their affected patients.

Nail Disease for the Primary Care Provider   1213

Lauren K. Biesbroeck and Philip Fleckman

> Nail disorders are commonly seen by both primary practitioners and dermatologists. Nail disease spans a broad variety of diagnoses, including infectious, inflammatory, and neoplastic disorders. Dermatophyte onychomycosis can have clinical findings that overlap with other disorders, mandating adequate diagnosis before treatment is initiated. Periungual verrucae typically respond to keratolytics or cryotherapy, but may require topical immunotherapy or intralesional injections. Any verruca recalcitrant

to treatment should undergo biopsy to rule out squamous cell carcinoma. Patients with longitudinal melanonychia or erythronychia involving a single digit should be evaluated by a dermatologist, with biopsy of nail matrix considered to rule out underlying malignancy.

Psoriasis and Cardiovascular Disease

1227

Kathryn T. Shahwan and Alexa B. Kimball

Psoriasis, a chronic inflammatory skin disease, has been linked to the metabolic syndrome and various manifestations of cardiovascular disease. Together, psoriasis and the metabolic syndrome constitute a proinflammatory state, and psoriasis shares many pathogenic features with the development of atherosclerotic plaques. Measures of early endothelial dysfunction and subclinical atherosclerosis, as well as corresponding serum biomarkers, may be useful tools to predict which patients are at greatest risk. Regular screening of patients with psoriasis for metabolic and cardiovascular risk factors is of utmost importance, and treatment goals should include management of modifiable risk factors and reduction in systemic inflammation.

Clinical Approach to Diffuse Blisters

1243

Tarannum Jaleel, Young Kwak, and Naveed Sami

Some blistering eruptions are self-limited, but others are life threatening, and prompt diagnosis and management are critical. The clinical presentation of vesicles and bullae suggests a broad differential and this article (1) highlights some common diagnoses that may be encountered by primary care physicians and subspecialists; (2) provides a possible systematic diagnostic approach to such patients, including history, physical examination, and relevant work-up.

Atopic Dermatitis: A Common Pediatric Condition and Its Evolution in Adulthood

1269

Deepti Gupta

Atopic dermatitis (AD) is a chronic and pruritic inflammatory skin disorder that has a relapsing course and can affect any age group. Patients with AD have higher rates of other allergic disorders, mental health disorders, and skin infections. An important feature of AD for practitioners to recognize is that the clinical presentation varies by age from infancy into adulthood. The goals of treatment and management of AD focuses on restoring and maintaining the skin barrier function, minimizing inflammation, breaking the itch-scratch cycle, and treating possible external triggers and secondary infections that may propagate AD.

Rheumatologic Skin Disease

1287

Andrea Kalus

In common rheumatologic diseases skin findings are an important diagnostic clue for astute clinicians. Skin manifestations can help identify systemic disease or may require therapy uniquely targeted at the cutaneous problem. This article discusses 3 common rheumatologic conditions seen in adults by dermatologists: cutaneous lupus, dermatomyositis, and morphea. The focus is on the cutaneous findings and clinical presentation. Some approaches to treatment are explored. Clues to help identify systemic disease are also highlighted.

Common Dermatologic Procedures 1305

Shelley Yang and Jeremy Kampp

Procedures are an essential component of dermatology practice. There is a wide variety of dermatologic procedures, including biopsies, excisions, curettage, cryosurgery, Mohs surgery, and more. This article reviews common dermatologic procedures, with a focus on the skin biopsy, a fundamental skill for all physicians who manage skin conditions. Common pitfalls, preoperative preparation, postoperative care, and select cosmetic procedures are also covered.

Skin Cancer Epidemiology, Detection, and Management 1323

Sumul Ashok Gandhi and Jeremy Kampp

Skin cancer, when defined as a single entity, is the most common malignancy in North America. Although attention has focused on melanoma, several other common cutaneous malignancies, such as basal and squamous cell carcinoma, and more rare neoplasms, like Merkel cell carcinoma, need to be considered when patients present with new or changing lesions. Identification of at-risk patients, incorporation of preventive actions, early detection, and prompt treatment remain the mainstays of care for all forms of cutaneous malignancy, regardless of type.

Approach to the Patient with a Suspected Cutaneous Adverse Drug Reaction 1337

Laura Swanson and Roy M. Colven

Cutaneous adverse drug reactions are common. They can present in a variety of forms with a broad spectrum of severity, morbidity, and mortality. It is crucial that the clinician be able to recognize signs and symptoms that suggest a more severe or complicated reaction so that appropriate work-up and treatment are initiated. This article provides a systematic approach to evaluating a patient with a suspected cutaneous adverse drug reaction. It also details the characteristics, work-up, and treatment of the common types of cutaneous adverse drug reactions.

Inpatient Consultative Dermatology 1349

Lauren K. Biesbroeck and Michi M. Shinohara

Skin disorders occur in one-third of inpatients, and dermatologists play a significant role in their diagnosis and management. Although there remain barriers, there are substantial benefits to involving dermatology, including opportunities for more extensive interaction and teaching with consulting services. A broad range of dermatoses are diagnosed in the inpatient setting, including drug eruptions, atypical or disseminated infections, and unusual causes of cutaneous ulcers. Eruptions occurring in immunosuppressed patients, in particular, can pose particular challenges. Dermatologists can aid in diagnosis with physical examination and judicious use of skin biopsies.

Teledermatology   1365

John D. Whited

This article provides an overview of teledermatology with an emphasis on the evidence most relevant to referring clinicians, who are often primary care clinicians. Discussion includes the different modalities used for teledermatology and their diagnostic reliability, diagnostic accuracy, impact on in-person dermatology visits, clinical outcomes, and user satisfaction.

Index   1381

Foreword

Dermatology

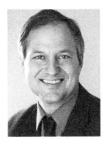

Douglas S. Paauw, MD, MACP
Consulting Editor

Dermatologic problems are ubiquitous. One of three people has a skin condition at any given time. In a recent Mayo Clinic study, dermatologic problems were the top reason for primary care visits, and 43% of patients had a skin problem within a 5-year study period.[1] Between 40% and 50% of Americans who live to age 65 will have either a basal or a squamous cell carcinoma diagnosed.[2] Dr Colven has done an excellent job in this issue of *Medical Clinics of North America* covering important topics in dermatology for the primary care physician. Articles to help with diagnosis of skin cancer, drug reactions, alopecia, blistering disorders, and nail disorders are helpful for the common questions we get in primary care. There is an article that reviews and guides us in approach and understanding of common dermatologic procedures. An article is devoted to inpatient consultative dermatology. The rest of the articles address dermatologic therapeutics, including an article devoted to correctly using topical dermatologic agents. I hope you enjoy this issue and find it helpful in improving the dermatologic care of your patients.

Douglas S. Paauw, MD, MACP
Division of General Internal Medicine
Department of Medicine
University of Washington School of Medicine
Seattle, WA 98195, USA

E-mail address:
DPaauw@medicine.washington.edu

http://dx.doi.org/10.1016/j.mcna.2015.08.003
0025-7125/15/$ – see front matter © 2015 Published by Elsevier Inc.
medical.theclinics.com

REFERENCES

1. St Sauver JL, Warner DO, Yawn B. Why patients visit their doctors: assessing the most prevalent conditions in a defined American population. Mayo Clin Proc 2013; 88(1):56–67.
2. Sun Protection. Cancer Trends Progress Report–2009/2010 Update. National Cancer Institute. Available at: http://progressreport.cancer.gov/prevention/sun_protection. Accessed August 22, 2015.

Preface

Dermatology

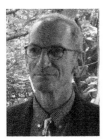

Roy M. Colven, MD
Editor

Like all of medicine, the specialty of dermatology is one that continues to expand and become more complex. The breadth of dermatology is already huge, and on top of that, names of conditions change, new diseases are identified, therapies for known skin diseases evolve, and new therapies enter the arena frequently. Moreover, skin disease is prevalent in all medical practices, and as health care providers, we are frequently asked about skin-related issues, whether disease or not, both in and out of our practices.

Globally, most skin disease is seen and managed by primary care providers, not dermatologists. Given the waiting times of most dermatology practices in North America, this arrangement *must* occur, as there is far more skin disease than there is capacity of skin disease expertise. In global regions where there are extreme shortages of specialists, general practitioners must become proficient in all areas of medicine, including dermatology.

This issue of *Medical Clinics of North America* is focused on assuring dermatologic proficiency. The topics here are chosen to help fill knowledge, practice, and performance gaps that many nondermatologists contend with on a regular basis. The guest editor's, as well as several of the senior authors', backgrounds as trained internists who later became academic dermatologists involved with training of internal medicine and dermatology residents, students of medicine, and practicing general physicians have guided these choices. Over many years, the same points of misunderstanding and patient management pitfalls have consistently arisen in the areas addressed in this volume.

The articles in this issue can be logically grouped, with calculated redundancy:

- Practical matters (topical therapy and skin procedures)
- Update in common diseases (skin cancer, atopic dermatitis, acne, nail diseases, and psoriasis)
- Systemic disease dermatology (rheumatologic skin diseases, psoriasis and its links to cardiovascular disease)

Med Clin N Am 99 (2015) xvii–xviii
http://dx.doi.org/10.1016/j.mcna.2015.08.002
0025-7125/15/$ – see front matter © 2015 Published by Elsevier Inc.

medical.theclinics.com

- Approaches to often vexing conditions (blisters, alopecia, hyperhidrosis, adverse drug reactions, and complex medical dermatology)
- Therapies in dermatology (topical, systemic nonbiologic, and biologic)
- Consultative support (teledermatology, consultative inpatient dermatology)

All of the authors are intimately involved with teaching and training in dermatology and so recognize the need to refresh and expand all health care providers' skills in managing skin-diseased patients.

We believe that you will find this issue interesting, practical, and most of all *immediately relevant* for your practice of medicine.

Roy M. Colven, MD
Division of Dermatology
University of Washington School of Medicine
Box 356524
1959 Northeast Pacific Street
BB 1353
Seattle, WA 98195, USA

E-mail address:
RColven@derm.washington.edu

Topical Therapy Primer for Nondermatologists

Jolene R. Jewell, MD, Sarah A. Myers, MD*

KEYWORDS

- Topical therapies • Corticosteroids • Antimicrobials • Retinoids
- Nondermatologist providers

KEY POINTS

- Many dermatologic conditions are effectively managed with topical therapies, including topical steroids, antimicrobials, retinoids, keratolytics, and antineoplastics.
- The proper active ingredient, potency, vehicle, quantity of medication, and patient instructions are critical when prescribing topical therapies.
- If a topical therapy is ineffective, clinicians should consider whether the medication is being used properly, whether the diagnosis is correct, and whether the topical may be contributing to the problem.

INTRODUCTION

Topical therapy is critical in the care of patients with cutaneous disease. This article offers a concise catalog of commonly used topical therapies and the included tables and cited publications serve as a toolkit for quick reference. Clinical vignettes are provided to reinforce the basic tenets of topical therapy and highlight basic guidelines for primary care providers.

PART I: TOPICAL MEDICATIONS
Topical Steroids

Regarded as the crux of dermatologic therapy, topical corticosteroids (TCS) are prescribed in up to 21% of dermatology office visits for atopic dermatitis, contact dermatitis, hand dermatitis, and many other cutaneous inflammatory conditions.[1] The proper use of TCS requires consideration of steroid potency, vehicle, and quantity of

Disclosures: The authors have no commercial or financial conflicts of interest or funding sources to disclose.
Department of Dermatology, Duke University Medical Center, DUMC 3852, Durham, NC 27710, USA
* Corresponding author.
E-mail address: sarah.myers@duke.edu

Med Clin N Am 99 (2015) 1167–1182
http://dx.doi.org/10.1016/j.mcna.2015.06.001
0025-7125/15/$ – see front matter © 2015 Elsevier Inc. All rights reserved.

medical.theclinics.com

medication. Despite standard Stoughton Vasoconstriction Assay–based potency classification, dermatologists often categorize prescription steroids as high, mid, or low potency.[2] TCS are pregnancy category C, thus low-potency steroids are reserved for severe dermatoses during pregnancy. **Table 1** highlights the topical steroids commonly prescribed by dermatologists.

TCS are generally well tolerated; however, side effect frequency and severity increase with prolonged use and steroid potency. Epidermal atrophy, folliculitis or steroid acne, perioral dermatitis, delayed wound healing, steroid rebound, tachyphylaxis, glaucoma, cataracts, and contact dermatitis are all reversible TCS side effects.[3] Striae development is irreversible, thus the risk of this specific adverse event should always be discussed with patients. Systemic side effects, such as hypothalamic-pituitary-adrenal axis suppression, iatrogenic Cushing syndrome, and growth retardation in children, can occur if TCS are used improperly.

Topical Antimicrobials

Acne, rosacea, periorificial dermatitis, tinea, candidal intertrigo, and scabies are frequently treated with topical antimicrobials. Most of the medications discussed here are available in generic formulations and some are available over the counter (OTC), as indicated in **Table 2**. When recommending an OTC medication, instruct patients to check ingredient lists because some brands manufacture similarly named products with different active ingredients.

Topical antimicrobials are often used for basic wound care; however, dermatologists generally recommend petrolatum use to maintain a moist wound-healing environment. A frequently cited randomized controlled trial from 1996 showed the absence of a statistically significant difference in infection rate when petrolatum versus bacitracin was used postoperatively. Further, petrolatum is cheaper than commercially available antibacterial ointments.[4] If an antibacterial ointment is indicated for a superficial skin infection, mupirocin is preferred because of lower risk of allergic contact dermatitis.

Topical Acne, Rosacea, and Psoriasis Medications

Mild to moderate comedonal and inflammatory acne can be effectively treated with topical medications. Many of the topicals listed in **Table 3** are used in conjunction with antimicrobials to improve efficacy and patient adherence. It should be emphasized that these treatments prevent new lesions from forming and thus need to be used on a regular basis for 6 to 8 weeks before efficacy can be assessed. Similarly, acne medications control acne and patients should be warned that their acne may flare if topicals are discontinued. Oral antibiotics and isotretinoin are typically reserved for severe nodulocystic acne with scarring or chest and back involvement. Treating pregnancy-related acne can be challenging because there are few pregnancy category B therapeutics, with the exception of azelaic acid, topical clindamycin, and topical erythromycin. Pregnant patients should be informed that OTC benzoyl peroxide and salicylic acid face washes are technically pregnancy category C.

It can be difficult to distinguish acne from rosacea in some patients. Dermatologists rely on the presence of comedones to suggest the diagnosis of acne rather than rosacea, and patients with rosacea tend to have more sensitive skin. Erythematotelangiectatic rosacea responds best to pulsed dye laser but some patients report significant improvement in flushing with topical brimonidine gel use.[8] Papulopustular rosacea responds well to topical metronidazole, azelaic acid, and newly available topical ivermectin. Ocular rosacea and severe inflammatory rosacea require oral antibiotic use. Phymatous rosacea responds poorly to topicals and often requires cosmetic surgery or laser treatment.[9]

Psoriatic plaques can be treated with topical steroids, but steroid-sparing agents have a special role in refractory disease and intertriginous sites. Unlike topical steroids, the topical calcineurin inhibitors (TCIs), tacrolimus and pimecrolimus, can be applied chronically for psoriasis or atopic dermatitis on the face, axillae, and inguinal folds without causing atrophy. Calcipotriene, a vitamin D analogue, is a similarly safe and effective alternative psoriasis therapeutic. Topical retinoids are traditionally reserved for acne treatment but tazarotene, specifically, is useful for thinning psoriatic plaques. Steroid-sparing medications can be expensive, thus generics should be prescribed when possible. If a generic medication is unavailable, often manufacturer coupons can be found online or via GoodRx.

Topicals for Actinic Keratoses and Nonmelanoma Skin Cancers

Treatment of actinic keratoses (AKs) is indicated because of the risk of progression to squamous cell carcinoma. Cryotherapy is most commonly used but field therapy with a topical can be helpful if a patient has numerous lesions in a localized area. 5-Fluorouracil is the most commonly used topical but all 4 medications in **Table 4** have similar reported efficacies for AK clearance if used properly.[10,11] Dermatologist recommendations on treatment frequency and duration vary but all patients should be warned regarding expected redness and irritation of the treated site. It can be helpful to show patients representative photographs of what they are likely to experience with adequate treatment. Exuberant reactions are common and can be managed by holding treatment for several days and starting a low-potency topical steroid. If field therapy for AKs is recommended, patients should follow up to ensure resolution of concerning lesions. If treatment of nonmelanoma skin cancers with topicals is being considered, a dermatology referral should be entertained.

PART II: CASES
Case 1

A 36-year-old man presents to clinic in February with an extremely pruritic rash on the upper back, arms, and lower legs, as shown in **Fig. 1**. He has been using topical diphenhydramine, which seemed to worsen his symptoms. You astutely diagnose the patient with asteatotic eczema and prescribe a 15-g tube of triamcinolone 0.1% cream for the patient to use twice daily. The patient leaves the clinic with his prescription but promptly calls your clinic the next day stating that the medication burns and he has already used the entire tube. What went wrong?

- Vehicle selection is a critical component of prescribing TCS and can greatly affect patient adherence, as shown in this case. Cream vehicles contain preservatives that can burn when applied to skin with impaired barrier function. The patient would have less burning if an ointment had been prescribed.
- An adequate amount of medication must be prescribed to treat the patient. As a general rule, it takes 30 g to coat an average-sized person from head to toe once. This patient would require 10 to 15 g per application to treat his rash on the back, arms, and legs. Topical steroids are used twice daily, thus he would need 30 g of triamcinolone per day. Commonly used topical steroids such as triamcinolone can be prescribed in 454-g (1 pound) jars.
- Topical diphenhydramine should have been discontinued. OTC topical antipruritics and analgesics can cause allergic and irritant contact dermatitis, which contribute to the patient's itching and burning.

Table 1
Topical corticosteroids commonly used by dermatologists

Potency	Generic Name	Concentration (%)	Vehicles	Brand Names (Vehicles)	Notes
High (class I/II)	Clobetasol propionate	0.05	Cream Foam Gel Lotion Ointment Shampoo Solution Spray	Clobex (lotion, shampoo, spray) Cormax (ointment, solution) Olux (foam) Temovate (cream, gel, ointment, solution)	Most potent topical steroid. Reserved for psoriasis, lichen sclerosus, discoid lupus, and other severe dermatoses. Foam, shampoo, and solution vehicles are useful for scalp psoriasis
	Halobetasol	0.05	Cream Ointment	Ultravate (cream, ointment)	—
	Betamethasone dipropionate	0.05	Cream Lotion Ointment	—	Available in combination products with calcipotriene or clotrimazole
	Fluocinonide	0.05 0.1	Cream Gel Ointment Solution	Lidex Vanos (cream)	Often referred to by brand name Lidex. Solution vehicle useful for scalp psoriasis. The 0.1% concentration only available in cream vehicle
Medium (class III/IV)	Triamcinolone	0.025 0.1 0.5	Cream Ointment Lotion	Trianex (0.05% ointment)	Most commonly used in 0.1% concentration. Lotion only available in 0.025% and 0.1%. Available in combination product with nystatin
	Betamethasone valerate	0.1	Cream Lotion Ointment Foam	Luxiq (0.12% foam)	Foam vehicle useful for scalp psoriasis. Do not confuse with betamethasone dipropionate, which is high potency
	Desoximetasone	0.05 0.25	Cream Gel Ointment Spray	Topicort	Preferred topical corticosteroid for patients with allergic contact dermatitis. Spray available in 0.25% and gel available in 0.05%

Low (class V/VI)	Fluocinolone	0.025 0.01	Body oil Cream Ointment Scalp oil Shampoo Solution	Capex (shampoo) Derma-Smoothe/FS (body oil, scalp oil) Synalar (cream, ointment, solution)	Oil vehicle useful for scalp psoriasis in patients with dry, coarse hair. Do not confuse with fluocinonide, which is high potency. 0.025% only available in cream and ointment
	Hydrocortisone valerate	0.2	Cream Ointment	Westcort	Note that hydrocortisone valerate at 0.2% is higher potency than hydrocortisone 1%
	Desonide	0.05	Cream Foam Gel Lotion Ointment	Desonate (gel) Desowen (cream, lotion, ointment) Verdeso (foam)	Often used in combination with ketoconazole 2% cream for seborrheic dermatitis
Least (class VII)	Hydrocortisone	0.5 1 2.5	Cream Lotion Ointment Solution	Hytone (1, 2.5% cream) Texacort (2.5% solution)	Lowest potency topical steroid. Available at 1% concentration in many OTC products, such as Cortizone-10 and Cortaid. The 2.5% concentration requires prescription

Abbreviation: OTC, over the counter.

Table 2
Topical antimicrobials commonly used by dermatologists

Antimicrobial Class	Generic Name	Concentration (%)	Vehicles	Brand Names (Vehicles)	Notes
Antibacterial	BPO	2.5–10	Cream Gel Pledget Wash	Numerous OTC preparations available, including PanOxyl, Clean and Clear, and AcneFree	Available in combination products with adapalene, clindamycin, and erythromycin. Bleaches towels/clothing if not rinsed thoroughly
	Clindamycin	1	Foam Gel Lotion Solution	Cleocin T (gel, lotion, solution) Clindagel (gel) Evoclin (foam)	Available in combination products with BPO and tretinoin. Use with BPO wash to prevent bacterial resistance[5]
	Dapsone	5	Gel	Aczone	Newer acne topical. There has been a case report of methemoglobinemia with topical dapsone use[6]
	Metronidazole	0.75 1	Cream Gel Lotion	MetroCream (cream) MetroGel (1% gel) MetroLotion (lotion) Noritate (cream)	Most commonly used for rosacea and periorificial dermatitis
	Mupirocin	2	Cream Ointment	Bactroban Centany (ointment)	Used TID and for MRSA decolonization. Preferred to because of decreased risk of allergic contact dermatitis
	Sulfacetamide-sulfur	10; 2–5	Cream Foam Lotion Suspension Wash	Klaron (10% lotion) Rosanil (10%/5% wash)	Used for acne, rosacea, and seborrheic dermatitis

				Brand names	Notes
Antifungal	Clotrimazole	1	Cream Solution	Lotrimin AF (cream) Fungicure (solution)	OTC. First-line use for candidal intertrigo because it also has some coverage for dermatophytes
	Econazole	1	Cream Foam	Ecoza (foam)	Can be more expensive than OTC antifungals depending on insurance
	Efinaconazole	10	Solution	Jublia	New topical therapy for onychomycosis, used daily for 48 wk
	Ketoconazole	1 2	Cream Gel Foam Shampoo	Extina (foam) Nizoral AD (1% shampoo) Nizoral (shampoo) Xolegel (gel)	Ketoconazole 1% shampoo is OTC, 2% requires a prescription
	Terbinafine	1	Cream Gel Spray	Lamisil AT (cream, gel, spray)	Fungicidal. First-line OTC topical for tinea pedis
Antiparasitic	Ivermectin	1	Cream	Soolantra	Increasingly being used for rosacea by dermatologists[7]
	Permethrin	1 5	Lotion Cream	Elimite (5% cream) Nix (1% lotion is OTC)	For scabies, recommend 5% cream from neck to toes overnight with repeat application in 14 d

Abbreviations: BPO, benzoyl peroxide; MRSA, methicillin-resistant *Staphylococcus aureus*; TID, 3 times a day.

Table 3
Topicals commonly used by dermatologists for acne, rosacea, and psoriasis

Dermatosis	Generic Name	Concentration (%)	Vehicles	Brand Names (Vehicles)	Notes
Acne	Tretinoin	0.025 0.05 0.1	Cream Gel Solution	There are numerous brand name products with varying concentrations and vehicles, the most commonly referred to is Retin-A. Recommend prescribing the generic	Advise patients to evenly apply a pea-sized amount to the entire face, 10–15 min after washing. May cause redness and scaling. Start 2–3 times per week and increase to nightly as tolerated
	Adapalene	0.1 0.3 (gel)	Cream Gel Lotion	Differin	Regarded as potentially less irritating than tretinoin, would use for patients with sensitive skin
	Tazarotene	0.05 0.1	Cream Gel Foam	Avage (0.1% cream) Fabior (0.1% foam) Tazorac (cream, gel)	Can be used for psoriasis as well
	Azelaic acid	15 20	Gel	Azelex (20%) Finacea (15%)	Pregnancy category B. Can be expensive because generic unavailable. Also used for rosacea
	Salicylic acid	2–3	Wash Shampoo	Numerous OTC washes available, including Neutrogena, Aveeno, and Clean and Clear	Can be used for warts at higher concentrations (17%–40%)
Rosacea	Brimonidine	0.33	Gel	Mirvaso	An alpha-2 agonist used qAM to decrease flushing associated with rosacea via vasoconstriction
Psoriasis	Calcipotriene	0.005	Cream Foam Ointment Solution	Calcitrene (ointment) Dovonex (cream, solution) Sorilux (foam)	Works well in combination with topical steroids for psoriasis vulgaris or as monotherapy for inverse psoriasis
	Tacrolimus	0.03 0.1	Ointment	Protopic	TCI commonly used for dermatitis or psoriasis on the face or intertriginous areas
	Pimecrolimus	1	Cream	Elidel	TCI commonly used for dermatitis or psoriasis on the face or intertriginous areas
	Ammonium lactate	12	Cream Lotion	Lac-Hydrin AmLactin (OTC)	Keratolytic. Used on scaly plaques. Also helpful for retention hyperkeratosis in elderly patients
	Urea	35 40 50	Cream Foam Gel Ointment Solution	Gordon's Urea (40% ointment)	Lower concentration creams are available OTC. Can be used for warts and nail removal as well. Irritating if used on normal skin

Abbreviations: qAM, every morning; TCI, topical calcineurin inhibitor.

Table 4
Topicals commonly used by dermatologists for AKs and nonmelanoma skin cancers

Generic Name	Concentration (%)	Brand Names	FDA Approved Use	Off-label Use	Notes
5-FU	0.5 1 2 5	Carac (0.5% cream) Efudex (2% solution, 5% cream) Fluoroplex (1% cream)	AKs • BID ×2–4 wk Superficial BCC • BID ×3–6 wk	SCC in situ • BID × 12 wk	Do not confuse with the topical steroid fluocinonide. Only 5% is FDA approved for treatment of superficial BCC
Diclofenac	3	Solaraze (gel)	AKs • BID ×60–90 d	—	There are 1%–2% diclofenac gels and solutions used for osteoarthritis
Imiquimod	2.5 3.75 5	Aldara Zyclara (2.5%, 3.75%)	AKs • BIW ×16 wk Superficial BCC • M-F qHS × 16 wk	—	Can also be used for genital warts. Requires longer treatment period than 5-FU
Ingenol mebutate	0.015 0.05	Picato (gel)	AK of face and scalp • 0.015% ×3 d Trunk and Ext • 0.05% ×2 d	—	The shortest treatment period of the topical antineoplastics

Abbreviations: BID, twice a day; BIW, twice a week; Ext, extremities; FDA, US Food and Drug Administration; FU, fluorouracil; M-F, Monday through Friday; qHS, every night at bedtime; SCC, squamous cell carcinoma.

Case 2

An 11-year-old girl with atopic dermatitis presents to clinic with worsening pruritus and rash on the popliteal fossae, as shown in **Fig. 2**. She is currently taking short, lukewarm showers once per day and applying fluocinonide 0.05% ointment twice daily. What other recommendations are appropriate at this time?

- Flares of atopic dermatitis can result from bacterial impetiginization or poor daily skin care. Bacterial impetiginization, if mild, can be treated with dilute bleach baths. Ask the patient to soak for 10 to 15 minutes in a warm tub full of water with one-quarter to one-half a cup of bleach 2 to 3 times per week. The patient may then shower to remove the bleach. If impetiginization is severe, bacterial culture and oral antibiotics may be indicated.
- Daily skin care for patients with atopic dermatitis should be emphasized at every appointment. Recommend daily, short, lukewarm showers with fragrance-free soaps. Immediately after bathing the patient should generously apply an emollient such as a fragrance-free cream, lotion, or petrolatum such as CeraVe,

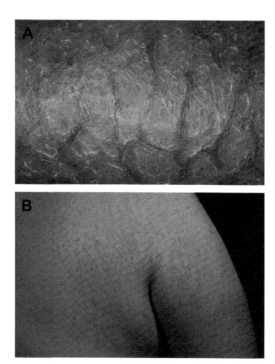

Fig. 1. Asteatotic eczema (eczema craquele). (*A*) The distal lower extremity has obvious inflammation and xerosis with adherent white scales (pseudoichthyosis) as well as criss-cross pattern of superficial cracks and fissures said to resemble a dried riverbed. (*B*) When widespread, there can be involvement of the trunk and proximal extremities. Along with the distal lower extremity, the posterior axillary line is a common site for asteatotic eczema. (*From* Reider N, Fritsch O. Other eczematous eruptions. In: Bolognia J, Jorizzo JL, Schaffer JV, editors. Dermatology. Philadelphia: Elsevier Saunders; 2012; with permission.)

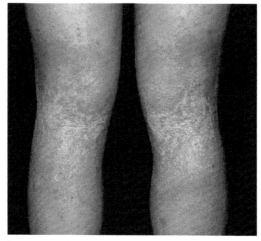

Fig. 2. Flexural involvement in childhood atopic dermatitis. (*From* James WD, Berger TG, Elston DM. Andrews' diseases of the skin: clinical dermatology. Philadelphia: Saunders; 2016; with permission.)

Cetaphil, Aquaphor, or Vaseline. Emollients should be repeated throughout the day as needed in combination with prescribed TCS. As flares resolve, the potency and frequency of TCS use should be decreased, especially in the body folds, because intertriginous skin is at particularly high risk for atrophy.

Case 3

A 42-year-old woman with chronic hand dermatitis presents to clinic with a flare of her eczema, as seen in **Fig. 3**. She has been using betamethasone valerate 0.1% cream twice daily every day for the past month. She reports that the topical steroid used to work but seems to have been less effective for the past week. What other treatment options could be considered?

- If betamethasone valerate 0.1% cream is ineffective, topical steroid potency could be increased to betamethasone dipropionate or clobetasol. The topical steroid vehicle could also be switched from cream to an ointment. More hydrophobic vehicles increase potency via occlusion and enhanced percutaneous absorption (ie, triamcinolone 0.1% ointment is more potent than triamcinolone 0.1% cream).
- When previously steroid-responsive dermatitis flares, clinicians should consider that the topical steroids themselves may be causing contact dermatitis. Recent patch testing results from the North American Contact Dermatitis Group indicates that the incidence of allergic contact dermatitis to TCS is nearly 3.9%.[12] In this situation, the patient could be switched to desoximetasone, an alternative, midpotency topical steroid that does not contain the common allergen propylene glycol.
- Tachyphylaxis should also be considered and the patient may benefit from taking a break of 4 to 7 days after every 2 weeks of treatment.

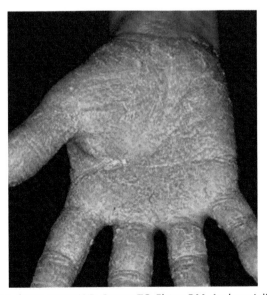

Fig. 3. Hand eczema. (*From* James WD, Berger TG, Elston DM. Andrews' diseases of the skin: clinical dermatology. Philadelphia: Saunders; 2016; with permission.)

Case 4

A 65-year-old woman with primary biliary cirrhosis presents with the nail examination shown in **Fig. 4**. Nail culture grows *Trichophyton rubrum*. She has tried ciclopirox on the nails nightly for 4 weeks without improvement. What treatment options are appropriate to discuss?

- Systemic treatment with terbinafine 250 mg daily for 6 weeks (fingernail treatment) or 12 weeks (toenail treatment) would not be recommended because the patient has known liver disease.
- The patient could continue ciclopirox for up to 48 weeks. Two double-blind, vehicle-controlled, parallel-group clinical trials show toenails with ∼5.5% to 8.5% complete clinical clearance and 29% to 36% mycologic clearance after completing 48 weeks of treatment.[13] The patient may have not used the medication long enough to see a result. Fingernails take 6 months and toenails take 12 to 18 months to grow completely. It is important to counsel patients that they will not see immediate results with onychomycosis treatment whether or not they use topical or systemic therapy.

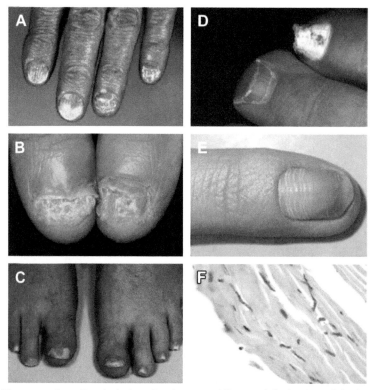

Fig. 4. Tinea unguium. Onycholysis, yellowing, crumbling, and thickening of the fingernails (*A*), thumb nails (*B*), and toenails (*C*) in the distal/lateral subungual variant. Diffuse (*D*) and striate (*E*) white discoloration of the toenail in the superficial white variant. Hyphae within formalin-fixed nail plate stained with periodic acid–Schiff (*F*). (*From* Elewski BE, Hughey LC, Sobera JO, et al. Fungal diseases. In: Bolognia J, Jorizzo JL, Schaffer JV, editors. Dermatology. Philadelphia: Elsevier Saunders; 2012; with permission.)

- She could switch to efinaconazole 10% solution and apply to the nails nightly for 48 weeks. Two recent phase III clinical trials show toenails with ~15% to 18% complete clinical clearance and 53% to 55% mycologic clearance 4 weeks after completing 48 weeks of treatment.[14] The efficacy of efinaconazole seems to be slightly greater than that of ciclopirox.

Case 5

A 66-year-old healthy man presents to clinic with yellow greasy scale with associated erythema and pruritus behind his ears, in his eyebrows, and on his scalp, as seen in **Fig. 5**. His wife is bothered by flakes falling on the patient's shirt and the cosmetic appearance. He is currently using his wife's shampoo because it smells good. What recommendations should be made?

- The patient has moderate seborrheic dermatitis, which is common, especially in the elderly and patients with neurologic conditions. He should discontinue his current shampoo and switch to either OTC antidandruff shampoo or prescription-strength ketoconazole 2% shampoo. Instruct the patient to let the shampoo sit on the scalp and face for 3 to 5 minutes before rinsing.
- A low-potency topical steroid (desonide 0.05% cream or hydrocortisone 2.5% cream), alone or mixed with ketoconazole 2% cream, can be applied behind ears and on eyebrows 1 to 2 times per day as needed to reduce redness and scaling.
- Despite his wife's concerns, if the patient is not bothered by the scaling, it could be argued that no treatment is necessary. Treatment of benign dermatoses such as seborrheic dermatitis is optional and many patients find using topical treatments cumbersome and unnecessary.

Case 6

An 18-year-old male teenager presents for follow up of acne shown in **Fig. 6**. He was last seen 4 weeks ago and was prescribed tretinoin 0.1% cream every night at bedtime, clindamycin 1% lotion every morning and an OTC benzoyl peroxide wash to use twice daily. He returns today because his skin is not improving and his acne medications are very irritating. What can be done to help?

- His follow-up appointment is too soon to evaluate the efficacy of his medications. If patients are tolerating their medications well, a follow-up in 2 to 3 months would be more appropriate. Acne medications take 6 to 8 weeks of regular use to see effect. It is important to emphasize that the tretinoin is to be used at night and applied to the entire face, not just on the individual acne lesions as spot treatment.
- His skin could be irritated for several reasons:
  - His tretinoin may be too strong. Options include decreasing the frequency of use to every other night, a trial of tretinoin 0.05% instead of 0.1%, or mixing a small amount of moisturizer with his current tretinoin cream to effectively dilute the concentration.
  - He may be using tretinoin immediately after washing his face or showering. Tretinoin can be very irritating if applied to a warm, flushed face. Instruct patient to wait 10 to 15 minutes after washing the face before applying tretinoin.
  - He may be irritated from using benzoyl peroxide twice daily. Advise him to use it only in the morning before he applies his topical clindamycin. He can use a gentle face cleanser in the evening.

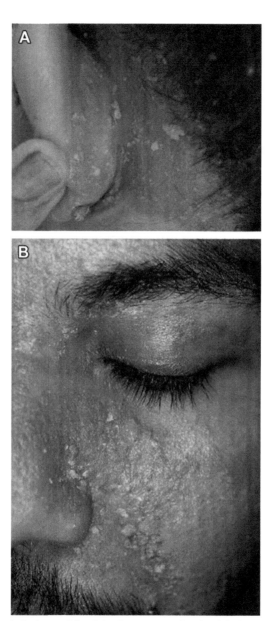

Fig. 5. Adult seborrheic dermatitis of the face, ear, and scalp. (*A*) Sharply demarcated pink plaque with white and greasy scale. Note the fissure in the retroauricular sulcus. (*B*) Sharply demarcated pink-orange thin plaques with yellow, greasy scale, especially in the melolabial fold. (*From* Reider N, Fritsch O. Other eczematous eruptions. In: Bolognia J, Jorizzo JL, Schaffer JV, editors. Dermatology. Philadelphia: Elsevier Saunders; 2012; with permission.)

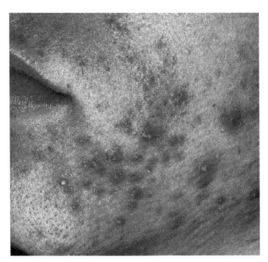

Fig. 6. Acne vulgaris, with papules and pustules, on the cheek. (*From* James WD, Berger TG, Elston DM. Andrews' diseases of the skin: clinical dermatology. Philadelphia: Saunders; 2016; with permission.)

SUMMARY

A representative assortment of topical therapies is discussed here with the goal of emphasizing the most commonly encountered diagnoses and treatments for nonder-matologists. When using topical therapies, carefully consider the proper active ingre-dient, potency, vehicle, and quantity of medication. If topical therapy is ineffective, question whether the medication is being used properly, whether the diagnosis is cor-rect, and whether the topical may be contributing to the problem. Examples of the topical contributing to the problem include tinea incognito exacerbated by topical ste-roid use and allergic contact dermatitis to topical steroid excipients. For some pa-tients, even maximum topical therapy is insufficient and systemic treatment is required. At this point, consultation with a dermatologist may be helpful.

REFERENCES

1. Stern RS. The pattern of topical corticosteroid prescribing in the United States, 1989–1991. J Am Acad Dermatol 1996;35(2 Pt 1):183–6.
2. Sandoval LF, Davis SA, Feldman SR. Dermatologists' knowledge of and prefer-ences regarding topical steroids. J Drugs Dermatol 2013;12(7):786–9.
3. Coondoo A, Phiske M, Verma S, et al. Side-effects of topical steroids: a long over-due revisit. Indian Dermatol Online J 2014;5(4):416–25.
4. Smack DP, Harrington AC, Dunn C, et al. Infection and allergy incidence in ambu-latory surgery patients using white petrolatum vs bacitracin ointment. A random-ized controlled trial. JAMA 1996;276(12):972–7.
5. Andriessen A, Lynde CW. Antibiotic resistance: shifting the paradigm in topical acne treatment. J Drugs Dermatol 2014;13(11):1358–64.
6. Swartzentruber GS, Yanta JH, Pizon AF. Methemoglobinemia as a complication of topical dapsone. N Engl J Med 2015;372(5):491–2.
7. Stein Gold L, Kircik L, Fowler J, et al. Long-term safety of ivermectin 1% cream vs azelaic acid 15% gel in treating inflammatory lesions of rosacea: results of two

40-week controlled, investigator-blinded trials. J Drugs Dermatol 2014;13(11): 1380–6.

8. Tanghetti EA, Jackson JM, Belasco KT, et al. Optimizing the use of topical brimonidine in rosacea management: panel recommendations. J Drugs Dermatol 2015; 14(1):33–40.

9. van Zuuren EJ, Kramer SF, Carter BR, et al. Effective and evidence-based management strategies for rosacea: summary of a Cochrane systematic review. Br J Dermatol 2011;165(4):760–81.

10. Micali G, Lacarrubba F, Nasca MR, et al. Topical pharmacotherapy for skin cancer: part I. Pharmacology. J Am Acad Dermatol 2014;70(6):965.e1–12 [quiz: 977–8].

11. Micali G, Lacarrubba F, Nasca MR, et al. Topical pharmacotherapy for skin cancer: part II. Clinical applications. J Am Acad Dermatol 2014;70(6):979.e1–12 [quiz: 9912].

12. Warshaw EM, Maibach HI, Taylor JS, et al. North American contact dermatitis group patch test results: 2011–2012. Dermatitis 2015;26(1):49–59.

13. Gupta AK, Fleckman P, Baran R. Ciclopirox nail lacquer topical solution 8% in the treatment of toenail onychomycosis. J Am Acad Dermatol 2000;43(4 Suppl): S70–80.

14. Elewski BE, Rich P, Pollak R, et al. Efinaconazole 10% solution in the treatment of toenail onychomycosis: two phase III multicenter, randomized, double-blind studies. J Am Acad Dermatol 2013;68(4):600–8.

The Role of Biologic Therapies in Dermatology

Ramin Fathi, MD*, April Wang Armstrong, MD, MPH

KEYWORDS

- Biologics • Dermatology • Etanercept • Adalimumab • Infliximab • Ustekinumab
- Secukinumab • IVIG

KEY POINTS

- Biologic therapies are molecules that target specific proteins implicated in immune-mediated disease and are frequently encountered in dermatology.
- Common biologic therapies encountered include tumor necrosis factor alpha inhibitors, interleukin (IL)-12/IL-23 inhibition, IL-17 inhibitors, rituximab, and intravenous immunoglobulin.
- Psoriasis is the most common indication for which biologics are used currently but several other dermatologic diseases seem to be responsive to biologic therapy.
- Understanding the mechanisms of action, labeled and off-label uses in dermatology, common adverse effects, and cost limitations helps to inform clinical decision making and improve patient outcomes.

INTRODUCTION

Advances in the understanding of disease pathophysiology for inflammatory skin diseases and in drug development have ushered in biologic therapies in dermatology. Biologic therapies are molecules that target specific proteins implicated in immune-mediated disease. In dermatology, the approved and emerging biologic therapies work extracellularly to alter T-cell activation and differentiation, block cytokines, or eliminate pathogenic B cells.[1] Biologic agents can be divided into 3 main groups: monoclonal antibodies, fusion proteins, and cytokines.[2] Depending on their mechanism of action, biologic medications have been used for different dermatologic indications. Notably, psoriasis is the skin disease for which biologics have been used most extensively.[3] However, biologics have also been used in, or are in development for, other inflammatory skin diseases. This article discusses the following biologic agents

Disclosures: Dr R. Fathi has no relevant disclosures. Dr A.W. Armstrong serves as investigator and/or consultant to AbbVie, Amgen, Celgene, Janssen, Merck, Lilly, Novartis, and Pfizer.
Department of Dermatology, University of Colorado Denver, 1665 Aurora Court, Room 3234, Mail Stop F703, Aurora, CO 80045, USA
* Corresponding author.
E-mail address: ramin.fathi@ucdenver.edu

Med Clin N Am 99 (2015) 1183–1194
http://dx.doi.org/10.1016/j.mcna.2015.07.008
0025-7125/15/$ – see front matter
medical.theclinics.com

used in dermatology with regard to their mechanism of action, clinical use, and adverse effects: tumor necrosis factor (TNF) alpha inhibitors, interleukin (IL)-12/IL-23 inhibition, IL-17 inhibitors, rituximab, and intravenous immunoglobulin (IVIG).

TUMOR NECROSIS FACTOR INHIBITORS

TNF plays a key role in chronic inflammatory diseases such as psoriasis and psoriatic arthritis. Biologic agents that inhibit TNF include a fusion protein, etanercept, and monoclonal antibodies such as infliximab and adalimumab.[4]

Differences exist in the mechanisms of action of various TNF inhibitors. Etanercept is a fully human fusion protein that is composed of a dimeric soluble p75 TNF receptor and a human immunoglobulin (Ig) G Fc fragment.[2] Infliximab is a chimeric IgG1-κ monoclonal antibody with human constant and murine variable regions that bind specifically to TNF-α.[2] Adalimumab is a fully human monoclonal IgG1 antibody that targets TNF-α.[2]

Etanercept, infliximab, and adalimumab are currently US Food and Drug Administration (FDA) approved in dermatology for plaque psoriasis and psoriatic arthritis.[2,5] The FDA-approved dose of etanercept for psoriasis is 50 mg twice weekly for 3 months, followed by 50 mg weekly for an unspecified amount of time.[5,6] Infliximab is an infusion dosed at 5 mg/kg at weeks 0, 2, and 6, then every 8 weeks.[6] The FDA-approved dose for adalimumab is an initial dose of 80 mg at week 0 that is followed by 40 mg every other week starting at week 1.[6]

The TNF inhibitors are used off label for several dermatologic conditions. Etanercept, infliximab, and adalimumab have been used for neutrophilic dermatoses (eg, aphthous stomatitis, Behçet disease, pyoderma gangrenosum), bullous dermatoses (eg, bullous pemphigoid, pemphigus vulgaris, cicatricial pemphigoid), granulomatous dermatoses (eg, generalized granuloma annulare, sarcoidosis), autoimmune connective tissue diseases (eg, dermatomyositis, scleroderma), and other disease (eg, graft-versus-host disease [GVHD], hidradenitis suppurativa, and pityriasis rubra pilaris).[5]

In general, when starting a patient on a TNF inhibitor, the following tests are ordered in our clinic: initial tuberculosis screening with a Purified protein derivative (PPD) or Quantiferon Gold test (but not both), complete blood count (rare cases of anemia and pancytopenia have been reported), comprehensive metabolic panel (liver function test abnormalities have been reported), hepatitis B surface antigen, hepatitis C virus (HCV) antibody, and possibly a human immunodeficiency virus (HIV) test. These tests are summarized in **Table 1**.

Absolute contraindications for the TNF inhibitors include a known hypersensitivity to the medication, concurrent use of anakinra (IL-1 receptor antagonist), and various infections.[5] These infections are described by the American College of Rheumatology as active bacterial infections or bacterial infections requiring antibiotic therapy, active tuberculosis or untreated latent tuberculosis, active herpes zoster infection, active life-threatening fungal infections, severe bacterial or viral upper respiratory tract infections, nonhealed infected skin ulcers, acute infection with hepatitis B virus (HBV) or HCV, untreated chronic HBV infection, or chronic HBV or HCV infection with significant liver injury (defined as Child-Pugh classes B or C).[7] In addition, infliximab should be avoided in patients who have a known hypersensitivity to murine proteins because it is a chimeric antibody.[5] Infliximab is also unique in that it is dosed intravenously, which can be inconvenient for patients.[4] A relative contraindication common to TNF inhibitors includes a family history of demyelinating disease. Infliximab is also relatively contraindicated in patients with high-grade congestive heart failure.[5]

Table 1
Biologics used in dermatology for FDA-approved indications

Biologic	FDA-approved Dermatologic Indication	Dosage	Monitoring Requirement
Etanercept	Plaque psoriasis Psoriatic arthritis	50 mg SC injection twice weekly for 3 mo; 50 mg weekly SC injection thereafter	Baseline tests: • CBC (repeat at 2–3 mo then every 6–12 mo) • CMP (repeat at 2–3 mo then every 6–12 mo) • PPD or Quantiferon gold (repeat yearly) • Hepatitis B surface antigen and core IgM antibody (repeat yearly) • HCV antibody • ±HIV and ANA
Infliximab	Plaque psoriasis Psoriatic arthritis	3–5 mg/kg per infusion at weeks 0, 2, and 6, then every 8 wk	Same as etanercept
Adalimumab	Plaque psoriasis Psoriatic arthritis	80 mg SC injection day 0, 40 mg SC injection day 7, then 40 mg SC injection every 14 d	Same as etanercept
Ustekinumab	Moderate to severe plaque psoriasis	45 mg ($\leq$100 kg) or 90 mg (>100 kg) by SC injection at weeks 0 and 4, then every 12 wk thereafter	Same as etanercept
Secukinumab	Moderate to severe plaque psoriasis	150 mg or 300 mg SC injection weekly for 5 consecutive weeks followed by SC injection once every 4 wk	Same as etanercept
Rituximab	Granulomatosis with polyangiitis Microscopic polyangiitis	• Rheumatoid arthritis dosing: 1000 mg every 2 wk × 2 doses • Lymphoma dosing: 375 mg/m^2 per week × 4 doses[5]	• CBC every 2 wk during treatment and every 1–3 mo thereafter[5] • Initial HBsAg and anti-HBc
IVIG[5]	GVHD Kawasaki disease	2 g/kg/cycle, divided into 3–5 equal doses, given over 3–5 consecutive days	• CBC • CMP • Immunoglobulin levels (in particular to exclude IgA deficiency) • Screen for rheumatoid factor and cryoglobulins because these patients are at increased risk for renal failure • Consider screening for hepatitis B and C as well as HIV

Abbreviations: ANA, antinuclear antibody; CBC, complete blood count; CMP, comprehensive metabolic panel; HBc, hepatitis B core antibody; HBsAg, hepatitis B surface antigen; SC, subcutaneous.

Several special issues deserve extra mention. The first includes a history of malignancy. Limited studies have failed to provide evidence for increased risk of recurrent or new cancer in patients treated with a TNF inhibitor who have a history of a prior malignancy. The paucity of data stems from exclusion of these patients from clinical trials. However, data from the British Society for Rheumatology Biologics Registry identified 177 patients treated with anti-TNF for rheumatoid arthritis (RA) with a prior malignancy and compared them with 117 patients with RA with prior malignancy being treated with traditional disease-modifying antirheumatic drugs (DMARDs). The rates of incident malignancy were 25.3 events/1000 person-years in the anti-TNF cohort compared with 38.3/1000 person-years in the DMARD cohort. Even with these data, the investigators recommended that these results should not be interpreted as indicating that it is safe to treat all patients with RA with prior malignancy with anti-TNF therapy.[8]

Screening for latent tuberculosis infection is another special issue and should be performed before the initiation of TNF-inhibitor therapy. Patients who have evidence of latent tuberculosis should initiate treatment of latent tuberculosis before starting a TNF inhibitor. Isoniazid for 9 months is the typical treatment. Although the duration of latent tuberculosis infection therapy before starting a TNF inhibitor has not been well established, most authorities suggest that patients receive at least 1 month of treatment before starting TNF-inhibitor therapy.[9]

HCV infection is also an issue commonly seen when starting a TNF inhibitor. Although HCV antibody is a commonly drawn laboratory test before the therapy, few data exist relating to the use of TNF inhibitors in patients infected with HCV. For example, one study examined 9 patients with RA infected with HCV who were treated with etanercept. At 3 months, no patient had evidence of increased hepatic inflammation. In addition, no significant viral load increases were observed in those with detectable HCV RNA. In addition, no reactivation was observed in those with undetectable HCV RNA.[10]

HIV is another issue commonly encountered with TNF inhibitors, especially considering that it is a risk factor for psoriasis. In general, anecdotal data suggest that TNF inhibition can be tolerated well by patients infected with HIV, provided that the patient is on an effective antiretroviral regimen before starting a TNF inhibitor.[11]

Several adverse effects are noted with the TNF inhibitors. Collectively, postmarketing case reports of the TNF inhibitors have reported rare adverse effects of nonmelanoma skin cancer, infections (specifically tuberculosis reactivation, invasive fungal infections, and hepatitis B reactivation), neurologic disease, congestive heart failure, autoimmune conditions, and hematologic toxicity (eg, leukopenia, neutropenia, thrombocytopenia, and pancytopenia).[5] The most common side effects associated with etanercept and adalimumab are injection site reactions. For patients receiving infliximab, infusion reaction needs to be monitored. Theoretically with all TNF inhibitors there is also an increased risk of developing neutralizing antidrug antibodies, but this risk seems to be highest with infliximab because it is a chimeric antibody.[5]

The risk of developing hematologic malignancies is a commonly discussed topic with the use of biologics. A black box warning for lymphoma and other malignancies accompanies the TNF inhibitors. TNF inhibitors have been used commercially for nearly 20 years. For example, etanercept was released for commercial use in late 1998. Since that time, numerous conflicting studies have discussed the risk of lymphoma associated their use. However, because TNF-inhibitor therapies are often reserved for patients with the most severe disease, there is likely to be a higher intrinsic risk of lymphoma in patients who require treatment with TNF inhibitors. Numerous large studies have found no increased risk of lymphoma in patients treated with TNF inhibitors compared with similar disease-equivalent cohorts.[12–14]

Although monotherapy with biologic agents is effective for many patients with psoriasis, some patients require combination therapy. Many trials have evaluated the efficacy and safety of combination therapies in moderate to severe psoriasis.[15] For example, etanercept or adalimumab with phototherapy may result in a greater reduction of disease severity than either alone. Etanercept and methotrexate in combination are more effective than monotherapy with either medication. Acitretin has been used to decrease the dosing of etanercept while maintaining similar levels of efficacy. Short-term cyclosporine has also been combined with etanercept of adalimumab to control psoriasis flares.[15]

INTERLEUKIN-12/INTERLEUKIN-23 INHIBITION

Ustekinumab is a fully human monoclonal antibody that binds the p40 subunit of IL-12 and IL-23.[4] IL-12 and IL-23 are implicated in the pathogenicity of psoriasis and other autoimmune inflammatory conditions. These key cytokines are secreted by antigen-presenting cells and are important mediators of the differentiation of naive T cells into T-helper (Th) 1 and Th17 cells. Th17 cells produce distinct cytokines that have essential functions in host defense, inflammation, and keratinocyte proliferation.[5]

Ustekinumab is approved for the treatment of moderate to severe psoriasis and psoriatic arthritis. It is administered based on weight at 45 mg (≤100 kg) or 90 mg (>100 kg) by subcutaneous (SC) injection at weeks 0 and 4, then every 12 weeks thereafter.[6] The same screening tests that were mentioned previously for initiation of TNF inhibitors are typically ordered for patients who are to start ustekinumab.

The safety and tolerability of ustekinumab have been studied extensively in clinical trials, and postmarketing studies are underway to further determine the long-term safety profile of the medication.[5] The most common adverse effects associated with ustekinumab are injection site reaction, headache, nasopharyngitis, and upper respiratory tract infections.[16] Ustekinumab has not been shown to increase the risk for serious infections, internal malignancy, or adverse cardiovascular events. A meta-analysis of the safety profile of ustekinumab showed no significant difference in serious infections or internal malignancies compared with placebo.[17] Recently, a multicenter, longitudinal, disease-based registry (Psoriasis Longitudinal Assessment and Registry [PSOLAR]) at dermatology centers examined 9154 patients treated with biologic agents and indicated that adalimumab and infliximab carry a higher risk of serious infection compared with nonbiologic therapies, whereas etanercept and ustekinumab do not.[18] In addition, at 5-years, there are no significant differences in rates of major adverse cardiovascular events between patients on ustekinumab and those in the general population.

When examining the efficacy of ustekinumab with a TNF inhibitor, a randomized controlled trial of 903 patients with moderate to severe psoriasis compared either 45 or 90 mg of ustekinumab (at weeks 0 and 4) with high-dose etanercept (50 mg twice weekly for 12 weeks) and found that the efficacy of ustekinumab was superior to etanercept over a 12-week period.[19] The primary end point was the proportion of patients with at least 75% improvement in the Psoriasis Area and Severity Index (PASI) at week 12. The efficacy and safety of a crossover from etanercept to ustekinumab were evaluated after week 12. There was at least 75% improvement in the PASI at week 12 in 67.5% of patients who received 45 mg of ustekinumab and 73.8% of patients who received 90 mg, compared with 56.8% of those who received etanercept ($P = .01$ and $P<.001$, respectively). Similarly, 65.1% of patients who received 45 mg of ustekinumab and 70.6% of patients who received 90 mg of ustekinumab had cleared or minimal disease according to the physician's global assessment, compared with 49.0% of patients who received etanercept (*P*<.001 for both comparisons). Among patients who did not have a response to etanercept, 48.9% had at least 75% improvement in the PASI within 12 weeks after crossover to ustekinumab.

INTERLEUKIN-17 INHIBITORS

The Th17 pathway is central to the pathogenesis of psoriasis, and the IL-17 molecule is key to the Th17 pathway. IL-17 consists of a class of cytokines that are important in activating the innate immune response and is considered the main driver against extracellular bacteria. Six cytokines belong to the IL-17 family, classified as IL-17A to IL-17F, with IL-17A and II-17F possessing the greatest amino acid sequence similarity (55%) and similar biological properties. Because of their pleiotropic activity on various tissue cells and innate immune cells, IL-17A is considered crucial in tissue inflammation. Increasing evidence suggests that IL-17A plays a key role in a large number of immune-mediated disorders, including psoriasis and psoriatic arthritis.[3]

At present, there are 3 biologic agents used to target IL-17A: secukinumab, brodalumab, and ixekizumab.[3] Secukinumab is a human IgG1(kappa) that neutralizes IL-17A. In January 2015, the FDA approved secukinumab to treat moderate to severe plaque psoriasis in adults who do not respond well to medication applied directly to the skin.[17,20] Secukinumab is given as an injection once a week for 5 consecutive weeks followed by an injection once every 4 weeks. It is approved at both 150-mg and 300-mg dosages.[17]

Ixekizumab is a humanized IgG4 monoclonal antibody (mAb) neutralizing IL-17A, a mechanism of action that is similar to secukinumab. Brodalumab is a human mAb blocking IL-17RA, the receptor subunit that is shared by IL-17A and IL-17F. Brodalumab and ixekizumab are currently being tested for the treatment of moderate to severe psoriasis in phase III clinical trials as of April 2015.[21,22]

At this time, initial laboratory work-up before initiating treatment with IL-17 inhibitors is similar to that for TNF inhibitors, and it is summarized in **Table 2**. The physiologic impact of long-term IL-17 antagonism needs to be shown in larger and longer clinical trials. There is a need for a better understanding of how IL-17 antagonism affects psoriatic arthritis. In addition, clinical implications of targeting the IL-17 versus IL-17 receptor needs to be better characterized.[3]

To date, the safety profile for secukinumab is acceptable. Nasopharyngitis is the most common adverse effect. Serious infection rates were not significantly different between those treated with secukinumab and those treated with placebo. Oral candidiasis has been noted in several subjects on secukinumab, and the effect seems to be dose dependent.[23] Findings from postmarketing studies will help inform clinicians and patients regarding long-term safety and rare adverse events. At this time, clinical studies for ixekizumab and brodalumab also showed acceptable safety profiles, and these biologics are pending FDA approval for use in patients with moderate to severe psoriasis.

RITUXIMAB

Rituximab is a chimeric murine-human IgG1 monoclonal antibody to CD20 that induces depletion of B cells. CD20 is a B cell–specific antigen expressed on the surface of B lymphocytes during differentiation from the pre–B-cell to the mature B-cell stage. CD20 is not found on plasma cells or stem cells. As a result, treatment with rituximab does not result in dramatic decreases of immunoglobulin levels. Rituximab's mechanisms of action include antibody-dependent cellular cytotoxicity, complement-mediated lysis,

Table 2
Biologics used in dermatology for selected non–FDA-approved indications

Biologic	Off-label Use	Dosage	Special Considerations
Etanercept	Pyoderma gangrenosum[33]	25–50 mg twice weekly	Effective in several case reports
Infliximab	Sarcoidosis[34]	3–10 mg/kg/dose at 0, 2, 6, and every 8–19 wk subsequently	9 of 10 patients reported subjective improvement of skin lesions; all 10 had objective improvement
	Pyoderma gangrenosum[35]	5 mg/kg/dose	Effective in placebo-controlled trial with 30 subjects
	Hidradenitis suppuritiva[36]	5 mg/kg/dose	Randomized, double-blind, placebo-controlled crossover trial
Adalimumab	Sarcoidosis[37]	80 mg initial loading dose followed by 40 mg once weekly	12-wk, double-blind placebo-controlled trial showed improvement in several cutaneous findings in the adalimumab-treated patients relative to placebo recipients
	Pyoderma gangrenosum[38]	80 mg initial loading dose, followed by 40 mg wk 1, then 40 mg every other week	May be effective after failure of other systemic therapies
	Hidradenitis suppuritiva[39]	160 mg initial loading dose followed by 40 mg once weekly	Higher doses needed than for psoriasis; large studies are pending
Ustekinumab	Subacute cutaneous lupus erythematosus[40]	45 mg (≤100 kg) or 90 mg (>100 kg) by SC injection at weeks 0 and 4, then every 12 wk thereafter	Multiple case reports showed efficacy in recalcitrant disease
Rituximab	Pemphigus vulgaris[26,41]	Lymphoma or RA dosing have been used. See **Table 1**	Several case reports and small series of efficacy. Recent report of improvement with combined anti-CD20 and IVIG. Needs controlled trials. Recent systematic review highlights clinical response within 6 wk of treatment
	Dermatomyositis[42]		Large, randomized, multicenter controlled trial sponsored by NIH showed efficacy
IVIG	Pyoderma gangrenosum[43]	2 g/kg/cycle over 3–5 consecutive days	Found effective in combination with systemic steroids and other immunosuppressant drugs in series of 7 cases
	Pemphigus vulgaris		Has been combined with rituximab for recalcitrant disease[44]
	Dermatomyositis[45]		Double-blind, placebo-controlled trial showed efficacy
	Toxic epidermal necrolysis[46,47]		Differing reports on efficacy of IVIG exist. Interpretation of literature is limited by lack of treatment regimen uniformity, lack of adequate control data, and size of studies performed

Abbreviation: NIH, US National Institutes of Health.

and direct disruption of signaling pathways and triggering of apoptosis. The contribution of each mechanism remains unclear, and different mechanisms may predominate in the treatment of different diseases.[24] However, within 6 months of therapy it is hoped that new B cells that do not produce the pathogenic antibodies will return to circulation.[25]

At present, rituximab is FDA approved for non-Hodgkin lymphoma, chronic lymphocytic leukemia, RA, granulomatosis with polyangiitis (Wegener granulomatosis), and microscopic polyangiitis.[17] Rituximab can be dosed in 2 different ways: lymphoma dosing (375 mg/m^2 per week for 4 doses) or RA dosing (1000 mg every 2 weeks for 2 doses).[5]

Rituximab is currently used off label for many conditions in dermatology. These conditions include pemphigus vulgaris, paraneoplastic pemphigus, epidermolysis bullosa acquisita, bullous pemphigoid, primary cutaneous B-cell lymphoma, dermatomyositis, acute and chronic GVHD, and systemic lupus erythematosus.[24] The use of rituximab for the pemphigus group of blistering diseases is worth extra discussion as it is currently the most common use of this drug in dermatology.[26] A large systematic review of patients receiving either the lymphoma or RA dosing showed that patients seem to experience an initial clinical response within 6 weeks of treatment. Most investigators also treat with conventional immunosuppressive therapies during and after rituximab therapy. However, relapse rates are 50% or more and many investigators conclude that additional rituximab or systemic therapies may be needed to maintain remission.[26]

In treatments with rituximab, infusion reactions are the most common adverse event. These reactions can be pretreated with acetaminophen, diphenhydramine, or methylprednisolone.[24] The incidence of serious adverse effects is low. In a study of rituximab for the treatment of RA, infections occurred in 35% of patients compared with 28% of the placebo group. Serious infections occurred in 2% of the rituximab group compared with 1% in the placebo group.[27] Because rituximab is a chimeric antibody, human antichimeric antibodies (HACA) can theoretically develop. One study showed that HACAs developed in less than 1% of patients treated for lymphoma, although the incidence may be higher in patients with autoimmune disorders.[28,29]

In addition, there is a risk of reactivation of the HBV infection. Reactivation of HBV can be idiopathic, asymptomatic, and rapid; rigorous reactivations can lead to fulminant liver failure and even death. The FDA issued a recommendation that all health care professionals screen patients on rituximab for HBV infection by measuring hepatitis B surface antigen and hepatitis B core antibody. In addition, patients with evidence of prior HBV infection should be monitored for clinical and laboratory signs of HBV reactivation during and for several months after completing rituximab therapy because reactivations may occur several months following completion of rituximab therapy.[17]

INTRAVENOUS IMMUNOGLOBULIN

IVIG is a fractioned blood product consisting of IgG antibodies that was first used in antibody deficiency disorders. It is increasingly being used for several inflammatory and autoimmune conditions.[30] IVIG is currently FDA approved in dermatology for GVHD and Kawasaki syndrome.[31] IVIG is also currently being used to treat a wide range of difficult-to-treat dermatologic diseases, including dermatomyositis, autoimmune bullous skin diseases, and toxic epidermal necrolysis.[30,31]

Before starting IVIG, a complete history and physical with emphasis on cardiopulmonary and renal status should be performed to assess patients at risk for fluid overload. Laboratory tests include a complete blood count and chemistries to assess liver and renal function. Immunoglobulin levels should be assessed, in particular IgA, because some patients have an increased risk of anaphylaxis. Screening for rheumatoid factor and cryoglobulins can be considered because patients with positive values are at increased risk for renal failure from IVIG. Consider screening for hepatitis B and C, along with HIV.[5]

Adverse effects of IVIG include infusion reactions that are generally mild and self-limiting, often occurring 30 to 60 minutes after onset of the infusion.[31] They include flushing, myalgia, headaches, fever, chills, lower backache, nausea or vomiting, chest tightness, wheezing, changes in blood pressure, and tachycardia. Rare episodes of anaphylaxis have occurred, particularly in IgA-deficient patients with anti-IgA antibodies.[31] Coombs-positive hemolysis and transient neutropenia have also been reported. Acute renal failure has also been reported and is thought to be related to an injury to the proximal tubule induced by high solute load. In addition, rare neurologic complications such as aseptic meningitis are seen 10 hours to 7 days after high-dose IVIG.[31]

SUMMARY

Biologic therapy has dramatically changed the way medicine, and specifically dermatology, is practiced today. The use of biologic agents in dermatology is evolving, with psoriasis being the most common indication for which biologics are used currently. However, several other dermatologic diseases seem to be responsive to biologic therapy, and continuing research and development efforts are elucidating the benefit-risk profiles of various biologic medications in these dermatologic conditions.[15]

Although biologic agents have revolutionized the management of dermatologic conditions, cost must also be considered when evaluating management options, especially compared with traditional agents. For example, the cost of 1 year of induction and maintenance treatment of psoriasis in 2014 was estimated to be $53,909 for ustekinumab, $46,395 for etanercept, and $39,041 for adalimumab.[32] Nonetheless, because of their efficacy, the cost of a biologic may be offset by significant reductions in the number of hospital stays, reduction in use of other systemic therapies, and increased satisfaction by patients.[32] Thus, understanding their mechanisms of action, labeled and off-label uses in dermatology, and common adverse effects helps to inform clinical decision making and improve patient outcomes.

REFERENCES

1. Bolognia JL, Jorizzo JL, Schaffer JV, editors. Dermatology. 3rd edition. Elsevier Health Sciences; 2012.
2. Brimhall AK, King LN, Licciardone JC, et al. Safety and efficacy of alefacept, efalizumab, etanercept and infliximab in treating moderate to severe plaque psoriasis: a meta-analysis of randomized controlled trials. Br J Dermatol 2008;159(2): 274–85.
3. Chiricozzi A, Krueger JG. IL-17 targeted therapies for psoriasis. Expert Opin Investig Drugs 2013;22(8):993–1005.
4. Mease PJ, Armstrong AW. Managing patients with psoriatic disease: the diagnosis and pharmacologic treatment of psoriatic arthritis in patients with psoriasis. Drugs 2014;74(4):423–41.
5. Wolverton SE. Comprehensive dermatologic drug therapy. 3rd edition. Elsevier Health Sciences; 2012. p. 1024.

6. Brezinski EA, Armstrong AW. Off-label biologic regimens in psoriasis: a systematic review of efficacy and safety of dose escalation, reduction, and interrupted biologic therapy. PLoS One 2012;7(4):e33486.

7. Singh JA, Furst DE, Bharat A, et al. 2012 update of the 2008 American College of Rheumatology recommendations for the use of disease-modifying antirheumatic drugs and biologic agents in the treatment of rheumatoid arthritis. Arthritis Care Res 2012;64(5):625–39.

8. Dixon WG, Watson KD, Lunt M, et al. Influence of anti-tumor necrosis factor therapy on cancer incidence in patients with rheumatoid arthritis who have had a prior malignancy: results from the British Society for Rheumatology Biologics Register. Arthritis Care Res 2010;62(6):755–63.

9. Gardam MA, Keystone EC, Menzies R, et al. Anti-tumour necrosis factor agents and tuberculosis risk: mechanisms of action and clinical management. Lancet Infect Dis 2003;3(3):148–55.

10. Marotte H, Fontanges E, Bailly F, et al. Etanercept treatment for three months is safe in patients with rheumatological manifestations associated with hepatitis C virus. Rheumatology (Oxford) 2007;46(1):97–9.

11. Cepeda EJ, Williams FM, Ishimori ML, et al. The use of anti-tumour necrosis factor therapy in HIV-positive individuals with rheumatic disease. Ann Rheum Dis 2008; 67(5):710–2.

12. Askling J, Fored CM, Baecklund E, et al. Haematopoietic malignancies in rheumatoid arthritis: lymphoma risk and characteristics after exposure to tumour necrosis factor antagonists. Ann Rheum Dis 2005;64(10):1414–20.

13. Askling J, Baecklund E, Granath F, et al. Anti-tumour necrosis factor therapy in rheumatoid arthritis and risk of malignant lymphomas: relative risks and time trends in the Swedish Biologics Register. Ann Rheum Dis 2009;68(5): 648–53.

14. Mariette X, Tubach F, Bagheri H, et al. Lymphoma in patients treated with anti-TNF: results of the 3-year prospective French RATIO registry. Ann Rheum Dis 2010;69(2):400–8.

15. Armstrong AW, Bagel J, Van Voorhees AS, et al. Combining biologic therapies with other systemic treatments in psoriasis: evidence-based, best-practice recommendations from the medical board of the national psoriasis foundation. JAMA Dermatol 2015;151(4):432–8.

16. Meng Y, Dongmei L, Yanbin P, et al. Systematic review and meta-analysis of ustekinumab for moderate to severe psoriasis. Clin Exp Dermatol 2014;39(6): 696–707.

17. US Food and Drug Administration. Available at: http://www.fda.gov. Accessed March 15, 2015.

18. Kalb RE, Fiorentino DF, Lebwohl MG, et al. Risk of serious infection with biologic and systemic treatment of psoriasis: results from the Psoriasis Longitudinal Assessment and Registry (PSOLAR). JAMA Dermatol 2015. [Epub ahead of print].

19. Griffiths CE, Strober BE, van de Kerkhof P, et al. Comparison of ustekinumab and etanercept for moderate-to-severe psoriasis. N Engl J Med 2010;362(2):118–28.

20. Available at: http://www.fda.gov/NewsEvents/Newsroom/PressAnnouncements/ucm430969.htm. Accessed January 21, 2015.

21. US National Institutes of Health. Study of efficacy and safety of brodalumab compared with placebo and ustekinumab in moderate to severe plaque psoriasis subjects (AMAGINE-2). 2015. Available at: https://clinicaltrials.gov/ct2/show/NCT01708603?term=brodalumab&rank=2. Accessed April 28, 2015.

22. US National Institutes of Health. Evaluation of ixekizumab using auto-injector or prefilled syringe in participants with moderate to severe plaque psoriasis (UN-COVER-A). 2015. Available at: https://clinicaltrials.gov/ct2/show/NCT01777191?term=Ixekizumab&rank=1. Accessed April 15, 2015.
23. Thaci D, Humeniuk J, Frambach Y, et al. Secukinumab in psoriasis: Randomized, controlled phase 3 trial results assessing the potential to improve treatment response in partial responders (STATURE). Br J Dermatol 2015. [Epub ahead of print].
24. Carr DR, Heffernan MP. Off-label uses of rituximab in dermatology. Dermatol Ther 2007;20(4):277–87.
25. Sehgal VN, Pandhi D, Khurana A. Biologics in dermatology: an integrated review. Indian J Dermatol 2014;59(5):425–41.
26. Ahmed AR, Shetty S. A comprehensive analysis of treatment outcomes in patients with pemphigus vulgaris treated with rituximab. Autoimmun Rev 2015; 14(4):323–31.
27. Emery P, Fleischmann R, Filipowicz-Sosnowska A, et al. The efficacy and safety of rituximab in patients with active rheumatoid arthritis despite methotrexate treatment: results of a phase IIB randomized, double-blind, placebo-controlled, dose-ranging trial. Arthritis Rheum 2006;54(5):1390–400.
28. Looney RJ, Anolik JH, Campbell D, et al. B cell depletion as a novel treatment for systemic lupus erythematosus: a phase I/II dose-escalation trial of rituximab. Arthritis Rheum 2004;50(8):2580–9.
29. McLaughlin P, Grillo-Lopez AJ, Link BK, et al. Rituximab chimeric anti-CD20 monoclonal antibody therapy for relapsed indolent lymphoma: half of patients respond to a four-dose treatment program. J Clin Oncol 1998;16(8):2825–33.
30. Cakmak SK, Cakmak A, Gonul M. A Klc, Gul U. Intravenous immunoglobulin therapy in dermatology: an update. Inflamm Allergy Drug Targets 2013;12(2):132–46.
31. Jolles S, Hughes J, Whittaker S. Dermatological uses of high-dose intravenous immunoglobulin. Arch Dermatol 1998;134(1):80–6.
32. Cheng J, Feldman SR. The cost of biologics for psoriasis is increasing. Drugs Context 2014;3:212266.
33. Patel F, Fitzmaurice S, Duong C, et al. Effective strategies for the management of pyoderma gangrenosum: a comprehensive review. Acta Dermato Venereologica 2015;95(5):525–31.
34. Doty JD, Mazur JE, Judson MA. Treatment of sarcoidosis with infliximab. Chest 2005;127(3):1064–71.
35. Brooklyn TN, Dunnill MG, Shetty A, et al. Infliximab for the treatment of pyoderma gangrenosum: a randomised, double blind, placebo controlled trial. Gut 2006; 55(4):505–9.
36. Grant A, Gonzalez T, Montgomery MO, et al. Infliximab therapy for patients with moderate to severe hidradenitis suppurativa: a randomized, double-blind, placebo-controlled crossover trial. J Am Acad Dermatol 2010;62(2):205–17.
37. Pariser RJ, Paul J, Hirano S, et al. A double-blind, randomized, placebo-controlled trial of adalimumab in the treatment of cutaneous sarcoidosis. J Am Acad Dermatol 2013;68(5):765–73.
38. Hinterberger L, Muller CS, Vogt T, et al. Adalimumab: a treatment option for pyoderma gangrenosum after failure of systemic standard therapies. Dermatol Ther 2012;2(1):6.
39. Kimball AB, Kerdel F, Adams D, et al. Adalimumab for the treatment of moderate to severe hidradenitis suppurativa: a parallel randomized trial. Ann Intern Med 2012;157(12):846–55.

40. Dahl C, Johansen C, Kragballe K, et al. Ustekinumab in the treatment of refractory chronic cutaneous lupus erythematosus: a case report. Acta dermato venereologica 2013;93(3):368–9.

41. Joly P, Mouquet H, Roujeau JC, et al. A single cycle of rituximab for the treatment of severe pemphigus. N Engl J Med 2007;357(6):545–52.

42. Oddis CV, Reed AM, Aggarwal R, et al. Rituximab in the treatment of refractory adult and juvenile dermatomyositis and adult polymyositis: a randomized, placebo-phase trial. Arthritis Rheum 2013;65(2):314–24.

43. Kreuter A, Reich-Schupke S, Stucker M, et al. Intravenous immunoglobulin for pyoderma gangrenosum. Br J Dermatol 2008;158(4):856–7.

44. Ahmed AR, Spigelman Z, Cavacini LA, et al. Treatment of pemphigus vulgaris with rituximab and intravenous immune globulin. N Engl J Med 2006;355(17): 1772–9.

45. Dalakas MC, Illa I, Dambrosia JM, et al. A controlled trial of high-dose intravenous immune globulin infusions as treatment for dermatomyositis. N Engl J Med 1993; 329(27):1993–2000.

46. Prins C, Kerdel FA, Padilla RS, et al. Treatment of toxic epidermal necrolysis with high-dose intravenous immunoglobulins: multicenter retrospective analysis of 48 consecutive cases. Arch Dermatol 2003;139(1):26–32.

47. Bachot N, Revuz J, Roujeau JC. Intravenous immunoglobulin treatment for Stevens-Johnson syndrome and toxic epidermal necrolysis: a prospective non-comparative study showing no benefit on mortality or progression. Arch Dermatol 2003;139(1):33–6.

Selected Disorders of Skin Appendages—Acne, Alopecia, Hyperhidrosis

Jay C. Vary Jr, MD, PhD

KEYWORDS

- Hyperhidrosis • Acne vulgaris • Alopecia areata • Female pattern hair loss
- Androgenetic alopecia • Telogen effluvium

KEY POINTS

- The etiology of hyperhidrosis can usually be determined by history and physical examination without the need for laboratory testing.
- Treatments for acne vulgaris are selected based on the type of the underlying acne and its pathogenesis.
- Alopecia areata (AA) is a common autoimmune condition for which resolution and relapse are common, but treatments can help minimize the manifestations.
- Female pattern alopecia is very common, and there are several options for treatment; however, large studies regarding treatments have not been done to show efficacy.
- Shedding of hair is often from telogen effluvium (TE), but other causes need to be ruled out in most cases.

INTRODUCTION

The skin appendages are composed of the eccrine and apocrine sweat glands, the hair follicles, the sebaceous glands, and the nails (**Fig. 1**). All of these are embryonically derived from buds of epidermis that grew down into the dermis to form these specialized structures. The eccrine glands are composed of secretory coils found deep in the dermis, which then transition through a long tubular portion, the eccrine duct, to empty directly onto the skin surface. These glands secrete a hypotonic saline solution in response to cholinergic stimulation and function to cool the skin surface to maintain thermal homeostasis. The eccrine glands are found in nearly all regions of the body surface but have the highest numbers in the skin of the palms, soles, and craniofacial areas. Pilosebaceous units are composed of hair follicles and sebaceous glands. Hairs are produced from the follicle and gain their color from melanocytes

Division of Dermatology, Department of Medicine, University of Washington, Box 354697, 4225 Roosevelt Way Northeast, 4th Floor, Seattle, WA 98105-6920, USA
E-mail address: jvary@uw.edu

Med Clin N Am 99 (2015) 1195–1211
http://dx.doi.org/10.1016/j.mcna.2015.07.003
0025-7125/15/$ – see front matter © 2015 Elsevier Inc. All rights reserved.

medical.theclinics.com

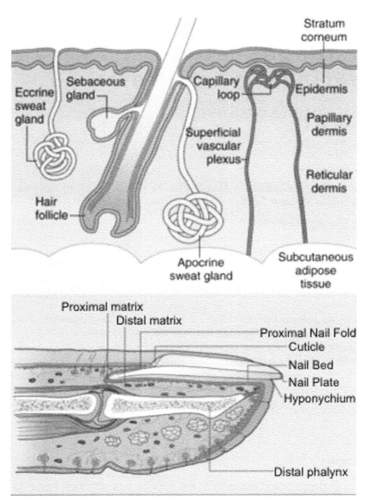

Fig. 1. Schematic showing the skin appendages and nail anatomy. (*Adapted from* Norris DA. Structure and function of the skin. In: Goldman L, Schafer AI, editors. Goldman's Cecil medicine. Philadelphia: Saunders; 2012. p. 2498–503, with permission; and Tosti A, Piraccini BM. Nail disorders. In: Bolognia JL, Jorizzo JL, Schaffer JV, editors. Dermatology. Elsevier Limited; 2011. p. 1129–47, with permission.)

located at the base of the follicle. Every hair follicle has an associated sebum-secreting sebaceous gland. Sebaceous glands are found throughout the skin surface, except the palms and soles, with the highest density being on the craniofacial skin and upper trunk. The glands are found independent of hair follicles around the lips, areolas, and genitals. Apocrine glands are specialized sweat glands that secrete a solution with higher oil content and are under adrenergic control. These glands are connected to pilosebaceous units along the milk line as well as the eyelids and ears, with the highest concentrations in the axillae and groin. Apoeccrine glands are also found in the axillae and groin and have similar anatomic characteristics as apocrine glands, but they function like eccrine glands, producing copious saline sweat under cholinergic control. Nails have a structure reminiscent of hair follicles but form a plate rather than a round hair. Hair and nails are formed of keratin proteins, similar to the epidermis.

This article discusses common representative diseases of the skin appendages. Nail disorders are not addressed here but are covered in a separate article in this journal issue.[1] The most common condition resulting from eccrine gland dysfunction is hyperhidrosis. Acne is a disease of the pilosebaceous unit. AA, female pattern hair loss (FPHL) and androgenetic alopecia (AGA), and TE are discussed with regard to hair follicles.

HYPERHIDROSIS

Although almost everyone sweats with exercise and emotional stimuli, when excessive it can impair quality of life. Hyperhidrosis is often recognized by patients and providers as a variation of normal, yet it negatively impacts the lives of about 1% to 3% of individuals.[2,3] Axillary hyperhidrosis often requires changes of clothing several times a day, and palmar hyperhidrosis can make shaking hands embarrassing, affecting social and work-related activities.

With an understanding of hyperhidrosis types and their underlying causes, patient history is usually all that is required to differentiate common primary hyperhidrosis from potentially worrisome causes. Primary hyperhidrosis is usually localized to the axilla, palmoplantar areas, and/or craniofacial areas; it is a functional problem occurring in anatomically normal-appearing eccrine glands.[4] Primary hyperhidrosis is always symmetric, usually starts in the second decade of life, and is often familial. Asymmetrical hyperhidrosis should prompt an investigation for a neurologic lesion. Primary hyperhidrosis is controlled by cortical input to the hypothalamus, whereas thermoregulatory sweating does not involve cortical direct inputs. Perhaps as a result, primary hyperhidrosis does not occur during sleep. This distinction is important for both the diagnosis and success of some topical treatments.

Generalized hyperhidrosis is usually secondary to other varied causes such as medications, endocrinopathies, infections, and malignancies.[5] An algorithm to differentiate primary from secondary hyperhidrosis and a nonexhaustive list of causes is given in **Fig. 2**. Among medications, sertraline and other selective serotonin reuptake inhibitors are among the most common pharmacologic causes. Neoplasms such as lymphoma, carcinoid tumor, and pheochromocytoma are important considerations and are common fodder for examination during medical school and beyond; however, they are uncommon. Specific testing for these conditions is only indicated if a review of systems supports accompanying specific symptoms and the complaint is of generalized rather than of localized sweating.

A few other less-common causes of localized hyperhidrosis deserve mention. Compensatory hyperhidrosis occurs in response to neurologic damage usually at a higher vertebral level. For example, after surgical sympathectomy for palmar hyperhidrosis, patients sometimes develop compensatory hyperhidrosis in areas innervated below the C3-5 level. Gustatory hyperhidrosis occurs symmetrically on craniofacial areas usually in response to spicy foods. This condition can be localized in Frey syndrome following damage to the auriculotemporal nerve; the regenerating parasympathetic fibers to the parotid gland can make incorrect connections resulting in unilateral sweating because of normal parotid salivation signals, even from anticipation of eating.

Treatment of hyperhidrosis is often multimodal and can include topical, injected, and oral therapies; surgical intervention; and even electrochemical treatments. The options presented in the following sections are in the typical order of use proceeding along an algorithm of treatment toward more risky and/or costly alternatives in more refractory cases.

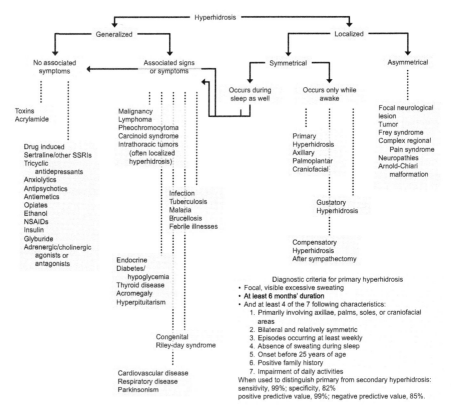

Fig. 2. Algorithm for diagnosis and a nonexhaustive list of causes of hyperhidrosis. NSAID, nonsteroidal antiinflammatory drugs; SSRI, selective serotonin reuptake inhibitors.

Topical Treatments

Over-the-counter antiperspirants typically contain zirconium or aluminum salts, while commercially available solutions of aluminum chloride (AlCl) are available as 12% formulations over the counter or 20% formulations by prescription. Higher concentrations of AlCl can be compounded, but the higher salt content of these preparations commonly causes irritation or burning, which can limit use. The metal salts precipitate with mucopolysaccharides in the eccrine duct causing obstruction and a short-lived necrosis of the secretory coils.[6] Initially, it is applied every night and rinsed off after 6 to 8 hours in the morning to reduce irritation somewhat. Nighttime application is key, because sweat glands of primary hyperhidrosis are less active during sleep, allowing the metal salts to remain in place. Compounding aluminum chloride with 2% to 4% salicylic acid gel has been reported to reduce irritation and improve penetration.[4] Hydrocortisone cream or baking soda can also help reduce irritation from AlCl.[6] Topical glycopyrrolate has also been used for hyperhidrosis and may be most effective for gustatory hyperhidrosis.

Oral Treatments

Oral treatments can offer significant benefit but are rarely tolerated at doses required for clinically meaningful effect. Eccrine gland secretion is under sympathetic nervous system control, but unlike most parts of the sympathetic system, the major direct stimulation of eccrine glands is by acetylcholine. As a result, the anticholinergic muscarinic antagonists glycopyrrolate (1–2 mg twice daily) and oxybutynin (5 mg twice daily) or the α_2 agonist clonidine (0.1 mg twice daily) have all shown efficacy in retrospective studies. Dry mouth or dry eyes are the most common limiting side effects, while oxybutynin can also have significant gastrointestinal and urinary side effects. Oxybutynin has shown efficacy specifically in sertraline-induced secondary hyperhidrosis as well.[7] Although these oral treatments are often not tolerated for long periods, they can help jump start topical treatment. For example, oral glycopyrrolate, 1 mg, dries the skin if used an hour before the nighttime AlCl application, thereby improving efficacy. After 3 days, the oral treatment often can be discontinued because it is often no longer needed.

Iontophoresis

Iontophoresis is an electrochemical treatment with efficacy in primary hyperhidrosis, although its mechanism of action is unclear. Commercially available devices apply a small current to metal plates onto which the palmar and/or plantar surfaces are placed. To improve contact with the skin and to provide a source of ions, tap water is usually added over the metal plates. These devices are sold for home use, often in a rent-to-own type model and are very cost effective after this initial investment. After use for 20 minutes every 2 to 3 days for the first few months, treatment can often be tapered to just 1 treatment every 2 to 3 weeks. Addition of glycopyrrolate or botulinum toxin to the tap water can also improve efficacy but usually results in dry mouth or significant cost, respectively.[7] Owing to the difficulty in getting adequate physical contact with the axillary vault, iontophoresis is not often used in this location.[8] Use is contraindicated in those with implantable electronic devices such as pacemakers or defibrillators, artificial joints, and in pregnant women.

Botulinum Toxin

The direct cholinergic stimulation of eccrine glands allows the use of injectable botulinum toxin for remissions of 4 to 6 months after each treatment. Following local anesthesia, 100 U are injected intradermally throughout each palm or 50 to 100 U per axilla, usually in a 1- to 2-cm grid of injections. Bilateral treatment is recommended because unilateral treatment can result in compensatory hyperhidrosis of the contralateral side. Side effects include pain, significant cost, and possible weakness of intrinsic hand muscles.[6]

Surgical Treatments

Surgical approaches include sympathectomy or physical destruction of axillary sweat glands. Sympathectomy procedures vary but involve creating an often irreversible break in the sympathetic innervation commonly at the T2-3 level, thereby blocking stimulation of palmar eccrine glands. Compensatory hyperhidrosis below this level is a common complication in addition to the perioperative risks.[4,8] This method is not recommended for plantar hyperhidrosis because some loss of sexual function is expected at these spinal levels.[8] For axillary hyperhidrosis, curettage or liposuction-cannula-assisted ablation of the glands can be fairly easily achieved given the deeper position of the axillary apoeccrine glands within the subcutaneous fat with lower risk than thoracic sympathectomy. Insertion of a liposuction cannula or curette into this layer via a small incision allows near-complete destruction of the glands in this space. Local hematoma, seroma, or necrosis can occur, as well as recurrence.[4,7,8]

ACNE

Pubertal acne vulgaris is a problem affecting nearly all people to some degree, such that it could be considered a normal part of maturity. The degree to which individuals are affected varies tremendously, however, resulting in wide estimates of prevalence from 35% to 90% in adolescence.[9] About 50% of those affected continue to have acne into adulthood, however.[10] Despite its commonality, those affected can have depression, anxiety, and social isolation because of severity, visibly obvious manifestations, and the adolescent age at which it is typically most severe.

An understanding of acne pathogenesis is critical to understanding which treatments are most appropriate for an individual. Acne is a disease of the pilosebaceous unit and is driven by the rich oily sebum from the sebaceous gland. The earliest defect identified in acne pathogenesis is the development of the microcomedone. This defect results from the overproduction of keratinocytes at the follicular ostium resulting in plugging of the opening. When this plug is superficial and exposed to the air, it oxidizes, and when it is observed from above, it has a dark appearance, commonly referred to as a blackhead. When this keratinous plug occurs lower in follicle and does not dilate the actual ostium, it is commonly referred to as a whitehead. These collections of open and closed comedones in the absence of other inflammation is referred to as comedonal acne (**Fig. 3**). As sebaceous gland production continues, the oil-rich sebum serves as a medium for bacterial growth for *Propionibacterium acnes* within the now isolated space of the follicle. As the follicle expands with sebum and often bacteria, the lipids and bacterial antigens are recognized by the innate immune system, resulting in inflammation. Erythema and influx of white blood cells result in inflammatory papules and pustules at the follicular sites referred to as inflammatory acne (**Fig. 4**). If overgrowth is exuberant, rupture of the follicle into the deep dermis or subcutaneous space results in deeper nodules and apparent cyst formation termed nodulocystic acne[10,11] (**Fig. 5**).

The underlying cause of microcomedone formation is still unclear, but the typical onset at puberty suggests a hormonal basis. Sebaceous gland production is clearly under androgenic stimulation primarily from dihydrotestosterone. Given this pathogenesis, treatments targeting comedones, sebaceous gland production, bacteria, and androgens are all used to treat the various forms of acne vulgaris.

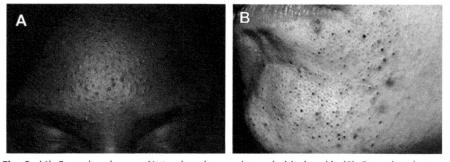

Fig. 3. (*A*) Comedonal acne. Note closed comedones (*whiteheads*). (*B*) Comedonal acne. Note open comedones (*blackheads*). (*Adapted from* [*A*] Brinster NK, Liu V, Diwan AH, et al. Dermatopathology: high-yield pathology. Philadelphia: Saunders; 2011, with permission; and [*B*] Benner N, Sammons D. Overview of the treatment of acne vulgaris. Osteopathic Family Physician 2013;5(5):185–90, with permission.)

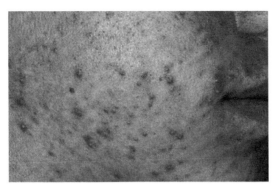

Fig. 4. Inflammatory acne. Note erythematous papules and pustules. (*Adapted from* Habif T, Campbell JL Jr, Chapman MS, et al. Skin disease: diagnosis and treatment. Elsevier; 2011. p. 102–19; with permission.)

Comedonal Acne

Comedolytics are the mainstay for all acne types because they target the earlier stage of the acne lesion and are the only type needed for comedonal acne. Comedolytics are not effective to treat already visible lesions but work to prevent formation of the micro-comedone. As a result, it takes 6 to 8 weeks to see a clinical effect with their use because visible and already developing lesions have to first resolve on their own. Comedolytics work by dislodging the early comedone or by normalizing epidermal differentiation at the follicular opening to prevent keratin plug formation. This mode of action may result in an initial peeling and xerosis for several weeks until the skin adapts to its new normal of treatment. Counseling patients about this initial dryness and inflammation and creating realistic expectations as to how quickly they should expect to see a result is critical to comedolytic success.

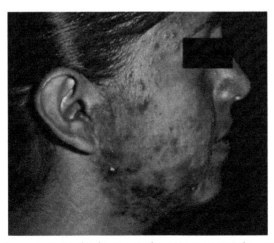

Fig. 5. Nodulocystic acne. Note the larger erythematous to purple papules and nodules along the jawline and scarring on the cheeks. (*From* Paller AS, Mancini AJ. Hurwitz clinical pediatric dermatology: a textbook of skin disorders of childhood and adolescence. Elsevier; 2011. p. 167–83; with permission.)

Comedolytics such as tea tree oil, salicylic acid, and benzoyl peroxide (BPO) are available over the counter, whereas topical retinoids, azelaic acid, and some BPO formulations are available on prescription only. Topical retinoids are the mainstay of acne treatment because they are highly effective at preventing comedone formation as well as improving penetration and efficacy of other treatments and are recommended as first-line treatment of all forms of acne vulgaris by the Global Alliance to Improve Outcomes in Acne Group.[10] The least expensive is tretinoin, which has moderate irritability. Adapalene is the least irritating but has substantially higher cost, even as a generic. Tazarotene is not only the most effective but also causes irritation to the skin and is the most expensive option of the 3 commonly used retinoids available in the United States. All are unstable in light and can cause some photosensitivity, so they are best used at night to increase efficacy and tolerability. As they promote differentiation of keratinocytes, the treated epidermis is slightly thinner. If the initial product is too strong or used too frequently, the difference in thickness of the older and newer epidermis is seen as a peeling layer of skin about a week after initiation, mimicking a sunburn peel. Conservative use of small amounts of retinoids just a few times a week for the first month can often minimize these effects, although application every night is the eventual application goal. Azelaic acid is usually better tolerated but is more costly and less effective than retinoids, so it is often not used as first-line treatment. Azelaic acid is produced by several plants and fungi including the yeast *Malassezia furfur,* which causes tinea versicolor. The slight bleaching effect seen in tinea versicolor is due to inhibition of melanin synthesis by azelaic acid, which can be useful in those with postinflammatory hyperpigmentation of acne lesions.

In addition to retinoids, or as a substitute because of cost or other considerations, over-the-counter products can be used. Tea tree oil, salicylic acid, and BPO all have roughly equal efficacy. Tea tree oil is sometimes associated with allergic contact dermatitis, and patients should be warned of this. Salicylic acid and BPO are usually well tolerated with xerosis as the main side effect, although BPO also bleaches towels, clothes, bedsheets, and even wall paint if it comes in contact. Clinicians should warn patients about this bleaching effect and inform them that linens made with BPO-resistant dyes are available.

Inflammatory Acne

The erythematous papules and pustules of acne result from an inflammatory response to the sebum and organisms found in more advanced lesions of acne. Topicals used for inflammatory acne work by reducing bacteria or more directly act on the inflammation. In addition to their comedolytic effects, BPO and azelaic acid both have some antibacterial effects and azelaic acid has some antiinflammatory activity as well, making these good options at addressing multiple types of acne. Topical antibiotics such as erythromycin, clindamycin, dapsone, or sulfur/sulfacetamide are also used for their direct effects on bacteria. Resistance to these occurs rapidly within several months, if used as monotherapy, however.[10,12–14] The addition of a nonspecific antibacterial agent such as BPO can prevent the proliferation of resistant bacteria resulting in synergy of activity. Combination products of BPO and clindamycin or erythromycin are commonly available as a result. Given the lack of head-to-head trials of topical dapsone compared with other topical antibiotics and its very high cost, it is not recommended as first-line therapy.

Oral antibiotics are highly effective for inflammatory acne and often result in visible improvement more quickly than most topical preparations. Tetracyclines, especially doxycycline and minocycline, are the most commonly used. Evidence shows that they not only target bacteria but also have substantial antiinflammatory activities.

Both are similarly effective and usually dosed at 50 to 100 mg orally twice daily, although some formulations of doxycycline (20 mg twice daily or 40 mg extended release once daily) allow use of subantimicrobial levels. These low dosages of doxycycline take advantage of the antiinflammatory activity with less selection for resistant organisms, although data have not conclusively shown that resistance does not occur.[13,14] Doxycycline is associated with slightly higher photosensitivity and GI upset than minocycline, but minocycline can also have vestibular effects when first initiated and can result in drug-induced lupus and skin deposition, resulting in hyperpigmentation with long-term use. Macrolides such as azithromycin are an alternative to tetracyclines with equal to possibly greater efficacy and less-frequent dosing. There is no standard dose of azithromycin, and many regimens have been published.[13] Systemic antibiotic use for extended periods inevitably results in production of resistant organisms not only in the skin but also in the GI tract and elsewhere, so long-term use should be avoided whenever possible to prevent the spread of resistant organisms in the environment. Monotherapy with a systemic antibiotic is rarely indicated, so topicals should be initiated concurrently with a goal of tapering off a systemic antibiotic after 3 months of use. All tetracyclines are contraindicated during pregnancy and lactation, whereas oral erythromycin or azithromycin is a safer alternative if needed.

Nodulocystic Acne

The deeper, often painful nodules and cystic lesions of acne are more likely to leave permanent scars than the superficial comedones and inflammatory papules seen in less-severe forms of acne. The most effective treatment of nodulocystic acne remains the oral retinoid isotretinoin. Isotretinoin is the closest thing to a cure for acne, in that after a 4- to 6-month course, acne is usually resolved or remains much milder in the future. In preventing formation of nodular and cystic lesions, it effectively halts potential scarring, the main long-term morbidity in severe acne. Isotretinoin, unlike topical retinoids, results in partial atrophy of sebaceous glands, and as a result, has significant cutaneous and systemic side effects—dry lips being the most obvious in nearly all during treatment. The most serious side effect is teratogenicity, and for this reason, isotretinoin is closely monitored in the United States through the iPledge program, with females of child-bearing potential having the most stringent preisotretinoin requirements and monitoring during therapy.[15] Other reported serious side effects are an increased risk of suicide among teenagers using it for acne, although this risk has not been substantiated after systematic review.[16] For these reasons, unless a clinician is experienced and a registered prescriber in the iPledge program, consideration of isotretinoin should generally involve a referral to a dermatologist.

Hormonal Treatments

As mentioned previously, sebaceous gland activity is promoted by androgenic hormones. Acne can be seen as a side effect from prescription of testosterone supplementation or from anabolic steroids used for bodybuilding. Unfortunately, many over-the-counter supplements for bodybuilding have been found to have anabolic steroids, so sudden onset of acne should prompt questioning about use of such supplements.[17] More commonly, either increased levels of endogenous steroids or an increased sensitivity to these androgens can result in acne in both men and women. Targeting androgens in men for the purposes of acne treatment is not recommended because of the risk of sexual and other side effects. In women, however, it can be highly effective with minimal side effects, although 4 to 6 months are needed for clinical efficacy. Clues to hormone-sensitive acne include flaring in the week before menses, onset in the mid-20s to 30s, and/or involvement of inflammatory or nodulocystic lesions on the chin and jawline predominantly. Oral contraceptive pills can be effective for acne, and several are approved by the US Food and Drug Administration (FDA) for this indication: ethinyl estradiol-norethindrone, ethinyl estradiol-norgestimate, and ethinyl estradiol-drospirenone. Spironolactone is also commonly used, although it is not approved by the FDA for acne. Spironolactone blocks the androgen receptor and also reduces testosterone production. Side effects include hypotension, hyperkalemia, and sometimes spotting between menses. Initially, diuresis and breast tenderness are common but transient. Due primarily to its antiandrogen effects, spironolactone is relatively contraindicated in pregnancy. An FDA warning was issued because of an increased risk of tumors based on studies done in rodents—benign thyroid, testicular, and liver tumors were seen as well as a dose-dependent increase of myelocytic leukemia[18] (http://www.accessdata.fda.gov/drugsatfda_docs/label/2008/012151s062lbl.pdf). Importantly, these were all at doses 20 to 500 times those given typically for acne. A Canadian study of a million women older than 55 years showed no increased incidence of breast cancer, and a Danish study followed up 1.3 million women aged 20 years and older with a similar lack of association with breast, ovarian, uterine, and cervical cancers.[19,20] Finasteride is likely effective but has a high risk of birth defects and should not be routinely used in premenopausal women. Cyproterone acetate is another likely effective option available in Canada and elsewhere, but not in the United States.

ALOPECIA

Hair loss is a very common complaint to both dermatologists and primary care physicians. There are dozens of potential causes of alopecia, and history and physical examination can usually narrow the differential diagnosis to one or a handful of possibilities to guide further testing and treatment. This section focuses only on scalp hair loss because alopecia in other sites without scalp involvement is unusual.

Historical elements that can help guide diagnosis include family history of hair loss; abrupt versus insidious onset; effluvium (shedding) versus gradual loss of hair without obvious effluvium; involvement of eyebrows, beard, or body hair; recent changes in medications; recent crash diets or other dietary changes; recent pregnancy; recent stressful physical or psychological events; and other symptoms such as pruritus or burning or scaling (dandruff).

Physical examination of patients with alopecia requires gross examination for pattern of hair loss, close examination of the scalp and follicular openings using a hand lens or dermatoscope, and a hair pull test. Generalized thinning of hair on the scalp versus patchy alopecia versus patterned alopecia can be assessed often upon walking in the examination room, but a thorough search through all areas of the scalp is required. Examining the width of a part on the central frontal scalp compared with the temporal or occipital scalp is often a more objective way to differentiate generalized thinning from patterned thinning. Use of magnification allows the presence or absence of follicular ostia to be easily seen in areas affected. Loss of ostia results from scarring alopecia, which is irreversible in humans and therefore critical to identify early in the disease course. Scarring should prompt a referral to a dermatologist because exact diagnosis and treatment are typically challenging. The presence and pattern of erythema and scale can more easily be assessed with magnification, as can the presence of miniaturized hairs of pattern alopecia. A hair pull test is done by grasping about 1 to 2 cm^2 of hairs and pulling rather firmly with fingertips to see how easily hairs are removed from their follicles. Normally, less than 5 telogen hairs should be removable on any one pull. Telogen hairs are often called club hairs because they have a small nearly spherical white bulb follicle at the end of the hair. Anagen follicles are much longer, appear similar to a rumpled sock at the end of the hair, and are never a normal finding without forcible removal (**Fig. 6**). If an attached follicular bulb is absent, it suggests that hair fragility is the major problem.

As shown in **Table 1**, the presence or absence of scarring and inflammation allows a paring of potential diagnosis to a more manageable list, which can be refined further using the historical elements and physical findings described above. Unfortunately, AA, pattern alopecias (FPHL and AGA), and TE account for the vast majority of patients with hair loss and are all typically nonscarring and noninflammatory. These conditions are selected for further discussion in the following sections, although a more in-depth review in this journal has been published previously.[21]

Alopecia Areata

One of the most distressing and common causes of hair loss is AA. AA can involve eyebrows, eyelashes, beard, or body hair, but scalp involvement is the most common reason patients seek medical attention, typically presenting with circular areas of complete or near-complete alopecia; it is generally noninflamed, although initially

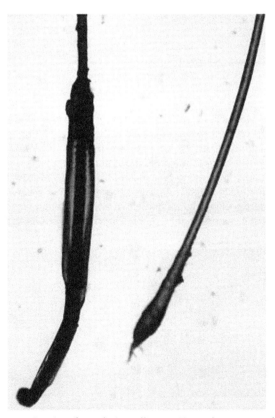

Fig. 6. Hair shaft examination from hair pull test. Note the anagen hair (*left*) has an attached rumpled inner root sheath still attached, while the telogen hair (*right*) is often referred to as a club hair because of its shape and lack of attached root sheath. (*From* James WD, Berger, T, Elston, D. Andrews' Diseases of the skin: clinical dermatology. Elsevier; 2011. p. 741–82; with permission.)

Table 1
Classification of alopecia diagnoses by presence of scarring and inflammation

	Scarring	Nonscarring
Inflammatory	• Lupus erythematosus (discoid or subacute cutaneous) • Lichen planopilaris • Frontal fibrosing alopecia • Chronic suppurative folliculitis • Folliculitis decalvans • Dissecting cellulitis of the scalp • Sarcoidosis • Favus • Acne keloidalis nuchae	• AA (early lesions) • Tinea capitis (can scar if very inflammatory, a kerion) • Syphilis • Early lupus
Noninflammatory	• Central centrifugal scarring alopecia (follicular degeneration syndrome) • Pseudopelade • Inactive burnt-out scarring alopecia • Scleroderma	• AGA • FPHL • AA • TE • Trichotillomania • Traction alopecia • Metabolic causes (thyroid, dietary deficiencies or excesses, etc) • Medications • Alopecia neoplastica • Congenital triangular alopecia

Adapted from Vary JC, O'Connor KM. Common dermatologic conditions. Med Clin North Am 2014;98(3):445–85; with permission.

patches sometimes have a light pink to peach color to the skin. Short 1- to 4-mm proximally tapered hairs termed exclamation point hairs are pathognomonic and often found near the expanding edges of patches (**Fig. 7**). Interestingly, the immune response leading to AA targets melanocytic antigens in follicles, so white hairs are often spared in those with graying hair. As hairs begin to regrow in affected areas, they often grow back white initially. Although there are other causes of patchy alopecia, AA is the only cause of patchy alopecia that spares white hairs. The lifetime risk of AA is about 2%, and it occurs slightly more commonly in adults than in children.[22,23]

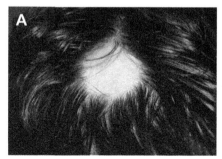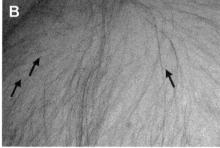

Fig. 7. (*A*) Alopecia areata. Note the isolated area of smooth alopecia. (*B*) Alopecia areata. Note the exclamation point hairs (*arrows*). (*Adapted from [A]* Calonje E, Brenn T, Lazar A, et al. McKee's pathology of the skin: with clinical correlations. Elsevier Limited; 2012. p. 967–1050, with permission; and [*B*] Sperling LC, Sinclair RD, El Shabrawi-Caelen L. Cicatricial alopecias. In: Bolognia JL, Jorizzo JL, Schaeffer JV, editors. Dermatology. Elsevier Limited; 2012. p. 1093–114, with permission.)

AA is more common in those with other autoimmune conditions such as autoimmune thyroid disease, type 1 diabetes, and vitiligo, although associations at the time of diagnosis are uncommon enough that laboratory screening is not indicated unless symptoms suggest otherwise. Like many autoimmune conditions, its cause is largely unknown and its course is unpredictable—spontaneous resolution with occasional recurrence is typical.[24] Treatment is aimed at allowing regrowth to occur in affected areas, although it is unclear if treatment affects the overall course of the condition. Localized treatment of individual patches may allow regrowth while a new area of involvement may develop elsewhere causing great frustration to the patient and provider. Although clinically uninflamed, histology reveals a lymphocytic inflammatory response that occurs at the base, or bulb, of terminal hair follicles, so application of topical steroids to the skin surface is not highly effective and takes months to see slow changes. A 1- to 2-cm grid of intralesional corticosteroid injection into the deep dermis of affected patches usually shows a response within 1 to 2 months, but repeated injections is usually necessary to allow continued growth.[22,25] Localized acne and atrophy are the only major sequelae of intralesional steroid injections and usually resolve with cessation of treatment if recognized early. Most patients are not concerned with atrophy if it remains well hidden under a thick coat of hair. Topical sensitizers and irritants such as squaric acid dibutyl ester, diphenylcyclopropenone, and anthralin can be effective as immunomodulatory agents but can be difficult to use and titrate initially. Systemic agents other than long-term prednisone are frustratingly less effective than for most other autoimmune conditions. Recent reports have been widely reported regarding success with the Janus kinase inhibitor, ruxolitinib, offering hope for new treatments.[26] Unfortunately, the cost of treatment approaches US $10,000 per month, making it untenable for use in its current oral form.

Androgenetic Alopecia/Female Pattern Hair Loss

Pattern hair loss is a very common condition affecting both men and women. AGA occurs in men, whereas FPHL is the preferred term in women, because many women do not clearly have an androgenic cause. Approximately 50% of men are affected to some extent by the age of 50 years by AGA.[27] As its name suggests, AGA's pathophysiology is driven by follicular sensitivity to androgens (principally dihydrotestosterone) as well as a genetic predisposition. AGA typically starts as bitemporal hairline recession and/or vertex thinning. As it progresses, the areas affected enlarge and may eventually connect with each other to create complete alopecia of the crown. The sides of the scalp and the occiput are always spared in AGA, reflecting a differing response to androgens in different locations of scalp hair (**Fig. 8**A). This situation is in direct contrast to follicles on the face, axilla, groin, and trunk that are often induced to grow visible hair in response to the same dihydrotestosterone. Contrary to popular belief, the hairs in AGA do not typically disappear, but rather become short, wispy, miniaturized hairs that are less-easily seen, giving the appearance of hairlessness.

FPHL is also quite common affecting 20% to 30% of women by the of age 50 years, although its manifestations are not as socially accepted as those of AGA in men, which often leads to a higher level of concern and distress.[27,28] Similar to AGA, FPHL spares the sides of the scalp and occiput, but FPHL results in thinning rather than hairline recession such that patients rarely appear bald but rather have a more easily seen scalp on the crown as the density of long hairs lessens (see **Fig. 8**B). A clear hormonal connection to FPHL remains controversial because some, but not all, FPHL responds to hormonally directed treatment, which is why the term AGA has fallen out of favor when describing women. Most women with FPHL have no evidence of

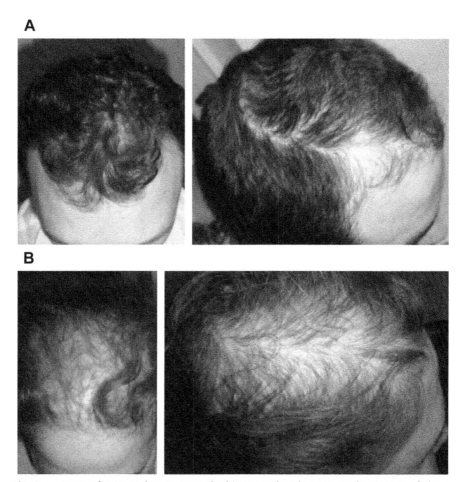

Fig. 8. Patterns of AGA and FPHL. Note the bitemporal and vertex predominance of alope-cia in AGA (*A*), while FPHL is associated with generalized thinning in the entire crown (*B*). (*Adapted from* Calonje E, Brenn T, Lazar A, et al. McKee's pathology of the skin: with clinical correlations. Elsevier Limited; 2012. p. 967–1050; with permission.)

hyperandrogenism such as hirsutism or irregular menses, and they will have normal hormone levels by routine laboratory testing. Women presenting with the male AGA pattern of recession are uncommon, however, and such atypical presentations should prompt laboratory testing to exclude polycystic ovarian syndrome, congenital adrenal hyperplasia, or hyperandrogenism from an ovarian or adrenal secreting tumor.[29,30]

The clinician makes the diagnosis of AGA and FPHL by recognizing the hair loss pattern and the presence of miniaturized hairs on examination and a suggestive family history (although the latter is not always present). Importantly, however, AGA and FPHL are very common, so the presence of all of the above does not exclude another coincident cause of alopecia. For example, a woman with FPHL who has lost 10% of the hair on her crown may not be aware of this until she also loses 20% of her scalp hair because of another problem such as hypothyroidism. Examination may confirm the presence of FPHL, but a secondary process may not be recognized if a diagnosis of FPHL is rendered too quickly.

Treatments for FPHL and AGA are often similar and include acceptance, changes in hairstyling, volumizing shampoos, aerosolized powders or fibers, hair transplant, and hairpieces. Medical treatments include topical and oral options. Minoxidil is an oral antihypertensive that, when used topically, can slow hair loss and sometimes promote regrowth. Minoxidil is relatively inexpensive and available without a prescription in the United States as both a 2% or 5% solution for women or men, respectively, and as a 5% foam for either gender. Local irritation is the most common side effect and is less when using the foam. Symptoms related to hypotension are occasional complaints of minoxidil, but were not more common than with vehicle alone in studies.[31] Patients should always be warned than an initial paradoxic hair loss occurs in the first weeks of use because of induction of a brief TE (see section on Telogen Effluvium), but this is a sign that the treatment is working and should not be stopped.

Antiandrogen medications such as spironolactone (discussed earlier in acne) and finasteride have also been used extensively for FPHL, although large controlled studies are still lacking to determine their efficacy. In males, spironolactone is not used for AGA given its propensity to cause gynecomastia with the extended courses required. The only oral FDA-approved medication for AGA in men is finasteride, which works by blocking type II 5α-reductase, thereby preventing formation of dihydrotestosterone. Side effects include reduced libido, erectile dysfunction, or decreased ejaculate volume, but discontinuation rates owing to these side effects have not been significant in studies.[32] Finasteride is not approved by the FDA for use in women, and given the high risk of feminization of male fetuses exposed to the medication, finasteride is contraindicated in pregnancy and should be used in premenopausal women with great caution.

Success with minoxidil, spironolactone, or finasteride is more likely with appropriate expectation setting in the following 2 areas: (1) it will be 6 months before any significant regrowth might be appreciable, if it occurs, and (2) ongoing use is required, because any hairs that have regrown or been spared will revert to a miniaturized state within a few months of stopping these medications.

Telogen Effluvium

The most common cause of diffuse shedding of hair is TE. Although it commonly occurs in men, it is far more common in women.[33,34] Each hair follicle undergoes a cycle with a growth phase (anagen) in which the follicle is fully developed and synthesizes a hair at a constant rate. This phase is followed by a brief catabolic phase (catagen) in which the lower portion of the follicle involutes. There is then a resting phase (telogen) in which the follicle lays dormant for about 3 months, yet it still is occupied with a hair with an involuted follicle at its end (a club hair). When the new anagen phase begins, a new hair is initiated and pushes out the telogen hair. This cycle lasts about 1000 days on the scalp, which contains about 100,000 hairs, thereby resulting in shedding of about 100 hairs a day normally. TE occurs when an increased number of hairs begin entering telogen synchronously; this commonly occurs postpartum when many follicles kept in anagen during pregnancy enter telogen at delivery, resulting in an effluvium 3 months later as they reenter anagen phase. Significantly stressful physical or psychological events can also trigger a brief TE. Chronic TE can occur from significant ongoing physical stress from crash diets or from ongoing psychological stress. People never go bald from TE because the hairs are only shed as new replacements are growing, however, significant thinning can occur.[33–35]

Diagnosis of TE is by a history of sudden-onset generalized effluvium with a clear trigger and/or exclusion of other causes (eg, chemotherapy) and a positive result of hair pull test of telogen hairs on examination. In about a third of cases, no obvious trigger is identifiable, making TE a diagnosis of exclusion in many cases.[36]

SUMMARY

This article reviewed some of the more common diseases of the skin appendages that are encountered in medicine: hyperhidrosis, acne, AA, FPHL, AGA, and TE. The pathophysiology behind the conditions and their treatments were discussed so that the clinician can make logical therapeutic choices for their affected patients.

REFERENCES

1. Biesbroeck LK, Fleckman P. Nail Disease for the Primary Care Provider. Med Clin N Am 2015, in press.
2. Adar R, Kurchin A, Zweig A, et al. Palmar hyperhidrosis and its surgical treatment: a report of 100 cases. Ann Surg 1977;186(1):34–41.
3. Strutton DR, Kowalski JW, Glaser DA, et al. US prevalence of hyperhidrosis and impact on individuals with axillary hyperhidrosis: results from a national survey. J Am Acad Dermatol 2004;51(2):241–8.
4. Hoorens I, Ongenae K. Primary focal hyperhidrosis: current treatment options and a step-by-step approach. J Eur Acad Dermatol Venereol 2012;26(1):1–8.
5. Walling HW. Clinical differentiation of primary from secondary hyperhidrosis. J Am Acad Dermatol 2011;64(4):690–5.
6. Reisfeld R, Berliner KI. Evidence-based review of the nonsurgical management of hyperhidrosis. Thorac Surg Clin 2008;18(2):157–66.
7. Lakraj AA, Moghimi N, Jabbari B. Hyperhidrosis: anatomy, pathophysiology and treatment with emphasis on the role of botulinum toxins. Toxins (Basel) 2013;5(4): 821–40.
8. Hornberger J, Grimes K, Naumann M, et al. Recognition, diagnosis, and treatment of primary focal hyperhidrosis. J Am Acad Dermatol 2004;51(2):274–86.
9. Stathakis V, Kilkenny M, Marks R. Descriptive epidemiology of acne vulgaris in the community. Australas J Dermatol 1997;38(3):115–23.
10. Thiboutot D, Gollnick H, Bettoli V, et al. New insights into the management of acne: an update from the Global Alliance to Improve Outcomes in Acne Group. J Am Acad Dermatol 2009;60(5 Suppl):S1–50.
11. Williams HC, Dellavalle RP, Garner S. Acne vulgaris. Lancet 2012;379(9813): 361–72.
12. Gamble R, Dunn J, Dawson A, et al. Topical antimicrobial treatment of acne vulgaris: an evidence-based review. Am J Clin Dermatol 2012;13(3):141–52.
13. Mays RM, Gordon RA, Wilson JM, et al. New antibiotic therapies for acne and rosacea. Dermatol Ther 2012;25(1):23–37.
14. Simonart T. Newer approaches to the treatment of acne vulgaris. Am J Clin Dermatol 2012;13(6):357–64.
15. Choi JS, Koren G, Nulman I. Pregnancy and isotretinoin therapy. CMAJ 2013; 185(5):411–3.
16. Kontaxakis VP, Skourides D, Ferentinos P, et al. Isotretinoin and psychopathology: a review. Ann Gen Psychiatry 2009;8:2.
17. Odoardi S, Castrignano E, Martello S, et al. Determination of anabolic agents in dietary supplements by liquid chromatography-high-resolution mass spectrometry. Food Addit Contam Part A Chem Anal Control Expo Risk Assess 2015; 32(5):635–47.

18. Food and Drug Administration, U.S. Aldactone (spironolactone) Prescribing Information. 2–14. Available at: http://www.accessdata.fda.gov/drugsatfda_docs/label/2008/012151s062lbl.pdf. Accessed August 10, 2015.

19. Biggar RJ, Andersen EW, Wohlfahrt J, et al. Spironolactone use and the risk of breast and gynecologic cancers. Cancer Epidemiol 2013;37(6):870–5.

20. Mackenzie IS, Macdonald TM, Thompson A, et al. Spironolactone and risk of incident breast cancer in women older than 55 years: retrospective, matched cohort study. BMJ 2012;345:e4447.

21. Vary JC, O'Connor KM. Common dermatologic conditions. Med Clin North Am 2014;98(3):445–85.

22. Gilhar A, Etzioni A, Paus R. Alopecia areata. N Engl J Med 2012;366(16):1515–25.

23. McMichael AJ, Pearce DJ, Wasserman D, et al. Alopecia in the United States: outpatient utilization and common prescribing patterns. J Am Acad Dermatol 2007;57(2 Suppl):S49–51.

24. Messenger AG, McKillop J, Farrant P, et al. British Association of Dermatologists' guidelines for the management of alopecia areata 2012. Br J Dermatol 2012;166(5):916–26.

25. Alkhalifah A, Alsantali A, Wang E, et al. Alopecia areata update: part I. Clinical picture, histopathology, and pathogenesis. J Am Acad Dermatol 2010;62(2):177–88 [quiz: 189–90].

26. Xing L, Dai Z, Jabbari A, et al. Alopecia areata is driven by cytotoxic T lymphocytes and is reversed by JAK inhibition. Nat Med 2014;20(9):1043–9.

27. Hamilton JB. Patterned loss of hair in man; types and incidence. Ann N Y Acad Sci 1951;53(3):708–28.

28. Norwood OT. Incidence of female androgenetic alopecia (female pattern alopecia). Dermatol Surg 2001;27(1):53–4.

29. Karrer-Voegeli S, Rey F, Reymond MJ, et al. Androgen dependence of hirsutism, acne, and alopecia in women: retrospective analysis of 228 patients investigated for hyperandrogenism. Medicine (Baltimore) 2009;88(1):32–45.

30. Futterweit W, Dunaif A, Yeh HC, et al. The prevalence of hyperandrogenism in 109 consecutive female patients with diffuse alopecia. J Am Acad Dermatol 1988;19(5 Pt 1):831–6.

31. Olsen EA, Whiting D, Bergfeld W, et al. A multicenter, randomized, placebo-controlled, double-blind clinical trial of a novel formulation of 5% minoxidil topical foam versus placebo in the treatment of androgenetic alopecia in men. J Am Acad Dermatol 2007;57(5):767–74.

32. Mella JM, Perret MC, Manzotti M, et al. Efficacy and safety of finasteride therapy for androgenetic alopecia: a systematic review. Arch Dermatol 2010;146(10):1141–50.

33. Whiting DA. Chronic telogen effluvium: increased scalp hair shedding in middle-aged women. J Am Acad Dermatol 1996;35(6):899–906.

34. Kligman AM. Pathologic dynamics of human hair loss. I. Telogen effuvium. Arch Dermatol 1961;83:175–98.

35. Harrison S, Sinclair R. Telogen effluvium. Clin Exp Dermatol 2002;27(5):389–95.

36. Shrivastava SB. Diffuse hair loss in an adult female: approach to diagnosis and management. Indian J Dermatol Venereol Leprol 2009;75(1):20–7 [quiz: 27–8].

Nail Disease for the Primary Care Provider

Lauren K. Biesbroeck, MD*, Philip Fleckman, MD

KEYWORDS

- Nail • Melanonychia • Onychomycosis • Paronychia • Subungual tumor • Wart

KEY POINTS

- Onychomycosis commonly affects the nail unit, and requires proper diagnosis before treatment is initiated.
- Periungual verrucae (warts) are common and often respond to typical destructive therapies. Recalcitrant lesions should be biopsied to rule out squamous cell carcinoma.
- Subungual tumors can present as longitudinal melanonychia or longitudinal erythronychia. Evaluation by a dermatologist and consideration of biopsy is necessary.

INTRODUCTION

Nail changes are a common presenting complaint of patients. Clinical evaluation can be challenging, and the differential diagnosis at times is broad. However, familiarity with several common diagnoses and their appropriate evaluation can improve care of the patient with a nail complaint.

INFECTIONS OF THE NAIL UNIT
Onychomycosis

Onychomycosis, or fungal infection of the nail plate, is a common disorder of nails, accounting for up to half of reported nail disease.[1,2] The prevalence in the general population is approximately 3%, with higher rates seen in elderly patients, patients with other concomitant diseases of the nails, and patients with comorbid medical conditions such as diabetes or peripheral vascular disease.[1,2] Accurate diagnosis of onychomycosis is critical. Not only can noninfectious conditions of the nail, such as psoriasis, lichen planus, and chronic trauma, mimic onychomycosis clinically, but onychomycosis caused by various fungal organisms can respond differently to antifungal agents.[1] In addition, treatment of onychomycosis often requires prolonged treatment

Disclosure Statement: The authors have nothing to disclose.
Division of Dermatology, University of Washington School of Medicine, 1959 Northeast Pacific Street, BB-1353, Box 356524, Seattle, WA 98195-6524, USA
* Corresponding author.
E-mail address: laurenkb@uw.edu

Med Clin N Am 99 (2015) 1213–1226
http://dx.doi.org/10.1016/j.mcna.2015.07.010
0025-7125/15/$ – see front matter © 2015 Elsevier Inc. All rights reserved.

with systemic antifungal medications, which may have adverse effects or medication interactions; therefore, appropriate treatment should be ensured.[3] The necessity for confirmation of clinical diagnosis is emphasized by the American Academy of Dermatology, which includes this as 1 of the 5 points in the American Board of Internal Medicine Foundation "Choosing Wisely" Program (www.choosingwisely.org).

Proper diagnosis of onychomycosis rests on collection of an adequate sample for evaluation. The most accurate diagnosis can be achieved by trimming the onycholytic portion of the affected nail plate as far proximally as possible. Subungual debris should be collected from the nail bed using a curette, as close as possible to the junction of the normal nail plate with the dystrophic, onycholytic plate.[1,4,5] Three methods can be used to confirm a diagnosis of onychomycosis from the specimen. Direct microscopy using potassium hydroxide (KOH) is an inexpensive, rapid method to confirm the presence of fungal hyphae. However, this study is operator dependent, with reported increased sensitivity with greater clinical experience.[6] Periodic acid-Schiff (PAS) staining of affected nail plates may offer greater sensitivity, but is more expensive and less rapid than KOH.[3] As neither KOH nor PAS staining can identify the exact infectious organism, speciation with culture of subungual debris is recommended. However, culture is slow, with a delay of up to 4 weeks or longer, and has sensitivity as low as 50%.[3] Molecular diagnostic methods such as polymerase chain reaction have recently been reported as a useful adjunct, with reported sensitivity of greater than 90%.[4] However, these techniques cannot differentiate true infectious organisms from nonviable or incidental contaminants, which may limit clinical utility.[1]

Most patients with onychomycosis have tinea unguium, or infection with dermatophyte organisms, which are common fungal organisms from the genera *Trichophyton*, *Epidermophyton*, and *Microsporum*. These organisms cause superficial fungal skin and appendageal infections such as onychomycosis, tinea corporis, tinea capitis, and tinea pedis. The most commonly implicated organisms in onychomycosis are from the *Trichophyton* genus.[1]

Dermatophyte onychomycosis has several clinical presentations, the most common of which is distal/lateral subungual onychomycosis (**Fig. 1**), caused by fungal invasion at the hyponychium or lateral nail folds, and presents clinically with onycholysis, nail plate thickening, and subungual debris. Superficial white onychomycosis (**Fig. 2**) is

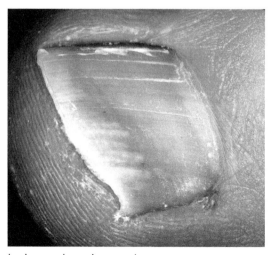

Fig. 1. Distal-lateral subungual onychomycosis.

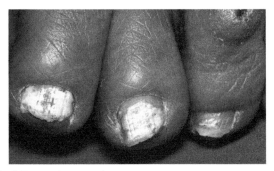

Fig. 2. Superficial white onychomycosis.

caused by infection of the superficial nail plate, and presents as a crumbling white surface to the nail. Proximal subungual onychomycosis (**Fig. 3**), caused by infection originating at the proximal nail fold (PNF), is the least common presentation, but is important because it can be a marker for lack of resistance to dermatophyte infection, such as with human immunodeficiency virus infection and other causes of immunosuppression.[1,7] Those with proximal subungual onychomycosis also have a tendency toward significant cutaneous dermatophyte infection elsewhere on the body.[8]

Onychomycosis can also be caused by other fungal species, including Candida and nondermatophyte molds. The exact prevalence of nondermatophyte onychomycosis is uncertain, and difficult to estimate because of lack of consistency in diagnostic methods between studies,[9] but seems to account for 10% to 20% of cases of onychomycosis worldwide.[1,9–11] The prevalence and relative frequency of implicated

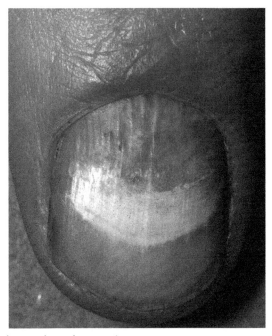

Fig. 3. Proximal subungual onychomycosis.

organisms vary based on geographic location.[9,11,12] Nondermatophyte molds, including *Acremonium, Scopularopsis, Aspergillus, Fusarium,* and *Scytalidium* species, while less common, should be recognized, as treatment choice may differ from that for dermatophyte infection. Nondermatophyte mold onychomycosis most commonly presents with distal-lateral subungual onychomycosis, which may be indistinguishable clinically from dermatophyte onychomycosis.[9,12] Candidal onychomycosis is uncommon; it can present more proximally in association with paronychia, or as onycholysis with onychauxis (thickening of the nail plate) and subungual debris (**Fig. 4**). Toenails are frequently spared, and most patients who have distal involvement of fingernails have concomitant Raynaud disease (or other causes of vascular insufficiency), or have been treated with oral corticosteroids or other immunosuppressant drugs.[1,13]

Treatment of onychomycosis must be individualized. Although many consider treatment of onychomycosis to be of primarily cosmetic concern, approximately half of patients with onychomycosis will experience some degree of pain or discomfort, which can in turn cause difficulty in donning appropriate footwear or in ambulation.[1] Indeed, pain and nail deformity resulting from onychomycosis have been reported as risk factors for falls in the elderly population.[14] In addition, dystrophic nails may cause disruption in the surrounding cutaneous barrier, which can be a nidus for the formation of chronic foot ulcer or an entry point for other infections such as cellulitis.[1,15] Onychomycosis of the fingernails interferes with touch, and fine motor function, such as fastening buttons and picking up thin objects, is more cosmetically apparent and more easily cured; for these reasons the treatment of fingernail onychomycosis should be encouraged.

Oral antifungal therapy is most effective means of clearing dermatophyte onychomycosis. Terbinafine is considered the first-choice oral agent for dermatophyte onychomycosis. Treatment includes 250 mg orally daily, for 6 weeks in fingernails and 12 to 16 weeks in toenails,[1,10] and is superior to alternative therapies such as itraconazole.[16] Treatment of nondermatophyte molds with oral itraconazole, either 200 mg

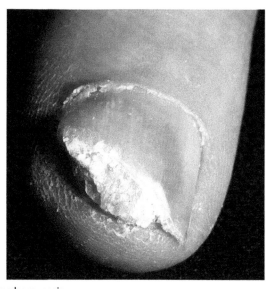

Fig. 4. *Candida* onychomycosis.

daily for 12 weeks, or pulse-dose treatment 400 mg daily for 1 week each month (2 months' duration for fingernail infection, 3 months for toenails) is considered first line.[1,10] Terbinafine shows high activity against infections with *Aspergillus* and *Scopulariopsis* species.[1,9] Itraconazole or fluconazole, dosed at 150 mg once weekly for a period of 6 months, are considered oral treatments of choice for *Candida* onychomycosis. Alternatively, avulsion and topical treatment is at least equally effective when a single nail is infected.[17] Treatment with systemic antifungals must be balanced with the rare but real risk of toxicity, especially liver toxicity, associated with the oral antifungal agents. In addition, azoles in particular are associated with numerous medication interactions, which may limit use in patients with numerous comorbidities. Despite the required prolonged treatment courses recurrence is common, with reported relapse rates ranging from 40% to 70%.[1]

Topical therapy is often desirable, especially considering the potential for adverse reactions and medication interactions with the oral antifungal agents. However, to date topical treatment regimens have been less effective. Until recently, ciclopirox lacquer was the only topical agent approved by the Food and Drug Administration (FDA) for the treatment of onychomycosis in the United States. Complete cure rates of 5.7% to 8.5%, despite prolonged treatment durations of up to 1 year, have been reported.[1,18] Two new topical agents, efinaconazole and tavaborole, have recently been approved by the FDA for treatment of onychomycosis. Reported complete cure rates for efinaconazole range from 15.2% to 18.5%,[18,19] and for tavaborole 6.5% to 9.1%.[18] Thus, despite the introduction of new topical agents with modestly increased efficacy, treatment success with topical agents still falls short of systemic treatment.

Other localized treatments, including photodynamic therapy, laser treatment, and surgical avulsion (in the case of dermatophyte onychomycosis) of affected nails, offer the possibility of treatment of onychomycosis without the risks associated with systemic treatment. However, to date the data on these therapies have been sparse and conflicting, and further studies are therefore required before they can be recommended.[1,20–22]

Pseudomonal Nail Infection

Pseudomonas is the most common organism implicated in bacterial infection of the nail.[23] *Pseudomonas* nail infection presents as blue-green discoloration beneath the nail, typically in association with onycholysis,[23,24] and often affects a single nail.[25] Risk factors include chronic nail trauma, chronic paronychia, exposure to wet work or moist environments, and concomitant nail disease such as psoriasis.[23–25] It is thought that onycholysis contributes to formation of a chronically moist environment beneath the nail plate, which is ideal for growth of *Pseudomonas* and eventuates in secondary infection.[23] Treatment can often be achieved with topical measures, including topical fluoroquinolone or aminoglycoside solutions or antiseptic soaks such as dilute acetic acid, dilute bleach, or chlorhexidine.[23–25] Alternatively, the onycholytic plate can be clipped back, which usually results in cure.

Acute Paronychia

Acute paronychia is an acute, typically bacterial, infection of the proximal and/or lateral nail folds, introduced by minor trauma to the skin that disrupts the cutaneous barrier. Patients typically present with pain, erythema, edema, and sometimes fluctuance involving a single digit.[26,27] Acute paronychia is most frequently caused by *Staphylococcus aureus*, with γ-hemolytic streptococci, *Eikenella corrodens*, and group A *Streptococcus* representing less frequent causes. Anaerobic bacteria, mixed infections, and *Candida albicans* can also be isolated.[28] Oral exposures (such as nail biting) may increase the risk for infection by oral flora such as *Eikenella*.[27] If no fluctuance is present on examination, treatment includes antistaphylococcal antibiotics and soaks with warm water, aluminum acetate (Burow solution), vinegar, or povidone-iodine solutions.[26,27] If fluctuance is present, incision and drainage are required.[26,27]

Periungual Verrucae

Verruca vulgaris (wart) is a common, human papillomavirus–mediated neoplasm of the skin, which commonly affects the periungual and subungual skin. Verrucae are the most common tumors of the nail unit, and tend to affect fingers more commonly than toes.[29] Periungual verrucae of the nail unit can present similarly to a wart on other cutaneous sites, with a keratotic papule and associated thrombosed capillaries, in addition to disruption of epidermal ridges (**Fig. 5**). Periungual verrucae can also present as periungual hyperkeratosis, a keratotic subungual nodule with onycholysis, or as erythronychia (redness of the nail plate). Verrucae do not typically involve the nail matrix epithelium, but PNF verrucae can lead to compression of the matrix and subsequent nail plate dystrophy.[29] Most periungual warts in children resolve spontaneously and are best left alone.

First-line therapy for periungual verrucae typically includes use of a keratolytic such as salicylic acid.[29,30] Successful treatment of verrucae with this method tends to take weeks to months of daily treatment, and occlusion (such as duct tape or adhesive bandage) is typically required.[30] Destructive treatment with cryotherapy is another commonly used first-line treatment. Paring of the hyperkeratotic portion of the wart along with longer freezing times leads to higher success rates.[29,30] Caution must be exercised at the PNF, as damage to the underlying matrix may result in permanent nail dystrophy.[29] Topical immunotherapy with squaric acid dibutylester or diphenylcyclopropenone has high success rates, but requires sensitization and weekly application of an immunotherapy agent to the wart.[29–31] Other topical agents, including imiquimod, podophyllotoxin, glutaraldehyde, and formaldehyde, or compounded topical cidofovir, can be used to clear verrucae.[29,30,32] Intralesional immunotherapy with *Candida* antigen or mumps antigen has a high success rate,[29,30] as does intralesional therapy with bleomycin, which can be successful even in refractory periungual

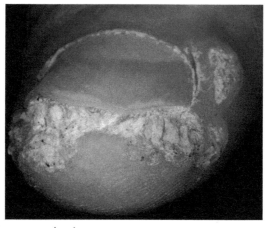

Fig. 5. Periungual verruca vulgaris.

verrucae.[29,30,33,34] Laser therapy with destructive CO_2 and erbium:YAG lasers have promising early data, but with the risk of scarring.[29,30] Laser therapy with pulsed-dye laser or Nd:YAG has a decreased risk of scarring, but additional studies are required to assess its efficacy.[29,30,35] Other surgical therapies such as excision, electrosurgery, and localized heat application are not recommended because of high potential for scarring and high recurrence rates.[29] In the authors' and others' opinion,[30] intralesional bleomycin is the most effective treatment for warts contiguous with the nail plate. Warts that do not respond to conventional therapy require biopsy, as squamous cell carcinoma of the nail unit can present as a keratotic lesion clinically indistinguishable from a wart.[29,36]

INFLAMMATORY DERMATOSES OF THE NAIL UNIT
Psoriasis

Of all inflammatory skin diseases, psoriasis most commonly affects the nail unit, with up to 90% of patients with psoriasis experiencing nail changes at some point during their lifetime.[37–39] Nail psoriasis presents differently depending on the portion of the nail unit that is affected. Nail matrix psoriasis leads to nail pitting (**Fig. 6**), leukonychia (white discoloration of the nail), or crumbling and destruction of the nail plate. Nail bed involvement leads to oil drop spots/salmon patches, splinter hemorrhages, nail bed hyperkeratosis, and thickening of the nail plate.[37–39] Because many of these findings can mimic onychomycosis, and onychomycosis commonly occurs in psoriatic nails, evaluation should always include proper fungal studies.[38–40] Recognition of psoriatic nail disease is important, as nail involvement is particularly common in patients with psoriatic arthritis, especially of the distal digits.[37,39,41] Treatment of nail psoriasis is indicated, especially as nail psoriasis can lead to decreased quality of life related to pain, functional impairment of the digit, and psychological distress.[37–39] Treatment choices must be individualized to take into consideration severity of nail involvement, severity of associated skin disease, presence of psoriatic arthritis, and potential adverse effects of the treatment. Topical treatments, including high-potency topical steroids, vitamin D analogues, topical retinoids, and others are available, but success is limited because of poor penetration of the nail plate and PNF. Other treatment options include intralesional

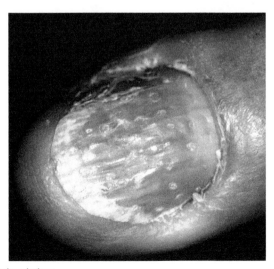

Fig. 6. Nail psoriasis: pitting.

corticosteroids, methotrexate, biologics, systemic retinoids, and apremilast, although use of systemic therapies must be considered carefully in light of the severity of disease and potential adverse effects.[37,39,40] Phototherapy is of limited efficacy because of poor penetration of ultraviolet light through the nail plate.[37]

Lichen Planus

Nail lichen planus can occur in association with either skin or mucosal lichen planus, or as isolated nail unit involvement.[37,42] Lichen planus typically affects numerous nails, but single-digit involvement can also occur. Nail matrix involvement can cause nail destruction, which presents as longitudinal ridging or fissuring, and can eventuate in scarring, which manifests as formation of dorsal pterygium. Nail bed involvement presents as onycholysis and subungual hyperkeratosis (**Fig. 7**).[37,38] Differential diagnosis includes nail psoriasis and onychomycosis, both of which can present in a similar fashion.[37] Early recognition and treatment of nail lichen planus is critical to lower the risk of permanent scarring. Treatment options include intralesional or systemic corticosteroids (either intramuscular or oral), which are typically used as first-line agents because topical therapies alone are usually ineffective. Treatment duration is undefined, but typically continued until normal nail growth is seen. Second-line therapies include azathioprine or systemic retinoids. Topical therapies including high-potency topical steroids or tacrolimus can be used as an adjunct. The cure rate for any treatment regimen is limited.[37,43]

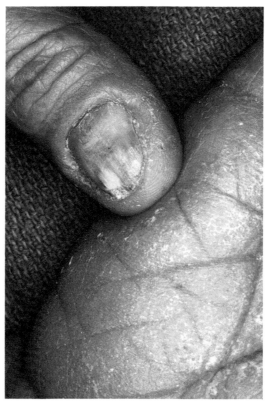

Fig. 7. Nail lichen planus.

Alopecia Areata

The nails are affected in approximately 20% of patients with alopecia areata.[38] Younger patients and those with more severe disease have nail changes more commonly.[38,44] Nail changes tend to present simultaneously with hair loss, but rarely can precede or follow hair changes by months or years.[44] Nail findings include pitting (typically smaller, more fine pits than in psoriasis, often in "rows of soldiers"), thinning of the nail plates, and longitudinal ridging, which when involving all 20 nails is termed trachyonychia or 20-nail dystrophy.[38,44] Treatment is conservative, as even with 20-nail dystrophy such nail changes often resolve spontaneously.[37]

Chronic Paronychia

In contrast to acute paronychia, chronic paronychia (CP) is not typically infectious in origin, but rather is considered a form of contact dermatitis related to chronic exposure to irritants or allergens.[45] Accordingly, CP is more common in patients with ongoing exposure to wet work and other irritants, such as food handlers, health care professionals, and cleaners.[45,46] Although *Candida* and bacteria can frequently be isolated from affected digits, they are thought to be a secondary colonizers rather than a primary infection. CP presents as erythema and edema of the PNF, with loss of the cuticle and, frequently, changes to the surface of the nail plate such as irregular transverse ridging.[45,46] Treatment of chronic paronychia includes use of potent topical steroid ointments or calcineurin inhibitors such as tacrolimus for PNF inflammation, along with drying agents beneath the PNF after exposure to water (such as 15% sulfacetamide in 50% ethanol) to roll beneath the free edge of the PNF.[47] In addition, avoidance of irritants or allergens is critical, including protection of the hands with rubber gloves (and white cotton gloves as a liner) while performing wet work.[45,46] Treatment of *Candida* colonization with systemic antifungals alone is less effective than conservative treatment,[45] but is occasionally necessary in severe cases (authors' personal observations).

NAIL UNIT NEOPLASMS
Longitudinal Melanonychia

Longitudinal melanonychia, or pigmented band of the nail plate, presents as a tan, brown, or black stripe that originates at the PNF and extends to the free edge of the nail plate (**Fig. 8**). Differential diagnosis includes inherited syndromes, systemic

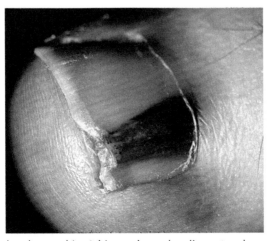

Fig. 8. Longitudinal melanonychia. A biopsy showed malignant melanoma.

disease (vitamin B_{12} deficiency and Addison disease), drug-related, trauma (with resultant intraungual hemorrhage or melanin deposition), fungal infection, melanocyte activation, benign subungual lentigo/melanotic macule, nevus, and melanoma.[48,49] The presence of pigmented bands on multiple nails is reassuring, and can be a normal finding in non-Caucasian populations.[48] Benign melanocyte activation can also be a result of drugs (particularly chemotherapy agents, antiretroviral agents, especially zidovudine, and antibiotics such as minocycline) or chronic trauma.[48] Worrisome signs for melanoma of the nail unit include pigment involving the PNF, cuticle, or hyponychium (Hutchinson sign), a widening band (wider proximally than distally), or irregular pigmentation or width of bands on dermoscopy.[48,49] When a single digit is involved, clinical differentiation of a benign lentigo or nevus from melanoma can be challenging or impossible, and biopsy of the affected nail matrix is frequently required.[48] Likewise, there are numerous pitfalls in the histologic diagnosis of nail matrix melanoma, and pathology should be interpreted by an experienced dermatopathologist.[49]

Longitudinal Erythronychia

Longitudinal erythronychia, or red band of the nail, is another common presenting nail complaint. Longitudinal erythronychia is commonly associated with splinter hemorrhages in the area of red discoloration.[49] The most common underlying diagnosis is a benign nail bed papilloma (formerly termed subungual acquired periungual fibrokeratoma),[50] but glomus tumor and Bowen disease (squamous cell carcinoma in situ) are also common histologic diagnoses. Other, less common entities include warty dyskeratoma, malignant melanoma, and basal cell carcinoma.[49] A subungual glomus tumor tends to be symptomatic with paroxysmal pain, cold sensitivity, and point tenderness.[51] The remainder of the neoplasms on the differential diagnosis tend to be asymptomatic, and without clinically specific differentiating features. Thus, nail bed/matrix exploration and biopsy is typically indicated.[49]

Subungual Exostosis

Subungual exostosis is a relatively common tumor of bone, which presents as a painful, hyperkeratotic nodule of the distal digit, frequently in association with onycholysis and deformity of the overlying nail plate (**Fig. 9**).[52,53] Children and young adults are affected most commonly.[52] Accurate diagnosis is critical, as clinical findings can mimic other tumors of the nail unit, including wart, glomus tumor, and squamous cell carcinoma.[53] Diagnosis can be confirmed by radiographic examination of the affected digit. Subungual exostoses are commonly symptomatic and progressive; surgical treatment with excision or curettage is therefore indicated.[52,53]

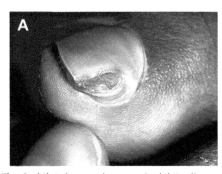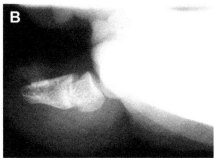

Fig. 9. (*A*) Subungual exostosis. (*B*) Radiograph of the digit showing subungual exostosis.

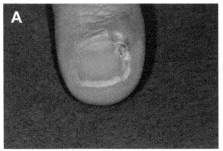
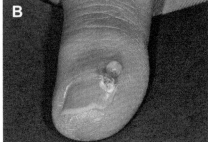

Fig. 10. (*A*) Digital myxoid cyst resulting in longitudinal grooving of the nail plate. (*B*) Myxoid material expressed after incision and drainage with large-bore needle.

Digital Mucous Cyst

Digital mucous (or myxoid) cyst (DMC) is a common cystic growth of the nail unit. DMC commonly presents as a rubbery nodule overlying the distal interphalangeal (DIP) joint or the PNF. When involving the PNF, compression of the nail matrix can result in longitudinal grooving of the nail plate (**Fig. 10**A). Digital mucous cysts are thought to be either reactive or caused by herniation of the synovium, and commonly occur overlying a joint affected by osteoarthritis. Treatment can be achieved by incision and drainage using a sterile large-bore needle (see **Fig. 10**B). Recurrences are common, but persistent cure can often be achieved after repeated treatments. Connection to the underlying joint is commonly found, and surgical excision and exploration by a hand surgeon may be necessary.[54] Alternatively, DMC can be left alone.

SUMMARY

Nail disorders are a common presenting complaint for both the primary care physician and the dermatologist. Nail diagnoses are broad in scope and include infectious, inflammatory, and neoplastic conditions. Onychomycosis is an especially common nail condition, and treatment should always be preceded by appropriate fungal studies for confirmation of diagnosis. Inflammatory conditions of the nail unit can mimic onychomycosis, and a dermatologist can assist with diagnosis and treatment recommendations. Likewise, subungual tumors often require biopsy, and should be evaluated by a dermatologist who is experienced in nail evaluation and treatment.

REFERENCES

1. Ameen M, Lear JT, Madan V, et al. British Association of Dermatologists' guidelines for the management of onychomycosis 2014. Br J Dermatol 2014;171(5): 937–58.
2. Gupta AK, Daigle D, Foley KA. The prevalence of culture-confirmed toenail onychomycosis in at-risk patient populations. J Eur Acad Dermatol Venereol 2015; 29(6):1039–44.
3. Jung MY, Shim JH, Lee JH, et al. Comparison of diagnostic methods for onychomycosis, and proposal of a diagnostic algorithm. Clin Exp Dermatol 2015;40(5): 479–84.
4. Petinataud D, Berger S, Contet-Audonneau N, et al. Molecular diagnosis of onychomycosis. J Mycol Med 2014;24(4):287–95.
5. Daniel CR, Elewski BE. The diagnosis of nail fungus infection revisited. Arch Dermatol 2000;136(9):1162–4.

6. Amir I, Foering KP, Lee JB. Revisiting office-based direct microscopy for the diagnosis of onychomycosis. J Am Acad Dermatol 2015;72(5):909–10.

7. Daniel CR, Norton LA, Scher RK. The spectrum of nail disease in patients with human immunodeficiency virus infection. J Am Acad Dermatol 1992;27(1):93–7.

8. Zaias N. Onychomycosis. Arch Dermatol 1972;105(2):263–74.

9. Gupta AK, Drummond-Main C, Cooper EA, et al. Systematic review of nondermatophyte mold onychomycosis: diagnosis, clinical types, epidemiology, and treatment. J Am Acad Dermatol 2012;66(3):494–502.

10. de Sá DC, Lamas AP, Tosti A. Oral therapy for onychomycosis: an evidence-based review. Am J Clin Dermatol 2014;15(1):17–36.

11. Bunyaratavej S, Prasertworonun N, Leeyaphan C, et al. Distinct characteristics of *Scytalidium dimidiatum* and non-dermatophyte onychomycosis as compared with dermatophyte onychomycosis. J Dermatol 2015;42(3):258–62.

12. Morales-Cardona CA, Valbuena-Mesa MC, Alvarado Z, et al. Non-dermatophyte mould onychomycosis: a clinical and epidemiological study at a dermatology referral centre in Bogota, Colombia. Mycoses 2014;57(5):284–93.

13. Hay RJ, Baran R, Moore MK, et al. Candida onychomycosis—an evaluation of the role of *Candida* species in nail disease. Br J Dermatol 1988;118(1):47–58.

14. Hay RJ, Baran R. Why should we care if onychomycosis is truly onychomycosis? Br J Dermatol 2015;172(2):316–7.

15. Roujeau JC, Sigurgeirsson B, Korting HC, et al. Chronic dermatomycoses of the foot as risk factors for acute bacterial cellulitis of the leg: a case-control study. Dermatology 2004;209(4):301–7.

16. Evans EG, Sigurgeirsson B. Double blind, randomised study of continuous terbinafine compared with intermittent itraconazole in treatment of toenail onychomycosis. The LION study group. BMJ 1999;318(7190):1031–5.

17. Tosti A, Piraccini BM, Lorenzi S. Onychomycosis caused by nondermatophytic molds: clinical features and response to treatment of 59 cases. J Am Acad Dermatol 2000;42(2 Pt 1):217–24.

18. Gupta AK, Daigle D, Foley KA. Topical therapy for toenail onychomycosis: an evidence-based review. Am J Clin Dermatol 2014;15(6):489–502.

19. Gupta AK, Elewski BE, Sugarman JL, et al. The efficacy and safety of efinaconazole 10% solution for treatment of mild to moderate onychomycosis: a pooled analysis of two phase 3 randomized trials. J Drugs Dermatol 2014;13(7):815–20.

20. Hollmig ST, Rahman Z, Henderson MT, et al. Lack of efficacy with 1064-nm neodymium:yttrium-aluminum-garnet laser for the treatment of onychomycosis: a randomized, controlled trial. J Am Acad Dermatol 2014;70(5):911–7.

21. Bhatta AK, Huang X, Keyal U, et al. Laser treatment for onychomycosis: a review. Mycoses 2014;57(12):734–40.

22. Simmons BJ, Griffith RD, Falto-Aizpurua LA, et al. An update on photodynamic therapies in the treatment of onychomycosis. J Eur Acad Dermatol Venereol 2015;29(7):1275–9.

23. Chiriac A, Brzezinski P, Foia L, et al. Chloronychia: green nail syndrome caused by Pseudomonas aeruginosa in elderly persons. Clin Interv Aging 2015;10:265–7.

24. Bae Y, Lee GM, Sim JH, et al. Green nail syndrome treated with the application of tobramycin eye drop. Ann Dermatol 2014;26(4):514–6.

25. Müller S, Ebnöther M, Itin P. Green nail syndrome (*Pseudomonas aeruginosa* nail infection): two cases successfully treated with topical nadifloxacin, an acne medication. Case Rep Dermatol 2014;6(2):180–4.

26. Osterman M, Draeger R, Stern P. Acute hand infections. J Hand Surg Am 2014; 39(8):1628–35 [quiz: 35].

27. Shafritz AB, Coppage JM. Acute and chronic paronychia of the hand. J Am Acad Orthop Surg 2014;22(3):165–74.
28. Brook I. Aerobic and anaerobic microbiology of paronychia. Ann Emerg Med 1990;19(9):994–6.
29. Tosti A, Piraccini BM. Warts of the nail unit: surgical and nonsurgical approaches. Dermatol Surg 2001;27(3):235–9.
30. Herschthal J, McLeod MP, Zaiac M. Management of ungual warts. Dermatol Ther 2012;25(6):545–50.
31. Choi Y, Kim DH, Jin SY, et al. Topical immunotherapy with diphenylcyclopropenone is effective and preferred in the treatment of periungual warts. Ann Dermatol 2013;25(4):434–9.
32. Padilla España L, Del Boz J, Fernández Morano T, et al. Successful treatment of periungual warts with topical cidofovir. Dermatol Ther 2014;27(6):337–42.
33. Soni P, Khandelwal K, Aara N, et al. Efficacy of intralesional bleomycin in palmoplantar and periungual warts. J Cutan Aesthet Surg 2011;4(3):188–91.
34. Bunney MH, Nolan MW, Buxton PK, et al. The treatment of resistant warts with intralesional bleomycin: a controlled clinical trial. Br J Dermatol 1984;111(2):197–207.
35. Kimura U, Takeuchi K, Kinoshita A, et al. Long-pulsed 1064-nm neodymium:yttrium-aluminum-garnet laser treatment for refractory warts on hands and feet. J Dermatol 2014;41(3):252–7.
36. Riddel C, Rashid R, Thomas V. Ungual and periungual human papillomavirus-associated squamous cell carcinoma: a review. J Am Acad Dermatol 2011; 64(6):1147–53.
37. Dehesa L, Tosti A. Treatment of inflammatory nail disorders. Dermatol Ther 2012; 25(6):525–34.
38. Haneke E. Non-infectious inflammatory disorders of the nail apparatus. J Dtsch Dermatol Ges 2009;7(9):787–97.
39. Schons KR, Knob CF, Murussi N, et al. Nail psoriasis: a review of the literature. An Bras Dermatol 2014;89(2):312–7.
40. Crowley JJ, Weinberg JM, Wu JJ, et al. Treatment of nail psoriasis: best practice recommendations from the Medical Board of the National Psoriasis Foundation. JAMA Dermatol 2015;151(1):87–94.
41. Villani AP, Rouzaud M, Sevrain M, et al. Symptoms dermatologists should look for in daily practice to improve detection of psoriatic arthritis in psoriasis patients: an expert group consensus. J Eur Acad Dermatol Venereol 2014;28(Suppl 5):27–32.
42. Goettmann S, Zaraa I, Moulonguet I. Nail lichen planus: epidemiological, clinical, pathological, therapeutic and prognosis study of 67 cases. J Eur Acad Dermatol Venereol 2012;26(10):1304–9.
43. Piraccini BM, Saccani E, Starace M, et al. Nail lichen planus: response to treatment and long term follow-up. Eur J Dermatol 2010;20(4):489–96.
44. Papadopoulos AJ, Schwartz RA, Janniger CK. Alopecia areata. Pathogenesis, diagnosis, and therapy. Am J Clin Dermatol 2000;1(2):101–5.
45. Tosti A, Piraccini BM, Ghetti E, et al. Topical steroids versus systemic antifungals in the treatment of chronic paronychia: an open, randomized double-blind and double dummy study. J Am Acad Dermatol 2002;47(1):73–6.
46. Rigopoulos D, Gregoriou S, Belyayeva E, et al. Efficacy and safety of tacrolimus ointment 0.1% vs. betamethasone 17-valerate 0.1% in the treatment of chronic paronychia: an unblinded randomized study. Br J Dermatol 2009;160(4):858–60.
47. Ray LF. Onycholysis. A classification and study. Arch Dermatol 1963;88:181–5.
48. Tosti A, Piraccini BM, de Farias DC. Dealing with melanonychia. Semin Cutan Med Surg 2009;28(1):49–54.

49. Perrin C. Tumors of the nail unit. A review. Part I: acquired localized longitudinal melanonychia and erythronychia. Am J Dermatopathol 2013;35(6):621–36.

50. Yasuki Y. Acquired periungual fibrokeratoma—a proposal for classification of periungual fibrous lesions. J Dermatol 1985;12(4):349–56.

51. Newman MJ, Pocock G, Allan P. Glomus tumour: a rare differential for subungual lesions. BMJ Case Rep 2015. Available online at: http://dx.doi.org/10.1136/bcr-2014.

52. Dacambra MP, Gupta SK, Ferri-de-Barros F. Subungual exostosis of the toes: a systematic review. Clin Orthop Relat Res 2014;472(4):1251–9.

53. Calligaris L, Berti I. Subungual exostosis. J Pediatr 2014;165(2):412.

54. Li K, Barankin B. Digital mucous cysts. J Cutan Med Surg 2010;14(5):199–206.

Psoriasis and Cardiovascular Disease

Kathryn T. Shahwan, MD, Alexa B. Kimball, MD, MPH*

KEYWORDS

- Psoriasis • Psoriatic arthritis • Metabolic syndrome • Cardiovascular disease
- Cerebrovascular disease

KEY POINTS

- Psoriasis patients have an increased risk of adverse cardiovascular events and related mortality.
- Psoriasis is associated with environmental risk factors, the metabolic syndrome, chronic kidney disease, venous thromboembolism, peripheral arterial disease, ischemic heart disease, heart failure, atrial fibrillation, and ischemic stroke.
- Psoriatic disease and atherosclerosis share similar pathogenic mechanisms and inflammatory pathways.
- Measures of subclinical atherosclerosis and related biomarkers may be useful to predict which patients are at the greatest risk for future cardiovascular events.
- Treatment goals should focus on targeting inflammation as well as careful screening and treatment of modifiable risk factors.

INTRODUCTION

Psoriasis is a chronic, waxing and waning, inflammatory skin disorder with hyperproliferation of keratinocytes resulting in indurated, erythematous, scaly, and often pruritic plaques.[1] The disease also has the potential to affect the joints, causing a destructive inflammatory arthropathy similar to rheumatoid arthritis and ankylosing spondylitis.[2] Like other chronic inflammatory disorders, psoriasis has been shown to result in systemic inflammation with an increase in acute phase reactants and inflammatory biomarkers. There is a strong genetic component, but environmental

Funding Sources: None.
Conflicts of Interest: A.B. Kimball has been a consultant and investigator for Amgen, Abbvie, Janssen, Novartis, Celgene and Pfizer, has been a consultant for Eli Lilly, and receives fellowship funding from Janssen. K.T. Shahwan receives fellowship funding from Janssen.
Clinical Unit for Research Trials and Outcomes in Skin (CURTIS), Department of Dermatology, Massachusetts General Hospital, Harvard Medical School, 50 Staniford Street, Suite 240, Boston, MA 02114, USA
* Corresponding author.
E-mail address: harvardskinstudies@partners.org

Med Clin N Am 99 (2015) 1227–1242
http://dx.doi.org/10.1016/j.mcna.2015.08.001
0025-7125/15/$ – see front matter © 2015 Elsevier Inc. All rights reserved.

factors can also trigger or worsen the disease.[1] Psoriasis has been shown to decrease quality of life significantly in its sufferers.[3] Treatment options include phototherapy, topical preparations including steroids, the vitamin D analog calcipotriene, calcineurin inhibitors, tar products, retinoids, nonbiologic disease-modifying drugs such as methotrexate and cyclosporine, and targeted biologic therapies including tumor necrosis factor (TNF)-α inhibitors, interleukin (IL)-12/23 inhibitors, and IL-17 inhibitors.[1]

Psoriasis is closely linked with the metabolic syndrome[4] and has been associated with an increased risk of various cardiovascular diseases, including renal insufficiency,[5] deep venous thromboses, pulmonary emboli,[6] peripheral arterial disease, coronary artery disease (CAD),[7] cardiomyopathy,[8] atrial fibrillation, and ischemic stroke.[9] Patients with psoriasis have significantly increased cardiovascular morbidity and mortality,[10] which results in a profound economic burden.[11] This review aims to explore the prevalence and characteristics of cardiovascular comorbidities in patients with psoriatic disease, the shared pathogenic mechanisms between psoriasis and atherosclerosis, useful clinical measures to predict future risk, the relationship of psoriasis treatments to cardiovascular outcomes, and the importance of screening for and treating modifiable risk factors.

PREVALENCE OF CARDIOVASCULAR COMORBIDITIES
Environmental Risk Factors

Although psoriasis is recognized as an independent risk factor for cardiovascular disease, patients with psoriasis have also been shown to have higher rates of classic environmental risk factors, such as smoking, alcohol use, and a sedentary lifestyle. Multiple observational studies have shown an association between smoking and psoriasis,[12–15] and a recent meta-analysis revealed that patients with psoriasis are 1.78 times more likely than the general population to be current smokers.[16] Similarly, in a systematic review examining the relationship between psoriasis and alcohol consumption, approximately 78% of the selected studies demonstrated an increased prevalence of alcohol abuse in patients with psoriasis.[17] Patients with severe psoriasis have also been shown to exercise less, with an odds ratio (OR) of 3.42 for a low level of physical activity based on the International Physical Activity Questionnaire–Short Form.[18]

The Metabolic Syndrome

The metabolic syndrome, which includes central obesity, dyslipidemia, hypertension, and insulin resistance, constitutes a proinflammatory, hypercoagulable state[19] and has long been associated with psoriatic disease.[4,20–22]

Obesity

In a meta-analysis performed by Armstrong and colleagues,[23] patients with mild psoriasis were 1.46 times more likely to be obese, and patients with severe psoriasis were 2.23 times more likely to be obese than controls. More important, psoriasis has been associated with increases in waist circumference[24,25] and waist-to-height ratio,[26] indicators of central obesity and abdominal visceral fat, which confer an even greater risk of cardiovascular disease.[27] Patients are also disproportionately affected by other miscellaneous obesity-related comorbidities, including obstructive sleep apnea,[28] nonalcoholic fatty liver disease,[29,30] and polycystic ovarian syndrome.[31]

Dyslipidemia

Interestingly, despite the clearly established relationship between psoriasis, the metabolic syndrome, and cardiovascular disease, studies evaluating the prevalence of dyslipidemia in psoriasis patients have had mixed results. In a systematic review by Ma and colleagues[32] of 25 observational studies, 80% of the studies demonstrated a significant correlation between psoriasis and lipid profile abnormalities including elevated triglyceride levels in 16%, high-density lipoprotein cholesterol level of less than 40 mg/dL in 12%, and unspecified hyperlipoproteinemia in 8%. Several studies also demonstrated a positive correlation between the severity of psoriasis and odds of dyslipidemia. In 20% of the studies, however, there were no differences in lipid levels between psoriasis patients and controls.

Hypertension

In contrast, psoriasis has been associated with hypertension consistently. In a recent meta-analysis, patients with psoriasis had significantly increased odds of hypertension (OR, 1.58; 95% CI, 1.42–1.76), and the prevalence was greatest in those with severe psoriasis and psoriatic arthritis.[33] Patients with psoriasis are more likely to have poor blood pressure control despite antihypertensive therapy,[34] and are significantly more likely to require multiple antihypertensive agents.[35] Ambulatory blood pressure monitoring has also revealed an increased prevalence of masked[36] and nocturnal hypertension[37] in patients with psoriasis, both of which have been associated with progression to sustained hypertension and increased cardiovascular morbidity.[38,39] Furthermore, longstanding hypertension has been associated with an increased risk of developing psoriasis,[40] and the use of beta-blockers[41–43] and angiotensin-converting enzyme inhibitors[44] have been linked with the development or exacerbation of psoriasis in several case reports and small observational studies. A large case control study, however, failed to detect an association between the use of antihypertensive medications and the development of psoriasis.[45]

Diabetes mellitus

There is also an increased prevalence of diabetes mellitus in psoriasis patients,[46–48] especially those with severe disease[49] or joint involvement.[50] Armstrong and colleagues[51] performed a systematic review and meta-analysis of observational studies that revealed that the ORs of diabetes in patients with psoriasis are 1.53 and 1.97 for mild and severe psoriasis, respectively. In addition, patients with psoriasis are 1.27 times more likely to develop incident diabetes.

Microvascular Disease

Research exploring the relationship between psoriasis and small vessel complications such as retinopathy and neuropathy is lacking; however, in one observational study the prevalence was comparable between psoriasis patients and controls.[24] There have been, however, data to suggest an association between psoriasis and chronic renal insufficiency. In a recent large nested cohort study, patients with moderate and severe psoriasis were 1.36 and 1.58 times more likely, respectively, than matched controls to develop stage III, IV, or V chronic kidney disease. This was after accounting for classic risk factors, suggesting that psoriasis may be an independent risk factor for the development of chronic kidney disease.[5]

Macrovascular and Cardiac Complications

Venous thromboembolism

Like other chronic inflammatory disorders, psoriasis has the ability to promote a hypercoagulable state, especially in combination with the metabolic syndrome. Accordingly, data from two large cohort studies—the Iowa Women's Health Study[15] and a Denmark national cohort study[6]—demonstrated a significantly increased risk of developing a deep vein thrombosis or pulmonary embolism in patients with psoriasis (hazard ratio, 1.39).[15] This effect was especially profound in patients with severe psoriasis, who had an incident rate of 3.2 compared with controls.[6]

Peripheral arterial disease

Individuals with psoriasis have an increased prevalence of peripheral arterial disease,[52–54] and this association was independent of traditional risk factors in a large database study.[52] In addition, patients with psoriatic arthritis have a significantly higher rate of peripheral vascular disease when compared with patients with other forms of inflammatory arthritis.[55]

Coronary artery disease and myocardial infarction

Perhaps most important to cardiovascular outcomes, patients with psoriatic disease are at an increased risk of CAD[7,56–58] and myocardial infarction (MI).[10,59–65] In a meta-analysis of observational studies performed by Horreau and colleagues,[7] there was a significant relationship between psoriasis, CAD, and MI, with pooled ORs of 1.19 to 1.84 and 1.25 to 1.57 for CAD and MI, respectively.

In studies that stratified patients by age and severity, the risk seemed to be greatest in younger patients and those with severe disease.[7] Although one large, case-control study failed to detect an increased risk in psoriasis patients overall, patients in their 30s were 5.48 times more likely than the general population to have a MI.[64] In another study, the OR for CAD in patients with Psoriasis Area and Severity Index score of greater than 10 were more than twice that of patients with Psoriasis Area and Severity Index score of less than 10 (6.48 and 2.97, respectively).[57] Furthermore, data from the US Nurses' Health Study demonstrated that women with psoriatic arthritis were significantly more likely to have a nonfatal MI than women with psoriasis alone,[65] suggesting that joint involvement may also confer greater risk.

Patients with psoriasis may also be more likely to have severe CAD than the general population; Picard and colleagues[58] demonstrated that in a group of patients with CAD undergoing coronary angiography, those with psoriasis were significantly more likely to have 3-vessel disease.

Cardiomyopathy

Heart failure is a well-known consequence of hypertension and ischemic heart disease, and a major cause of cardiovascular morbidity and mortality. Psoriatic disease has been linked to cardiomyopathy in several case reports,[66,67] and observational studies have revealed an association with subclinical left ventricular dysfunction.[68,69] In addition, a recent large cohort study demonstrated a significant severity-dependent relationship between psoriasis and new-onset clinical heart failure, with hazard ratios of 1.22 for mild and 1.53 for severe disease.[8] Similarly, the prevalence of congestive heart failure in patients with psoriatic arthritis has been estimated to be 1.5 times that of the general population based on a recent study.[56]

Atrial fibrillation and cerebrovascular disease

Atrial fibrillation, a common arrhythmia that carries a 5-fold increase in risk of ischemic stroke,[70] is also more prevalent in patients with psoriasis.[9,71] One cohort study revealed that psoriasis patients younger than 50 years of age had a relative risk of 1.5 and 2.98 for mild and severe disease, respectively. Patients 50 years of age and older had a smaller but still significant relationship, with a relative risk of 1.16 and 1.29 for mild and severe psoriasis.[9] As expected, psoriasis patients with atrial fibrillation also have a higher risk of subsequent thromboembolic stroke. In a cohort study of patients with nonvalvular atrial fibrillation who had not been treated with anticoagulation, those with psoriasis had significantly higher rates of thromboembolism and related mortality, which exceeded that predicted by their $CHA_2DSVASc$ score by 2.6 to 3.4 times.[71] The relationship between psoriatic arthritis and atrial fibrillation remains unclear.

In contrast, studies examining the relationship between psoriasis and overall stroke risk have had varied results. The systematic review by Horreau and colleagues[7] that was discussed previously also examined rates of cerebrovascular events in psoriasis patients; although a meta-analysis of cross-sectional studies revealed an increased risk of stroke, especially in younger patients and those with severe disease, a meta-analysis of cohort studies failed to confirm this relationship. Three other meta-analyses of cohort studies, however, did demonstrate a significantly increased risk of cerebrovascular events in psoriasis patients.[10,60,63] In a retrospective cohort study, patients with psoriasis had a 27% increase in the risk of incident stroke.[72] Psoriatic arthritis was shown to confer an even greater risk of cerebrovascular events in a retrospective cohort study in which these patients had a hazard ratio of 1.82 compared with patients with psoriasis alone.[73]

PATHOPHYSIOLOGIC MECHANISMS AND BIOMARKERS

The pathogenesis of psoriasis shares substantial similarities with that of atherosclerosis. In psoriasis, cytokine dysregulation and inflammation cause aberrant dermal angiogenesis,[74] as well as rapid keratinocyte proliferation, incomplete terminal differentiation, and inadequate cell-to-cell adhesion resulting in erythema and scaling with disruption of the normal skin barrier.[75] Similarly, the pathogenesis of atherosclerosis involves systemic inflammation, dysregulated cytokine signaling, endothelial expression of adhesion molecules, recruitment and endothelial invasion of inflammatory cells including macrophages, production of foam cells by the consumption of oxidized lipoprotein particles,[76] and release of metalloproteinases and procoagulants, which allow for degradation of the vessel matrix and formation of atherosclerotic plaques.[75]

Environmental and genetic factors both serve as triggers of inflammation in psoriasis and atherosclerosis. As discussed previously, psoriasis is frequently associated with central obesity, hypertension, insulin resistance, smoking, and alcohol use, all of which can contribute to the shared inflammatory cascade. Oxidative stress and increased homocysteine levels may also play a role.[77] Although genetic factors underlie both psoriasis and atherosclerosis, genome studies have failed to reveal shared susceptibility loci.[78] Psoriasis has been associated with polymorphisms of the ApoE4 gene, however, which may explain partially the link between psoriasis and metabolic dysfunction.[75] Expression of Wnt5a, a protein involved in obesity and insulin resistance, is also increased in psoriasis patients, independent of body mass index.[79] In addition, skin biopsies of psoriasis lesions have displayed aberrant gene transcription of anti-inflammatory proteins (monocyte chemoattractant protein-1 and macrophage-derived chemokine) and modulators of lipid metabolism (peroxisome proliferator activated receptor -α and liver X receptor-α), all of which have been implicated in atherosclerosis.[80] Dysregulated ATF-3 and ATF-4 gene expression has also been implicated in both conditions.[81]

The inflammatory pathways of psoriasis and atherosclerosis involve T helper (Th)1, Th17, regulatory T cells,[82] and natural killer T cells[83] with downstream expression of cytokines.[77] Cytokines that have been implicated in the shared pathogenesis of these diseases include cathelicidin (LL-37),[84,85] IL-17,[86] IL-18,[87] IL-20,[88] IL-2, IL-6, IL-7, IL-8, IL-12, IL-15, IL-23, interferon-γ, and TNF-α,[77] and each has its own corresponding role in the activation and homeostasis of inflammatory cells, expression of endothelial adhesion molecules, induction of keratinocyte and vascular smooth muscle proliferation, and stimulation of other cytokines, chemokines, growth factors, and acute phase reactants.[77]

Given the strikingly similar pathophysiology between the two conditions, there has been recent interest in evaluating for the presence of early pathogenic vascular changes in patients with psoriasis. Results of such studies have revealed that psoriatic disease is associated with multiple measures of endothelial dysfunction and subclinical atherosclerosis, including significant increases in carotid intima media thickness,[89–97] epicardial fat thickness,[96,98] coronary artery calcification,[90] arterial inflammation by PET scan,[99,100] aortic strain and stiffness parameters,[92,93,101] aortic root diameter,[102] and peripheral arterial stiffness,[103] as well as significant decreases in aortic propagation velocity,[95] coronary flow reserve,[104–107] and brachial artery flow mediated dilation.[93,97,108] In addition, various biomarkers have been found to correlate with these measures including platelet CD62 expression,[102] neutrophil-to-lymphocyte ratio, platelet-to-lymphocyte ratio,[95] apolipoprotein (apo)B/apoA-I ratio,[12] and levels of leptin,[12,91] resistin,[91] calprotectin,[109] fibrinogen, C3 complement,[92] C-reactive protein,[92,101,103] YKL-40,[92] CD40L,[108] TNF-α, osteoprotegerin,[97] oxidized low-density lipoprotein cholesterol, nitric oxide,[110] and ADMA,[104,106] suggesting these may have predictive value.

EFFECT OF PSORIASIS THERAPIES ON CARDIOVASCULAR OUTCOMES

Since inflammation is the driving link between psoriasis and cardiovascular disease, it is plausible that targeting inflammation would improve cardiovascular outcomes. Unfortunately, traditional anti-inflammatory agents, such as systemic corticosteroids, nonsteroidal anti-inflammatory drugs, and cyclooxygenase-2 inhibitors,[111,112] as well as the systemic immunomodulator cyclosporine,[77,113] have been associated with an increased risk of hypertension, dyslipidemia, homocysteinemia, and adverse cardiovascular events.

In studies of other systemic therapies, including methotrexate, retinoids, and biologic drugs, results have been somewhat controversial but overall show promising results for decreasing cardiovascular risk. A cohort study comparing cardiovascular outcomes in psoriasis patients treated with systemic therapies (including methotrexate, cyclosporine, alefacept, efalizumab, adalimumab, etancercept, and infliximab) with a control group treated with ultraviolet B phototherapy revealed no significant difference in risk of MI between the two groups; however, the authors did not analyze the medications individually and cyclosporine was included in the dataset.[114] Subsequently, a meta-analysis of 6 studies in patients with psoriasis or psoriatic arthritis revealed a significant protective effect of all systemic medications on relative risk of cardiovascular disease.[111]

Nonbiologic Systemic Therapies

Methotrexate and oral retinoids are commonly used systemic medications in the treatment of psoriatic disease. Methotrexate, a folate analog that inhibits dihydrofolate reductase, has been shown to improve the risk of ischemic heart disease and stroke[73,115,116] in patients with psoriasis, despite increasing serum homocysteine levels.[117] In a retrospective cohort study, the greatest protective effect was seen in patients who had received a low cumulative dose and in those who had received folate supplementation.[115]

Cardiovascular outcomes associated with systemic retinoids have not been well-studied, but in a case control study they did not confer any cardioprotective effect.[116] In addition, in a cohort study of psoriasis patients taking etretinate, a retinoid which has since been taken off the US market, the incidence of cardiovascular events was similar to that of the control group.[118]

Biologic Therapies

Targeted biologic therapies, including TNF-α inhibitors and inhibitors of the shared subunit of IL-12 and IL-23, have proven to be extremely effective in the treatment of psoriasis and psoriatic arthritis. Recent studies have focused on whether they might also confer a protective effect on cardiovascular outcomes by decreasing systemic inflammation.[119] The newest class, IL-17 inhibitors, has yet to be studied in depth with respect to cardiovascular disease.

Tumor Necrosis Factor-α Inhibitors

In a meta-analysis including randomized controlled trials of TNF-α inhibitors, the risk of cardiovascular events in the short-term treatment period was similar to that of the general population.[119] In a large retrospective cohort study, patients treated with TNF-α inhibitors, oral medications, or phototherapy had a significantly reduced risk of MI compared with patients treated with topical medications. The greatest decrease in risk was seen in patients treated with TNF-α inhibitors; however, this difference was not significant when compared with the oral/phototherapy group.[120] There was no change in the results when patients were stratified by duration of treatment[121] or gender.[122] When they were stratified by ethnicity, results were similar in the Caucasian group; however, in the non-Caucasian group only the TNF-α inhibitors were superior to topical therapies.[123] When patients with skin involvement alone were separated from those with psoriatic arthritis, only the patients with psoriasis alone experienced a significant improvement in risk of MI with TNF-α inhibitors.[124] Furthermore, TNF-α inhibitors have been associated with improvements in aortic pulse wave velocity,[109] brachial artery intima media thickness,[125] and carotid intima media thickness[109,125,126] in patients with psoriatic disease. In a retrospective cohort study, treatment with etanercept for 24 weeks did not result in any changes in lipid profiles[127]; however, it was likely too short of a time period to detect a difference and further studies evaluating the effects of biologics on metabolic parameters are warranted.

Interleukin-12/23 inhibitors

The effect of IL-12/23 inhibitors, such as ustekinumab and briakinumab, on cardiovascular outcomes is somewhat controversial. In a meta-analysis of early randomized controlled trials, the incidence of adverse cardiovascular events was greater in the treatment group than in the control group, although this was not significant.[119] The lack of significance may have been due to inadequate power and a short follow-up period, however, and one commenter pointed out that the number needed to harm was 83, which could be considered clinically significant.[128] A subsequent meta-analysis of phase II and phase III clinical trials did not reveal any increase in cardiovascular risk associated with ustekinumab.[129] Furthermore, in a group of 753 patients who were followed for 5 years, only 10 major adverse cardiovascular events occurred and all were in patients with multiple preexisting cardiovascular risk factors.[130] Later, however, Tzellos and colleagues[131] performed a meta-analysis employing the Peto 1-step method, which did reveal a significant association between IL-12/23 inhibitors and major cardiovascular events (OR, 4.23; 95% CI, 1.07–16.75).

SCREENING AND TREATMENT OF RISK FACTORS

Screening, counseling, and treatment of modifiable cardiovascular risk factors in patients with psoriasis is paramount. Accordingly, the National Psoriasis Foundation released guidelines in 2008. Blood pressure, body mass index, waist circumference, heart rate, lipid profile, and fasting blood glucose should be evaluated and treated according to the American Heart Association guidelines at as early as 20 years of age and at least by age 40 in patients with psoriasis. These patients should also avoid smoking and excess alcohol use, engage in moderate physical activity several times weekly, maintain a body mass index of less than 25 kg/m^2, and eat a healthy, balanced diet.[132]

Unfortunately, multiple cross-sectional studies have demonstrated that the prevalence of screening for cardiovascular risk factors in psoriasis patients is currently inadequate,[133–135] and a high percentage of physicians lack awareness of the association between psoriasis and cardiovascular disease.[134] In addition, a large retrospective registry study revealed that hypertension and dyslipidemia are more likely to go untreated in patients with psoriasis,[136] which may have a significant impact on cardiovascular outcomes.

Intriguingly, treatment of dyslipidemia has been shown to improve the severity of psoriasis in several trials. Statins are known to have anti-inflammatory effects, and a pilot study of simvastatin revealed a significant improvement in skin lesions.[137] Similarly, a large case-control study demonstrated that patients on statin medications had a lower risk of psoriasis.[42] Thiazolidinediones have also been studied; a meta-analysis of four randomized trials revealed that treatment with pioglitazone resulted in a significant improvement in Psoriasis Area and Severity Index score compared with placebo, whereas treatment with rosiglitazone resulted in a nonsignificant improvement.[138]

Weight loss has also been shown to improve the severity of psoriasis, whether achieved through diet or bariatric surgery.[139,140] In one study, weight loss in psoriasis patients also correlated with improved blood pressures, lipid profiles, glucose levels, and hemoglobin A1C levels; there was no change, however, in peripheral arterial tonometry measures.[141] Obese patients with psoriasis have also been shown to have a diminished response to systemic treatments, and weight loss during treatment may improve this response.[139]

Although the evidence presented suggests that treatment of cardiovascular risk factors has the potential to improve psoriasis, further studies examining the impact of these interventions on cardiovascular morbidity and mortality are needed.

SUMMARY

Psoriasis is a systemic inflammatory disease that confers significant risk of metabolic derangements and adverse cardiovascular outcomes. Early detection and treatment of modifiable risk factors and modulation of the systemic inflammatory response are important treatment goals. Studies have shown that there is a significant lack of awareness of the relationship between psoriasis and cardiovascular disease, so future considerations should focus on education of and collaboration with health care providers, especially those in primary care, and development of updated, rigorous screening guidelines. In addition, targeted biologic therapies such as TNF-α inhibitors have shown immense promise in targeting the systemic inflammation associated with psoriatic disease, but whether they will impact long-term cardiovascular outcomes remains to be seen.

REFERENCES

1. Boehncke WH, Schön MP. Psoriasis. Lancet 2015 [pii:S0140-6736(14) 61909-7]. [Epub ahead of print].
2. Oliveira Mde F, Rocha Bde O, Duarte GV. Psoriasis: classical and emerging comorbidities. An Bras Dermatol 2015;90(1):9–20.

3. Rapp SR, Feldman SR, Exum ML, et al. Psoriasis causes as much disability as other major medical diseases. J Am Acad Dermatol 1999;41(3 Pt 1):401–7.
4. Baeta IG, Bittencourt FV, Gontijo B, et al. Comorbidities and cardiovascular risk factors in patients with psoriasis. An Bras Dermatol 2014;89(5):735–44.
5. Wan J, Wang S, Haynes K, et al. Risk of moderate to advanced kidney disease in patients with psoriasis: population based cohort study. BMJ 2013; 347:f5961.
6. Ahlehoff O, Gislason GH, Lindhardsen J, et al. Psoriasis carries an increased risk of venous thromboembolism: a Danish nationwide cohort study. PLoS One 2011;6(3):e18125.
7. Horreau C, Pouplard C, Brenaut E, et al. Cardiovascular morbidity and mortality in psoriasis and psoriatic arthritis: a systematic literature review. J Eur Acad Dermatol Venereol 2013;27(Suppl 3):12–29.
8. Khalid U, Ahlehoff O, Gislason GH, et al. Psoriasis and risk of heart failure: a nationwide cohort study. Eur J Heart Fail 2014;16(7):743–8.
9. Ahlehoff O, Gislason GH, Jørgensen CH, et al. Psoriasis and risk of atrial fibrillation and ischaemic stroke: a Danish Nationwide Cohort Study. Eur Heart J 2012;33(16):2054–64.
10. Armstrong EJ, Harskamp CT, Armstrong AW. Psoriasis and major adverse cardiovascular events: a systematic review and meta-analysis of observational studies. J Am Heart Assoc 2013;2(2):e000062.
11. Kimball AB, Guérin A, Tsaneva M, et al. Economic burden of comorbidities in patients with psoriasis is substantial. J Eur Acad Dermatol Venereol 2011; 25(2):157–63.
12. Asha K, Sharma SB, Singal A, et al. Association of carotid intima-media thickness with leptin and apoliprotein B/apoliprotein A-I ratio reveals imminent predictors of subclinical atherosclerosis in psoriasis patients. Acta Med (Hradec Kralove) 2014;57(1):21–7.
13. Dowlatshahi EA, Kavousi M, Nijsten T, et al. Psoriasis is not associated with atherosclerosis and incident cardiovascular events: the Rotterdam Study. J Invest Dermatol 2013;133(10):2347–54.
14. Menegon DB, Pereira AG, Camerin AC, et al. Psoriasis and comorbidities in a southern Brazilian population: a case-control study. Int J Dermatol 2014;53(11): e518–25.
15. Lutsey PL, Prizment AE, Folsom AR. Psoriasis is associated with a greater risk of incident venous thromboembolism: the Iowa Women's Health Study. J Thromb Haemost 2012;10(4):708–11.
16. Armstrong AW, Harskamp CT, Dhillon JS, et al. Psoriasis and smoking: a systematic review and meta-analysis. Br J Dermatol 2014;170(2):304–14.
17. Brenaut E, Horreau C, Pouplard C, et al. Alcohol consumption and psoriasis: a systematic literature review. J Eur Acad Dermatol Venereol 2013;27(Suppl 3): 30–5.
18. Torres T, Alexandre JM, Mendonça D, et al. Levels of physical activity in patients with severe psoriasis: a cross-sectional questionnaire study. Am J Clin Dermatol 2014;15(2):129–35.
19. Kaur J. A comprehensive review on metabolic syndrome. Cardiol Res Pract 2014;2014:943162.
20. Karoli R, Fatima J, Shukla V, et al. A study of cardio-metabolic risk profile in patients with psoriasis. J Assoc Physicians India 2013;61(11):798–803.
21. Torres T, Bettencourt N, Mendonça D, et al. Complement C3 as a marker of cardiometabolic risk in psoriasis. Arch Dermatol Res 2014;306(7):653–60.

22. Mok CC, Ko GT, Ho LY, et al. Prevalence of atherosclerotic risk factors and the metabolic syndrome in patients with chronic inflammatory arthritis. Arthritis Care Res (Hoboken) 2011;63(2):195–202.

23. Armstrong AW, Harskamp CT, Armstrong EJ. The association between psoriasis and obesity: a systematic review and meta-analysis of observational studies. Nutr Diabetes 2012;2:e54.

24. Casagrande SS, Menke A, Cowie CC. No association between psoriasis and diabetes in the U.S. population. Diabetes Res Clin Pract 2014;104(3):e58–60.

25. Jensen PR, Zachariae C, Hansen P, et al. Normal endothelial function in patients with mild-to-moderate psoriasis: a case-control study. Acta Derm Venereol 2011;91(5):516–20.

26. Duarte GV, Silva LP. Correlation between psoriasis' severity and waist-to-height ratio. An Bras Dermatol 2014;89(5):846–7.

27. Pouliot MC, Despres JP, Lemieux S, et al. Waist circumference and abdominal sagittal diameter: best simple anthropometric indexes of abdominal visceral adipose tissue accumulation and related cardiovascular risk in men and women. Am J Cardiol 1994;73:460–8.

28. Karaca S, Fidan F, Erkan F, et al. Might psoriasis be a risk factor for obstructive sleep apnea syndrome? Sleep Breath 2013;17(1):275–80.

29. van der Voort EA, Koehler EM, Dowlatshahi EA, et al. Psoriasis is independently associated with nonalcoholic fatty liver disease in patients 55 years old or older: results from a population-based study. J Am Acad Dermatol 2014;70(3):517–24.

30. Abedini R, Salehi M, Lajevardi V, et al. Patients with psoriasis are at a higher risk of developing nonalcoholic fatty liver disease. Clin Exp Dermatol 2015 [Epub ahead of print].

31. Moro F, De Simone C, Morciano A, et al. Psoriatic patients have an increased risk of polycystic ovary syndrome: results of a cross-sectional analysis. Fertil Steril 2013;99(3):936–42.

32. Ma C, Harskamp CT, Armstrong EJ, et al. The association between psoriasis and dyslipidaemia: a systematic review. Br J Dermatol 2013;168(3):486–95.

33. Armstrong AW, Harskamp CT, Armstrong EJ. The association between psoriasis and hypertension: a systematic review and meta-analysis of observational studies. J Hypertens 2013;31(3):433–42 [discussion: 442–3].

34. Takeshita J, Wang S, Shin DB, et al. Effect of psoriasis severity on hypertension control: a population-based study in the United Kingdom. JAMA Dermatol 2015; 151(2):161–9.

35. Armstrong AW, Lin SW, Chambers CJ, et al. Psoriasis and hypertension severity: results from a case-control study. PLoS One 2011;6(3):e18227.

36. Bacaksiz A, Erdogan E, Sonmez O, et al. Ambulatory blood pressure monitoring can unmask hypertension in patients with psoriasis vulgaris. Med Sci Monit 2013;19:501–9.

37. Bacaksiz A, Akif Vatankulu M, Sonmez O, et al. Non-dipping nocturnal blood pressure in psoriasis vulgaris. Wien Klin Wochenschr 2012;124(23–24):822–9.

38. Yano Y, Bakris GL. Recognition and management of masked hypertension: a review and novel approach. J Am Soc Hypertens 2013;7(3):244–52.

39. Friedman O, Logan AG. Can nocturnal hypertension predict cardiovascular risk? Integr Blood Press Control 2009;2:25–37.

40. Wu S, Han J, Li WQ, et al. Hypertension, antihypertensive medication use, and risk of psoriasis. JAMA Dermatol 2014;150(9):957–63.

41. Waqar S, Sarkar PK. Exacerbation of psoriasis with beta-blocker therapy. CMAJ 2009;181(1–2):60.

42. Wolkenstein P, Revuz J, Roujeau JC, et al. French Society of Dermatology. Psoriasis in France and associated risk factors: results of a case-control study based on a large community survey. Dermatology 2009;218(2):103–9.

43. Cohen AD, Bonneh DY, Reuveni H, et al. Drug exposure and psoriasis vulgaris: case-control and case-crossover studies. Acta Derm Venereol 2005;85(4): 299–303.

44. Cohen AD, Kagen M, Friger M, et al. Calcium channel blockers intake and psoriasis: a case-control study. Acta Derm Venereol 2001;81(5):347–9.

45. Brauchli YB, Jick SS, Curtin F, et al. Association between beta-blockers, other antihypertensive drugs and psoriasis: population-based case-control study. Br J Dermatol 2008;158(6):1299–307.

46. Bang CN, Okin PM, Køber L, et al. Psoriasis is associated with subsequent atrial fibrillation in hypertensive patients with left ventricular hypertrophy: the Losartan Intervention For Endpoint study. J Hypertens 2014;32(3):667–72.

47. Kupetsky EA, Rincon F. The prevalence of systemic diseases associated with dermatoses and stroke in the United States: a cross-sectional study. Dermatology 2013;227(4):330–7.

48. Shapiro J, Cohen AD, Weitzman D, et al. Psoriasis and cardiovascular risk factors: a case-control study on inpatients comparing psoriasis to dermatitis. J Am Acad Dermatol 2012;66(2):252–8.

49. Dregan A, Charlton J, Chowienczyk P, et al. Chronic inflammatory disorders and risk of type 2 diabetes mellitus, coronary heart disease, and stroke: a population-based cohort study. Circulation 2014;130(10):837–44.

50. Armesto S, Santos-Juanes J, Galache-Osuna C, et al. Psoriasis and type 2 diabetes risk among psoriatic patients in a Spanish population. Australas J Dermatol 2012;53(2):128–30.

51. Armstrong AW, Harskamp CT, Armstrong EJ. Psoriasis and the risk of diabetes mellitus: a systematic review and meta-analysis. JAMA Dermatol 2013;149(1): 84–91.

52. Prodanovich S, Kirsner RS, Kravetz JD, et al. Association of psoriasis with coronary artery, cerebrovascular, and peripheral vascular diseases and mortality. Arch Dermatol 2009;145(6):700–3.

53. Kaye JA, Li L, Jick SS. Incidence of risk factors for myocardial infarction and other vascular diseases in patients with psoriasis. Br J Dermatol 2008;159(4):895–902.

54. Kimball AB, Robinson D Jr, Wu Y, et al. Cardiovascular disease and risk factors among psoriasis patients in two US healthcare databases, 2001-2002. Dermatology 2008;217(1):27–37.

55. Han C, Robinson DW Jr, Hackett MV, et al. Cardiovascular disease and risk factors in patients with rheumatoid arthritis, psoriatic arthritis, and ankylosing spondylitis. J Rheumatol 2006;33(11):2167–72.

56. Armstrong AW, Harskamp CT, Ledo L, et al. Coronary artery disease in patients with psoriasis referred for coronary angiography. Am J Cardiol 2012;109(7): 976–80.

57. Al-Mutairi N, Al-Farag S, Al-Mutairi A, et al. Comorbidities associated with psoriasis: an experience from the Middle East. J Dermatol 2010;37:146–55.

58. Picard D, Bénichou J, Sin C, et al. Increased prevalence of psoriasis in patients with coronary artery disease: results from a case-control study. Br J Dermatol 2014;171(3):580–7.

59. Levesque A, Lachaine J, Bissonnette R. Risk of myocardial infarction in Canadian patients with psoriasis: a retrospective cohort study. J Cutan Med Surg 2013;17(6):398–403.

60. Xu T, Zhang YH. Association of psoriasis with stroke and myocardial infarction: meta-analysis of cohort studies. Br J Dermatol 2012;167(6):1345–50.
61. Lin HW, Wang KH, Lin HC, et al. Increased risk of acute myocardial infarction in patients with psoriasis: a 5-year population-based study in Taiwan. J Am Acad Dermatol 2011;64(3):495–501.
62. Ahlehoff O, Gislason GH, Charlot M, et al. Psoriasis is associated with clinically significant cardiovascular risk: a Danish nationwide cohort study. J Intern Med 2011;270(2):147–57.
63. Samarasekera EJ, Neilson JM, Warren RB, et al. Incidence of cardiovascular disease in individuals with psoriasis: a systematic review and meta-analysis. J Invest Dermatol 2013;133(10):2340–6.
64. Brauchli YB, Jick SS, Miret M, et al. Psoriasis and risk of incident myocardial infarction, stroke or transient ischaemic attack: an inception cohort study with a nested case–control analysis. Br J Dermatol 2009;160:1048–56.
65. Li WQ, Han JL, Manson JE, et al. Psoriasis and risk of nonfatal cardiovascular disease in U.S. women: a cohort study. Br J Dermatol 2012;166:811–8.
66. Jha PK, Das SR, Musleh GS, et al. Psoriasis-induced postoperative cardiac failure. Ann Thorac Surg 2005;79(4):1390–1.
67. Pietrzak A, Brzozowska A, Lotti T, et al. Future diagnosis, today's treatment - cardiomyopathy in the course of psoriasis: a case report. Dermatol Ther 2013; 26(6):489–92.
68. Ikonomidis I, Makavos G, Papadavid E, et al. Similarities in coronary function and myocardial deformation between psoriasis and coronary artery disease: the role of oxidative stress and inflammation. Can J Cardiol 2015;31(3): 287–95.
69. Shang Q, Tam LS, Yip GW, et al. High prevalence of subclinical left ventricular dysfunction in patients with psoriatic arthritis. J Rheumatol 2011;38(7):1363–70.
70. Poli D, Antonucci E. Epidemiology, diagnosis, and management of atrial fibrillation in women. Int J Womens Health 2015;7:605–14.
71. Ahlehoff O, Gislason G, Lamberts M, et al. Risk of thromboembolism and fatal stroke in patients with psoriasis and nonvalvular atrial fibrillation: a Danish nationwide cohort study. J Intern Med 2015;277(4):447–55.
72. Chiang CH, Huang CC, Chan WL, et al. Psoriasis and increased risk of ischemic stroke in Taiwan: a nationwide study. J Dermatol 2012;39(3):279–81.
73. Chin YY, Yu HS, Li WC, et al. Arthritis as an important determinant for psoriatic patients to develop severe vascular events in Taiwan: a nation-wide study. J Eur Acad Dermatol Venereol 2013;27(10):1262–8.
74. Armstrong AW, Voyles SV, Armstrong EJ, et al. Angiogenesis and oxidative stress: common mechanisms linking psoriasis with atherosclerosis. J Dermatol Sci 2011;63(1):1–9.
75. Raychaudhuri SP. A cutting edge overview: psoriatic disease. Clin Rev Allergy Immunol 2013;44(2):109–13.
76. Feige E, Mendel I, George J, et al. Modified phospholipids as anti-inflammatory compounds. Curr Opin Lipidol 2010;21(6):525–9.
77. Ghazizadeh R, Shimizu H, Tosa M, et al. Pathogenic mechanisms shared between psoriasis and cardiovascular disease. Int J Med Sci 2010;7(5):284–9.
78. Gupta Y, Möller S, Zillikens D, et al. Genetic control of psoriasis is relatively distinct from that of metabolic syndrome and coronary artery disease. Exp Dermatol 2013;22(8):552–3.
79. Gerdes S, Laudes M, Neumann K, et al. Wnt5a: a potential factor linking psoriasis to metabolic complications. Exp Dermatol 2014;23(6):438–40.

80. Mehta NN, Li K, Szapary P, et al. Modulation of cardiometabolic pathways in skin and serum from patients with psoriasis. J Transl Med 2013;11:194.
81. Sobolev VV, Starodubtseva NL, Piruzyan AL, et al. Comparative study of the expression of ATF-3 and ATF-4 genes in vessels involved into atherosclerosis process and in psoriatic skin. Bull Exp Biol Med 2011;151(6):713–6.
82. Armstrong AW, Voyles SV, Armstrong EJ, et al. A tale of two plaques: convergent mechanisms of T-cell-mediated inflammation in psoriasis and atherosclerosis. Exp Dermatol 2011;20(7):544–9.
83. Simoni Y, Diana J, Ghazarian L, et al. Therapeutic manipulation of natural killer (NK) T cells in autoimmunity: are we close to reality? Clin Exp Immunol 2013; 171(1):8–19.
84. Kahlenberg JM, Kaplan MJ. Little peptide, big effects: the role of LL-37 in inflammation and autoimmune disease. J Immunol 2013;191(10):4895–901.
85. Reinholz M, Ruzicka T, Schauber J. Cathelicidin LL-37: an antimicrobial peptide with a role in inflammatory skin disease. Ann Dermatol 2012;24(2):126–35.
86. Karbach S, Croxford AL, Oelze M, et al. Interleukin 17 drives vascular inflammation, endothelial dysfunction, and arterial hypertension in psoriasis-like skin disease. Arterioscler Thromb Vasc Biol 2014;34(12):2658–68.
87. Sedimbi SK, Hägglöf T, Karlsson MC. IL-18 in inflammatory and autoimmune disease. Cell Mol Life Sci 2013;70(24):4795–808.
88. Logsdon NJ, Deshpande A, Harris BD, et al. Structural basis for receptor sharing and activation by interleukin-20 receptor-2 (IL-20R2) binding cytokines. Proc Natl Acad Sci U S A 2012;109(31):12704–9.
89. Troitzsch P, Paulista Markus MR, Dörr M, et al. Psoriasis is associated with increased intima-media thickness–the Study of Health in Pomerania (SHIP). Atherosclerosis 2012;225(2):486–90.
90. Yiu KH, Yeung CK, Zhao CT, et al. Prevalence and extent of subclinical atherosclerosis in patients with psoriasis. J Intern Med 2013;273(3):273–82.
91. Robati RM, Partovi-Kia M, Haghighatkhah HR, et al. Increased serum leptin and resistin levels and increased carotid intima-media wall thickness in patients with psoriasis: is psoriasis associated with atherosclerosis? J Am Acad Dermatol 2014;71(4):642–8.
92. Alpsoy S, Akyuz A, Erfan G, et al. Atherosclerosis, some serum inflammatory markers in psoriasis. G Ital Dermatol Venereol 2014;149(2):167–75.
93. Brezinski EA, Follansbee MR, Armstrong EJ, et al. Endothelial dysfunction and the effects of TNF inhibitors on the endothelium in psoriasis and psoriatic arthritis: a systematic review. Curr Pharm Des 2014;20(4):513–28.
94. Altekin ER, Koç S, Karakaş MS, et al. Determination of subclinical atherosclerosis in plaque type psoriasis patients without traditional risk factors for atherosclerosis. Turk Kardiyol Dern Ars 2012;40(7):574–80.
95. Yurtdaş M, Yaylali YT, Kaya Y, et al. Neutrophil-to-lymphocyte ratio may predict subclinical atherosclerosis in patients with psoriasis. Echocardiography 2014; 31(9):1095–104.
96. Bulbul Sen B, Atci N, Rifaioglu EN, et al. Increased epicardial fat tissue is a marker of subclinical atherosclerosis in patients with psoriasis. Br J Dermatol 2013;169(5):1081–6.
97. Puato M, Ramonda R, Doria A, et al. Impact of hypertension on vascular remodeling in patients with psoriatic arthritis. J Hum Hypertens 2014;28(2): 105–10.
98. Balci A, Celik M, Balci DD, et al. Patients with psoriasis have an increased amount of epicardial fat tissue. Clin Exp Dermatol 2014;39(2):123–8.

99. Rose S, Dave J, Millo C, et al. Psoriatic arthritis and sacroiliitis are associated with increased vascular inflammation by 18-fluorodeoxyglucose positron emission tomography computed tomography: baseline report from the Psoriasis Atherosclerosis and Cardiometabolic Disease Initiative. Arthritis Res Ther 2014;16(4):R161.

100. Mehta NN, Yu Y, Saboury B, et al. Systemic and vascular inflammation in patients with moderate to severe psoriasis as measured by [18F]-fluorodeoxyglucose positron emission tomography-computed tomography (FDG-PET/CT): a pilot study. Arch Dermatol 2011;147(9):1031–9.

101. Balta I, Balta S, Demirkol S, et al. Aortic arterial stiffness is a moderate predictor of cardiovascular disease in patients with psoriasis vulgaris. Angiology 2014; 65(1):74–8.

102. Saleh HM, Attia EA, Onsy AM, et al. Platelet activation: a link between psoriasis per se and subclinical atherosclerosis–a case-control study. Br J Dermatol 2013; 169(1):68–75.

103. Yiu KH, Yeung CK, Chan HT, et al. Increased arterial stiffness in patients with psoriasis is associated with active systemic inflammation. Br J Dermatol 2011; 164(3):514–20.

104. Atzeni F, Sarzi-Puttini P, Sitia S, et al. Coronary flow reserve and asymmetric dimethylarginine levels: new measurements for identifying subclinical atherosclerosis in patients with psoriatic arthritis. J Rheumatol 2011;38(8):1661–4.

105. Gullu H, Caliskan M, Dursun R, et al. Impaired coronary microvascular function and its association with disease duration and inflammation in patients with psoriasis. Echocardiography 2013;30(8):912–8.

106. Atzeni F, Turiel M, Boccassini L, et al. Cardiovascular involvement in psoriatic arthritis. Reumatismo 2011;63(3):148–54.

107. Osto E, Piaserico S, Maddalozzo A, et al. Impaired coronary flow reserve in young patients affected by severe psoriasis. Atherosclerosis 2012;221(1): 113–7.

108. Erturan I, Köroğlu BK, Adiloğlu A, et al. Evaluation of serum sCD40L and homocysteine levels with subclinical atherosclerosis indicators in patients with psoriasis: a pilot study. Int J Dermatol 2014;53(4):503–9.

109. Angel K, Provan SA, Fagerhol MK, et al. Effect of 1-year anti-TNF-α therapy on aortic stiffness, carotid atherosclerosis, and calprotectin in inflammatory arthropathies: a controlled study. Am J Hypertens 2012;25(6):644–50.

110. Profumo E, Di Franco M, Buttari B, et al. Biomarkers of subclinical atherosclerosis in patients with autoimmune disorders. Mediators Inflamm 2012;2012: 503942.

111. Roubille C, Richer V, Starnino T, et al. The effects of tumour necrosis factor inhibitors, methotrexate, non-steroidal anti-inflammatory drugs and corticosteroids on cardiovascular events in rheumatoid arthritis, psoriasis and psoriatic arthritis: a systematic review and meta-analysis. Ann Rheum Dis 2015;74(3): 480–9.

112. White WB, West CR, Borer JS, et al. Risk of cardiovascular events in patients receiving celecoxib: a meta-analysis of randomized clinical trials. Am J Cardiol 2007;99(1):91–8.

113. Flammer AJ, Ruschitzka F. Psoriasis and atherosclerosis: two plaques, one syndrome? Eur Heart J 2012;33(16):1989–91.

114. Abuabara K, Lee H, Kimball AB. The effect of systemic psoriasis therapies on the incidence of myocardial infarction: a cohort study. Br J Dermatol 2011; 165(5):1066–73.

115. Prodanovich S, Ma F, Taylor JR, et al. Methotrexate reduces incidence of vascular diseases in veterans with psoriasis or rheumatoid arthritis. J Am Acad Dermatol 2005;52(2):262–7.
116. Lan CC, Ko YC, Yu HS, et al. Methotrexate reduces the occurrence of cerebrovascular events among Taiwanese psoriatic patients: a nationwide population-based study. Acta Derm Venereol 2012;92(4):349–52.
117. Refsum H, Helland S, Ueland PM. Fasting plasma homocysteine as a sensitive parameter of antifolate effect: a study of psoriasis patients receiving low-dose methotrexate treatment. Clin Pharmacol Ther 1989;46(5):510–20.
118. Stern RS, Fitzgerald E, Ellis CN, et al. The safety of etretinate as long-term therapy for psoriasis: results of the etretinate follow-up study. J Am Acad Dermatol 1995;33(1):44–52.
119. Ryan C, Leonardi CL, Krueger JG, et al. Association between biologic therapies for chronic plaque psoriasis and cardiovascular events: a meta-analysis of randomized controlled trials. JAMA 2011;306(8):864–71.
120. Wu JJ, Poon KY, Channual JC, et al. Association between tumor necrosis factor inhibitor therapy and myocardial infarction risk in patients with psoriasis. Arch Dermatol 2012;148(11):1244–50.
121. Wu JJ, Poon KY, Bebchuk JD. Association between the type and length of tumor necrosis factor inhibitor therapy and myocardial infarction risk in patients with psoriasis. J Drugs Dermatol 2013;12(8):899–903.
122. Wu JJ, Poon KY. Association of gender, tumor necrosis factor inhibitor therapy, and myocardial infarction risk in patients with psoriasis. J Am Acad Dermatol 2013;69(4):650–1.
123. Wu JJ, Poon KY. Association of ethnicity, tumor necrosis factor inhibitor therapy, and myocardial infarction risk in patients with psoriasis. J Am Acad Dermatol 2013;69(1):167–8.
124. Wu JJ, Poon KY. Tumor necrosis factor inhibitor therapy and myocardial infarction risk in patients with psoriasis, psoriatic arthritis, or both. J Drugs Dermatol 2014;13(8):932–4.
125. Jókai H, Szakonyi J, Kontár O, et al. Impact of effective tumor necrosis factor-alfa inhibitor treatment on arterial intima-media thickness in psoriasis: results of a pilot study. J Am Acad Dermatol 2013;69(4):523–9.
126. Di Minno MN, Iervolino S, Peluso R, et al. Carotid intima-media thickness in psoriatic arthritis: differences between tumor necrosis factor-α blockers and traditional disease-modifying antirheumatic drugs. Arterioscler Thromb Vasc Biol 2011;31(3):705–12.
127. Lestre S, Diamantino F, Veloso L, et al. Effects of etanercept treatment on lipid profile in patients with moderate-to-severe chronic plaque psoriasis: a retrospective cohort study. Eur J Dermatol 2011;21(6):916–20.
128. Bigby M. The use of anti-interleukin-12/23 agents and major adverse cardiovascular events. Arch Dermatol 2012;148(6):753–4.
129. Reich K, Langley RG, Lebwohl M, et al. Cardiovascular safety of ustekinumab in patients with moderate to severe psoriasis: results of integrated analyses of data from phase II and III clinical studies. Br J Dermatol 2011;164(4):862–72.
130. Kimball AB, Papp KA, Wasfi Y, et al, PHOENIX 1 Investigators. Long-term efficacy of ustekinumab in patients with moderate-to-severe psoriasis treated for up to 5 years in the PHOENIX 1 study. J Eur Acad Dermatol Venereol 2013; 27(12):1535–45.
131. Tzellos T, Kyrgidis A, Zouboulis CC. Re-evaluation of the risk for major adverse cardiovascular events in patients treated with anti-IL-12/23 biological agents for

chronic plaque psoriasis: a meta-analysis of randomized controlled trials. J Eur Acad Dermatol Venereol 2013;27(5):622–7.

132. Kimball AB, Gladman D, Gelfand JM, et al. National Psoriasis Foundation clinical consensus on psoriasis comorbidities and recommendations for screening. J Am Acad Dermatol 2008;58(6):1031–42.

133. Alamdari HS, Gustafson CJ, Davis SA, et al. Psoriasis and cardiovascular screening rates in the United States. J Drugs Dermatol 2013;12(1):e14–9.

134. Parsi KK, Brezinski EA, Lin TC, et al. Are patients with psoriasis being screened for cardiovascular risk factors? A study of screening practices and awareness among primary care physicians and cardiologists. J Am Acad Dermatol 2012; 67(3):357–62.

135. Adler BL, Krausz AE, Tian J, et al. Modifiable lifestyle factors in psoriasis: screening and counseling practices among dermatologists and dermatology residents in academic institutions. J Am Acad Dermatol 2014;71(5):1028–9.

136. Ahlehoff O, Skov L, Gislason G, et al. Pharmacological undertreatment of coronary risk factors in patients with psoriasis: observational study of the Danish nationwide registries. PLoS One 2012;7(4):e36342.

137. Shirinsky IV, Shirinsky VS. Efficacy of simvastatin in plaque psoriasis: a pilot study. J Am Acad Dermatol 2007;57(3):529–31.

138. Malhotra A, Shafiq N, Rajagopalan S, et al. Thiazolidinediones for plaque psoriasis: a systematic review and meta-analysis. Evid Based Med 2012; 17(6):171–6.

139. Debbaneh M, Millsop JW, Bhatia BK, et al. Diet and psoriasis, part I: impact of weight loss interventions. J Am Acad Dermatol 2014;71(1):133–40.

140. Halawi A, Abiad F, Abbas O. Bariatric surgery and its effects on the skin and skin diseases. Obes Surg 2013;23(3):408–13.

141. Jensen P, Zachariae C, Christensen R, et al. Effect of weight loss on the cardiovascular risk profile of obese patients with psoriasis. Acta Derm Venereol 2014;94(6):691–4.

Clinical Approach to Diffuse Blisters

Tarannum Jaleel, MD, Young Kwak, MD, Naveed Sami, MD*

KEYWORDS

- Blisters • Vesicles • Diffuse blisters • Vesiculobullous
- Autoimmune bullous disorders • Bullous drug eruptions

KEY POINTS

- A thorough history is essential because it may provide clues for both internal and external triggers of certain vesiculobullous eruptions. Medications are an important cause of bullous eruptions, which have the potential to be life threatening (eg, Stevens-Johnson syndrome/toxic epidermal necrolysis).
- Immunocompromised patients often have more severe and atypical manifestations of infectious vesiculobullous disease (eg, herpetic infections) and require more aggressive therapy.
- Specialized tests such as direct immunofluorescence and serologies are helpful in diagnosing certain autoimmune blistering diseases.
- Appropriate further testing should be considered because specific bullous eruptions are strongly associated with systemic diseases (eg, myeloproliferative disorders, connective tissue diseases, systemic vasculitides, inflammatory bowel disease, and certain infections).

At some point during their careers, it is likely that most physicians will encounter a patient who presents with blisters. The clinical presentation of vesicles and bullae suggests a broad differential and confusion often arises in how to approach such patients, especially if a dermatology service is not readily accessible. In most circumstances, these tend to be acute presentations. Although some blistering eruptions may be self-limited, others are life threatening, and prompt diagnosis and management are critical. This article (1) provides a systematic diagnostic approach to such patients, including history, physical examination, and relevant work-up (**Fig. 1**); and (2) introduces some common blistering diseases that may be encountered by primary care physicians and subspecialists.

Funding Sources: None.
Conflicts of Interest: None.
Department of Dermatology, University of Alabama at Birmingham, 1520 3rd Avenue South, EFH 414, Birmingham, AL 35294-0009, USA
* Corresponding author.
E-mail address: nsami@uab.edu

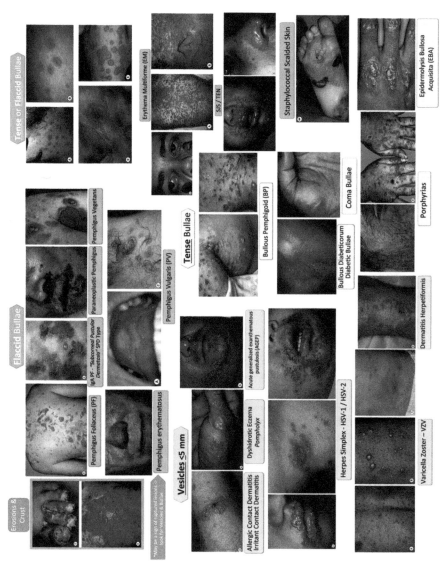

Fig. 1. Diagnostic approach for common vesiculobullous eruptions. Assoc., associated; IgA, immunoglobulin A; SJS, Stevens-Johnson syndrome; TEN, toxic epidermal necrolysis.

PATIENT HISTORY

During the initial encounter, a thorough history can play a vital role in determining the cause of a bullous eruption. There are many pertinent points in a history that help exclude possibilities, especially if the blistering eruption is atypical. Many of these variables are discussed here.

The age of onset can be crucial because certain bullous diseases are more common in specific age groups. Inherited blistering disorders such as epidermolysis bullosa begin in childhood, and may continue into adulthood.[1] Acquired processes such as autoimmune bullous disorders (ABDs) and bullous diseases secondary to systemic disease or external triggers can present in all age groups, but presentation may vary between children and adults.[2] For example, herpes zoster frequently presents in adults, whereas primary varicella presents more often in children.[3,4] Another example, staphylococcal scalded skin syndrome (SSSS), is more common in young children.

The timing of a rash can help identify acute causes, and tends to be related to particular triggers. Vesicles and bullae in the setting of external triggers, such as new medications, contact with chemicals/allergens, and infections, are acute in onset and tend to resolve after removal of the trigger. However, some ABDs and eruptions secondary to systemic disease are usually subacute to chronic with intermittent exacerbations and remissions.[2] As with any presenting illness, it is important to inquire about modifying factors that the patient may have observed in exacerbated and possibly accelerated progression of blisters. For example, photoaggravation of disease is seen in bullous lupus,[5] porphyria cutanea tarda,[6] and phytophotodermatitis,[7] whereas cold, wet environments worsen chilblains.[8]

A comprehensive review of systems is important because some diseases have particular prodromal symptoms that tend to continue as the blisters present and progress. Although diabetic bullae are asymptomatic,[9] bullous pemphigoid and contact dermatitis can be preceded by intense pruritus.[2,10] Necrotizing fasciitis and sepsis are frequent complications of bullous cellulitis associated with organisms like *Vibrio vulnificus*.[11] Immunosuppressed patients occasionally have atypical presentations, such as disseminated zoster.[3]

PHYSICAL EXAMINATION

Vesicles are elevated, fluid-filled, well-circumscribed clefts in the skin less than 1 cm in diameter, whereas bullae are greater than or equal to 1 cm in diameter (see **Fig. 1**). Although vesicles and bullae are the primary lesions, secondary changes such as crusting and erosions are concomitant in most blistering disorders. Herpes simplex and zoster, dyshidrotic eczema, and dermatitis herpetiformis present with a predominantly vesicular eruption, although in the dermatitis herpetiformis the eruption is often intensely itchy such that vesicles are excoriated before being recognized as blistering. Tense bullae (subepidermal split) are frequently seen in bullous pemphigoid, and flaccid bullae (intraepidermal split) in pemphigus vulgaris. Occasionally, only large erosions are present in cases of pemphigus foliaceous because the superficial bullae rupture before presentation. Nikolsky sign (shearing of epidermis with lateral pressure) is often seen with toxic epidermal necrolysis (TEN), SSSS, and pemphigus. Other commonly associated findings, such as erythematous urticarial plaques (eg, bullous pemphigoid), palpable purpura (eg, small vessel vasculitis), or targetoid macules (eg, erythema multiforme), can help facilitate a diagnosis.[12]

The configuration and pattern of blisters in a particular area can often provide clues to the diagnosis. Grouped vesicles are strongly suggestive of herpetic infections.[3] Geometric shapes and/or linear patterns are usually seen in the setting of phytophotodermatitis and contact dermatitis.[7,10] Annular configurations of bullae can suggest linear immunoglobulin (Ig) A bullous disease,[13] which is often described as resembling a string of pearls.

The area of distribution has important diagnostic implications, and includes the observation of key features such as the body areas involved (eg, acral/perioral/perineal), localized versus diffuse, photoexposed surfaces, and mucosal or conjunctival involvement. Localized distributions are seen in herpes zoster (dermatomal),[3] porphyria cutanea tarda (hands),[6] phototoxic drug eruptions (face, neck, and dorsal arms),[14] and diabetic bullae (areas of trauma, typically shins).[9,14] Mucosal involvement is seen in pemphigus and some variants of pemphigoid.[15,16]

DIAGNOSTIC TESTING

Initial diagnostic testing is ordered based on history and physical examination. In acute settings, diagnosis often relies on a bedside clinical assessment. If there are multiple possibilities, a skin (punch) biopsy of a new vesicle or the edge of an intact blister is recommended. Direct immunofluorescence (DIF) testing of a biopsy from perilesional skin along with serologic testing for relevant antibodies is helpful in differentiating various autoimmune bullous diseases. Special stains for infections can also be performed on biopsies. However, swabbing the skin for cultures and viral polymerase chain reaction (PCR) is easier, faster, and may provide more information. Additional pertinent blood tests can be performed based on the initial results to help identify any systemic causes.[12]

BLISTERING CONDITIONS CAUSED BY EXTERNAL TRIGGERS
Allergic Contact Dermatitis

Background
Allergic contact dermatitis (ACD) is the result of a type IV, delayed type, hypersensitivity response to specific allergens in the setting of prior sensitization. Subsequent reexposure to an allergen at low concentrations is often sufficient to elicit a response.[10,17,18]

History
Patients with ACD present with significant pruritus accompanying a rash, which usually develops within days of exposure to a specific allergen. It is important to inquire about changes to a patient's daily routine, including new hobbies or occupations, or the recent use of new products. Location of the rash may help determine the cause. For example, a rash around the neck and earlobes may indicate an allergy to nickel, which is present in some jewelry. A detailed history can help identify the cause of less common presentations such as eyelid dermatitis, which may be caused by a new nail polish.[10,17,18]

Physical examination
ACD typically presents as a well-demarcated pruritic eruption. Blisters and vesicles are often seen in an acute setting, whereas eczematous erythematous patches and plaques are more typical in the chronic setting. Geometric configurations, such as linear streaks caused by poison ivy dermatitis, are a key examination clue to ACD. Diffuse patchy eruptions well away from the primary contact reaction may be associated with autosensitization (the so-called id reaction). Occasionally, ACD and systemic autosensitization may result in erythroderma.[10,17,18]

Differential diagnosis
Irritant contact dermatitis (discussed later), dyshidrotic eczema, and bullous tinea pedis. Erythroderma that is caused by mycosis fungoides, medications, or other causes.

Diagnostic study/biopsy
ACD is generally diagnosed by history and physical examination. In some cases, a biopsy may help exclude other diagnoses. The histology usually shows spongiotic dermatitis with a mixed inflammatory infiltrate including eosinophils. Patch testing is the gold standard to identify an allergen. The top 10 common allergens are presented in **Table 1**.[10,17,18]

Treatment
The primary treatment is avoidance of the allergen, and provision of information regarding products containing identified allergens. It may take several weeks for the eruption to resolve despite allergen avoidance. Medium-potency to high-potency topical steroids may be used in localized cases. A systemic corticosteroid taper over 2 to 3 weeks may be indicated in severe cases. This treatment is typically reserved for contact dermatitis involving involvement of body surface areas of greater than 20%.[10,18]

Irritant Contact Dermatitis

Background
Irritant contact dermatitis (ICD) results from a local caustic reaction to chemicals. Chronic repetitive exposure to various mild irritants, such as soaps and cleansers, leads to breakdown of the skin barrier, and can present with various morphologies ranging from erythema and scaling to vesicles and bullae.[19,20]

History
Onset often is not abrupt, and the condition is usually chronic with intermittent flares. Affected areas tend to be painful rather than pruritic. Patients usually have a history of repetitive chronic exposure to low-grade irritants such as soaps and solvents. Bullae are more likely with exposure to strong irritants such as alkali or acids.[20]

Physical examination
Patients usually present with well-defined vesicular, bullous, or scaly erythematous patches corresponding with sites of contact. For example, ICD of the hands frequently presents with vesicles and scaly erythematous patches on the lateral aspects of

Table 1
Top 10 allergens as identified by the North American Contact Dermatitis Group

Test Substance	Allergic Reactions (%)	Relevant Reactions: Definite, Probable, Possible Combined (%)
Nickel sulfate	19	57
Myroxylon pereirae (balsam of Peru)	12	87
Fragrance mix 1	11.5	86
Quaternium-15	10	89
Neomycin sulfate	10	28
Bacitracin	9	39
Formaldehyde	9	91
Cobalt chloride	8.5	48
Methyldibromoglutaronitrile/ phenoxyethanol	6	75
p-Phenylenediamine	5	56

From Mowad CM, Marks JG. Allergic contact dermatitis. In: Bolognia JL, Jorizzo JL, Schaeffer JV, editors. Dermatology. London: Saunders; 2012; with permission.

fingers in the setting of chronic exposure to soaps and cleansers. Prolonged contact with irritants may eventually cause thickening of skin and fissuring. Involved areas can be painful and thus limit activity.[20] ACD to leather gloves can have similar appearance with localized lesions at sites of contact.[14]

Differential diagnosis
Excluding ACD can be difficult without patch testing. Also consider tinea manuum or pustular psoriasis with localized lesions on the hands. Dyshidrotic eczema (pompholyx) is a chronic and recurrent palmoplantar dermatosis with a similar clinical appearance, and is a result of atopic dermatitis with a component of ICD and/or ACD.[7,20] However, this entity is a diagnosis of exclusion and external triggers must be addressed.

Diagnostic study/biopsy
Diagnosis is based on clinical history. Biopsy can be helpful but is not definitive, and usually shows a spongiotic dermatitis with occasional necrotic keratinocytes and a lymphocytic infiltrate.[19]

Treatment/further work-up
The focus of treatment is the restoration of the skin barrier and removal of the trigger. In general, topical steroids, barrier creams, and avoidance of irritants are critical in management. Treatments in the setting of exposure to alkali or acid products are agent dependent.[19]

Phototoxic Bullous Eruption (Phytophotodermatitis)

Background
Phototoxic bullous eruptions are caused by contact with agents containing furocoumarins. Furocoumarins are toxic to skin on conversion by ultraviolet (UV) light. Phytophotodermatitis is a result of UV exposure to plant sources of furocoumarins.[7,21]

History and physical examination
The eruption begins 30 minutes to 2 hours after UV exposure and progresses to burning, erythema, vesicles, and blisters over the following 2 to 3 days. The clinical appearance is distinctive, with vesicles in a linear or geometric pattern, and bulla with concomitant erythema. The rash usually resolves with hyperpigmentation that can persist for several months. Of note, some cases show recurrence in the identical site on exposure to UV several months after the initial presentation. Patients may present at any stage, and diagnosis may be difficult when asymptomatic or with only residual hyperpigmentation. It is important to obtain a history regarding exposures within 2 to 3 days before initial presentation to plants (ie, celery, lime, or rue), medications (application of insect repellants or consumption of psoralens), and fragrances containing bergamot compounds.[7,21]

Differential diagnosis
Photoallergic contact dermatitis, bullous lupus, porphyria cutanea tarda, photoallergic drug-induced photosensitivity, and pseudoporphyria.

Diagnostic study/biopsy
A biopsy can be helpful when the diagnosis is unclear, and usually shows epidermal hyperkeratosis, spongiosis with necrotic keratinocytes, and occasionally intraepidermal and subepidermal blistering. The inflammatory infiltrate can vary with neutrophils and a perivascular lymphohistiocytic infiltrate with occasional eosinophils (in the acute setting). Later stages may show melanophages with pigment incontinence, increased melanin, melanocytic hyperplasia with variable acanthosis, hyperkeratosis, and hypergranulosis.[7,21]

Treatment/further work-up

Treatment in the acute setting depends on the severity of involvement. Topical steroids with antihistamines can be considered initially. Oral corticosteroids may be required for severe involvement. Strict, long-term sun avoidance is also necessary to avoid flares.[7,21]

Bullous Arthropod Bite Reactions

Background

An exaggerated bite response to mosquitoes, fleas, scabies, and bed bugs can sometimes be seen in children or in individuals with myeloproliferative disorders such as chronic lymphocytic leukemia.[14,22]

History

Patients present with an acute onset of blisters associated with intense pruritus localized to the affected site. Patients may not always recall a history of bug bites, but they have usually been outdoors.[14,22]

Physical examination

Bites usually present as grouped pink papules, but in some cases progress to vesicles or blisters. In cases associated with hematological malignancies, large bullae and necrosis can be seen (**Fig. 2**).[14,22]

Differential diagnosis

Bullous impetigo, bullous erythema multiforme, bullous Sweet syndrome, and localized ABDs such as bullous pemphigoid.

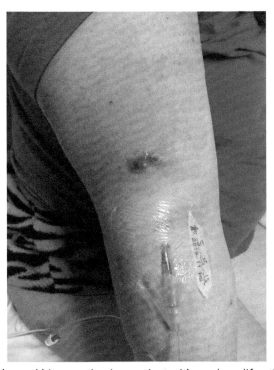

Fig. 2. Bullous arthropod bite eruption in a patient with myeloproliferative disorder.

Diagnostic study/biopsy

Biopsy shows a superficial and deep perivascular infiltrate with eosinophils along with possible epidermal necrosis at the bite site. Eosinophilic spongiosis is seen in the early phase, and may progress to subepidermal blisters.[14,22]

Treatment

Supportive care with antihistamines and topical corticosteroids for symptomatic control. Consider systemic corticosteroids if previous treatments are not sufficient. Counsel on insect avoidance and the use of insect repellants and protective clothing.[14,22]

AUTOIMMUNE BULLOUS DISORDERS

ABDs are a group of diseases with autoantibody formation to various components of the epidermis and basement membrane.[5] For example, autoantibodies targeting desmosomes in the epidermis result in an intraepidermal split presenting as flaccid bullae and erosions (mucosal and skin), as seen in pemphigus (see **Fig. 1**). Autoantibodies against hemidesmosomes and other components of the basement membrane zone result in a subepidermal split leading to disorders including pemphigoid, as detailed in **Table 2**.[1,2,12,15,16,23–25] Diagnosis requires a combination of clinical, histopathologic, immunofluorescence, and serologic findings. In performing a skin biopsy, a well-developed new vesicle or the edge of an intact blister should be sampled. The level of split, along with concomitant histologic findings, is essential to the diagnosis. DIF evaluation of perilesional skin is helpful in differentiating an ABD from a non-ABD and between various ABDs. In some cases, such as dermatitis herpetiformis, sampling of normal skin directly adjacent to vesicles and bullae is necessary in order to detect sufficient antibodies to make the diagnosis. Special stains can also be used to detect organisms. Various serologic tests are also commercially available to confirm the diagnosis of various ABDs (see **Table 2**). Appropriate early treatment and management are critical given the significant disease morbidity and mortality.[12]

BULLOUS ERUPTIONS ASSOCIATED WITH INTERNAL DISEASES
Bullous Diabeticorum

Background

Diabetic patients can develop bullae on distal extremities, most commonly at sites of trauma. Although the cause is unclear, these bullae are exacerbated by concomitant microangiopathy.[9,14]

History

Blisters are sudden in onset and generally asymptomatic, but patients may experience a prodrome of burning in the affected area before onset. Patients tend to have other diabetic complications, such as diabetic neuropathy and systemic organ involvement (ie, nephropathy, retinopathy).[9,14]

Physical examination

Tense bullae are typically distributed on the distal extremities (most commonly feet and legs), and usually have no surrounding inflammation or erythema. The fluid within the bullae is usually clear and viscous in consistency.[9,14]

Differential diagnosis

Friction blisters, pseudoporphyria, bullous pemphigoid, and edema bullae.

Table 2
Autoimmune bullous diseases: clinical characteristics, work-up, and management

Disease	Level of Split	Clinical Characteristics	DDX	Work-up	Treatment
Pemphigus: • PV • PF • Other subtypes (see **Fig. 1**)	Intraepidermal (suprabasal)	• Mean age of onset usually 50–60 y, but may affect all ages • Present with painful erosions and flaccid bullae, most commonly on torso • Tend to heal slowly with hyperpigmentation • Pruritus less common • PF: may have only erosions and crusts • PV: oral mucosa is most commonly affected and predominant finding is painful erosions • PV may involve other mucosal surfaces (conjunctiva, pharynx, larynx, esophagus, nasal, anal, genital) • Other symptoms: hoarseness and dysphagia • Clinical course: chronic with intermittent flares	• Acute herpetic flare, EM, SJS • Mucosal forms of pemphigoid may present with similar mucosal erosions and blisters • Consider paraneoplastic pemphigus in recalcitrant cases	• H&E: Intraepidermal acantholysis • DIF: perilesional skin with antibodies to keratinocyte cell surface • IIF and ELISA: IgG autoantibodies against DSG 1 and 3 correlate with disease activity • PF: autoantibodies to DSG1 (predominantly skin) • PV: autoantibodies to DSG3 (predominantly mucosal) ± DSG1 (skin)	• Prompt treatment is critical because it is potentially fatal • Initial treatment: systemic corticosteroids with slow transition to steroid-sparing agents to minimize adverse effects of corticosteroids • Supportive measures during flares: pain management, nonadherent dressings, topical steroids • Some commonly used steroid-sparing agents: azathioprine, MMF, cyclophosphamide, MTX, IVIg, rituximab, plasmapheresis

(continued on next page)

Table 2
(continued)

Disease	Level of Split	Clinical Characteristics	DDX	Work-up	Treatment
BP	Subepidermal (hemidesmosome)	• Typically affects the elderly • Very pruritic • Rarely with pain in oral cavity, dysphagia, or dysuria secondary to mucosal involvement • Diverse skin manifestations: before progressing to bullae formation, may present with pruritus and no skin lesions, excoriations, erythematous eczematous plaques, and/or urticarial erythematous plaques • Some patients may present only with urticarial plaques with excoriations • Although mucosal involvement is rare, erosions and ulcers can involve the oral cavity and genitalia • Lesions distributed symmetrically on lower trunk and lower extremities • Clinical course: chronic with frequent exacerbations and remissions	• Nonbullous phase: urticaria, urticarial vasculitis • Bullous phase: EBA, bullous lupus, LABD, drug-induced, bullous EM, bullous bite reaction, edema bullae, bullous diabeticorum	• H&E: bullous phase, subepidermal blister with predominant eosinophils in a mixed inflammatory infiltrate • H&E: nonbullous phase, subepidermal cleft + epidermal spongiosis and/or dermal eosinophils • DIF: Perilesional skin shows antibodies against epidermal basement membrane (hemidesmosome components) • Salt-split skin[a]: IgG autoantibodies bind to epidermal side of blister • Commercial ELISA serologic tests are available to check for autoantibodies to BP antigens (180 and 230)	• Potent topical steroids: useful in mild and moderate nonprogressive disease • Systemic steroids: initial mainstay of treatment of severe progressive disease • Chronic systemic treatment can vary depending on severity of disease and comorbidities. These can include tetracyclines (± nicotinamide), dapsone, azathioprine, MTX, MMF, rituximab
Bullous lupus	Subepidermal (sub–lamina densa)	• Female predilection, affecting individuals aged 20–40 y • Acute onset and can be the first sign of SLE • Can be accompanied by other systemic manifestations of SLE	• Subepidermal ABDs (BP, inflammatory EBA) • Phototoxic drug reactions • PCT	• H&E: lesional skin from intact blister shows subepidermal blister with neutrophils • DIF: granular deposition of autoantibodies along the BMZ	• Dapsone along with other immunosuppressants • Rituximab has been used with some success in recalcitrant cases

		Clinical features	ABDs	Workup	Treatment
		• Often presents in the spring and summer with more sun exposure • Vesicles and bullae develop within existing lupus lesions or de novo with predilection for sun-exposed areas such as face, trunk, and arms • Lesions tend to heal with no scarring or milia	• Can be mistaken for SJS/TEN if involvement is extensive and leading to desquamation		• Serologies: autoantibodies to type 7 collagen, ANA, anti-dsDNA, anti-Sm, anti-Ro/SS-A, anti-La/SS-B
EBA	Subepidermal (sub–lamina densa)	• Rare chronic condition with slow onset affecting trauma-prone skin and mucous membranes • Can occur at any age • Has been associated with inflammatory bowel disease • Presents with tense bullae on trauma-prone sites (eg, knuckles, wrists, extensor surfaces, hands and feet) and tend to heal with milia, and scarring • Scarring alopecia may develop with scalp involvement • Inflammatory subtype of EBA tends to be more acute and generalized, and blisters may also involve flexural as well as intertriginous areas • Mucosal involvement: oral, nasal, conjunctival, laryngeal, pharyngeal, esophageal, urogenital, anal • Mucosal lesions can lead to irreversible scarring and dysfunction	• ABDs: BP, LABD, bullous lupus	• H&E: subepidermal blister with a mixed inflammatory infiltrate • DIF: autoantibody IgG along the BMZ in a U-serrated pattern • Salt-split skin[a]: autoantibody binding to the dermal side of the salt-split skin • ELISA: detect autoantibodies to type VII collagen • Age-specific cancer screening recommended	• Systemic corticosteroids, dapsone, colchicine, and other conventional immunosuppressants

(continued on next page)

Table 2
(continued)

Disease	Level of Split	Clinical Characteristics	DDX	Work-up	Treatment
Pemphigoid gestationis	Subepidermal	• Rare pruritic blistering condition seen in late pregnancy or early postpartum • Present acutely with pruritic urticarial plaques progressing to grouped vesicles and tense bullae • May be present predominantly around the umbilicus/abdomen, and can progress to involve the entire body, especially around the time of delivery • Concurrent erythematous plaques and papules are also present • Occasionally, the neonate has vesicles and blisters caused by maternal transfer of antibodies (IgG) • Most cases resolve a few weeks after delivery, but may flare around menstruation, with use of oral contraceptives, or with recurrent pregnancies • Associated with an increased risk of Graves disease and antithyroid antibodies may be present on evaluation • Precautions should be taken because of a higher risk of prematurity and small-for-gestational-age size	• PEP/PUPPP • Urticaria	• H&E: subepidermal vesicle with eosinophils on lesional skin • DIF: most commonly shows C3 deposition along the BMZ • Monitor newborn for bullae	• Topical corticosteroids + antihistamines (category B) for minor disease • Oral corticosteroids for severe disease • Unusual for disease to persist after delivery • Provide counseling because the disease may flare with oral contraceptives and subsequent pregnancies

| Dermatitis herpetiformis | Subepidermal | • Seen in genetically predisposed individuals with gluten sensitivity and most patients have some form of gastrointestinal involvement (celiac disease)
• Chronic, lifelong condition with intermittent flares and remissions correlating with gluten consumption. Spontaneous remission is rare
• Significant pruritus
• Diarrhea and abdominal pain may be present in patients with celiac disease
• Symmetrically distributed grouped erythematous papules, vesicles, and plaques with surrounding erythema most commonly on extensor surfaces (dorsal forearms, elbows, knees), buttocks, and back
• Secondary excoriations and hemorrhagic crusting also present in most cases caused by severe pruritus | • ABDs: LABD, EBA, BP
• Infections (herpetic)
• Drug-induced blisters
• Folliculitis
• Pityriasis lichenoides | • H&E: biopsy of a vesicle with a subepidermal blister and predominant neutrophils along the dermal papillae
• DIF: uninvolved adjacent skin shows granular autoantibody IgA deposition along the dermal papillae
• Serologies: positive for antiendomysial and antitransglutaminase (tissue and epidermal) autoantibodies
• May be associated with other autoimmune diseases; consider monitoring of blood glucose and thyroid function
• Referral to gastroenterology for celiac disease and surveillance for lymphoma | • Significant improvement can be seen with avoidance of gluten and use of dapsone |

Abbreviations: ANA, antinuclear antibodies; anti-Sm, anti-Smith; Anti-SSA, Anti-Sjogren's Syndrome A; Anti-SSB, Anti-Sjogren's Syndrome B; BMZ, basement membrane zone; BP, bullous pemphigoid; C3, complement 3; DDX, differential diagnosis; DIF, direct immunofluorescence; dsDNA, double-stranded DNA; DSG, desmoglein; EBA, epidermolysis bullosa acquisita; ELISA, enzyme-linked immunosorbent assay; EM, erythema multiforme; H&E, hematoxylin and eosin; IVIg, intravenous immunoglobulin; La, Anti-SSB; LABD, linear IgA bullous disease (see text); IgA, immunoglobulin A; IgG, immunoglobulin G; IIF, indirect immunofluorescence; MMF, mycophenolate mofetil; MTX, methotrexate; PCT, porphyria cutanea tarda; PEP, polymorphic eruption of pregnancy; PF, pemphigus foliaceus; PUPPP, pruritic urticarial papules and plaques of pregnancy; PV, pemphigus vulgaris; Ro, Anti-SSA; SJS, Stevens-Johnson syndrome; SLE, systemic lupus erythematosus; TEN, toxic epidermal necrolysis.

a Specimens incubated in 5 mL of NaCl (1 mol/L) at 4°C for24 hours. Epidermis then separated from dermis and specimens processed in same manner and treated with IgG and C3 conjugates as in DIF. BP shows floor pattern and EBA shows roof pattern; correlates with autoantibodies against hemidesmosomal proteins versus collagen 7, respectively.

Diagnostic study/biopsy
Biopsy shows primarily subepidermal blisters in active lesions, and intraepidermal splits in older lesions. Friction blisters show a split below the stratum granulosum and are usually seen in the setting of repetitive trauma. DIF is negative.[9,14]

Treatment
Supportive care, treatment with an aluminum acetate solution, and prevention of infection.[9,14]

Chilblains

Background
Chilblains occur with exposure of acral surfaces (hands and feet) to cold, wet environments. It is an aberrant response in predisposed individuals, and has an unknown pathogenesis.[8,26]

History
Chilblains are commonly seen in women, children, and elderly living in cold climates with no central heating. It is a chronic condition affecting acral surfaces, and may involve the ears and nose. There is usually an associated burning pain and occasionally pruritus.[8,26]

Physical examination
The eruptions usually present as violaceous to erythematous macules, papules, or patches on volar surfaces of the distal toes and fingers, ears, and nose. Severe cases may progress to blistering and ulceration.[8,26]

Differential diagnosis
Cryoglobulinemia, myelomonocytic leukemia, hemolytic anemia, chilblain lupus erythematosus, Raynaud phenomenon, and several other cold-induced eruptions should be considered. Second-degree and third-degree frostbite also have a similar acral distribution with bullae.[8,26]

Diagnostic study/biopsy
Biopsy shows papillary dermal edema with a superficial and deep lymphocytic infiltrate, and can be helpful in distinguishing from other entities, such as chilblain lupus. Laboratory evaluation is necessary to rule out systemic causes.[8,26]

Treatment
Calcium channel blockers (amlodipine and nifedipine), cold weather clothing, and avoidance of cold and wet environments are recommended. Hydroxychloroquine can be considered if associated with systemic lupus erythematosus.[8,26]

Coma Bullae

Background
Coma bullae were previously referred to as barbiturate bullae. Although the exact cause is unknown, they are frequently seen with prolonged immobilization caused by loss of consciousness (ie, neurologic and endocrine disorders, medications, illicit drug use),[14,27] thus pressure-induced injury may play a role in pathogenesis.

History
Blisters generally develop acutely at sites of greatest pressure within 48 to 72 hours of loss of consciousness, and tend to be asymptomatic.[14,27]

Physical examination
Tense blisters develop over bony prominences and areas of greatest pressure, and eventually result in erosions.[14,27]

Differential diagnosis
Bullous diabeticorum and friction blisters.

Diagnostic study/biopsy
Biopsy shows a subepidermal split along with eccrine sweat gland necrosis, which helps to distinguish coma bullae from other blistering entities. Additional findings of rhabdomyolysis and compression neuropathy may be seen in some patients.[14,27]

Treatment
Avoidance of pressure to sites with bullae to prevent further progression, supportive wound care, toxicology evaluation, and review of medications.[14,27]

Edema Bullae

Background
Edema bullae develop because of sudden acute swelling in patients with underlying comorbidities such as congestive heart failure, renal disease, liver disease, or thrombosis leading to lower extremity edema and/or anasarca.[12,14]

History
Bullae usually develop acutely and are asymptomatic. In patients with conditions leading to chronic fluid overload, acute exacerbations can cause increased edema of the lower extremities that may be painful.[14,27]

Physical examination
Tense bullae with clear to serosanguineous fluid and minimal surrounding inflammation as well as concomitant edema are usually seen. This condition predominantly occurs in acutely ill hospitalized patients receiving excessive intravenous fluids, or in the setting of anasarca. Bullae may be localized to the distal lower extremities (dorsal foot and ankle) in patients with heart or kidney disease who acutely develop increased swelling from baseline.[14,27]

Differential diagnosis
Bullous diabeticorum, bullous pemphigoid, and medication-induced bullous eruptions, including drug-induced ABDs (discussed later).

Diagnostic study/biopsy
Biopsy usually shows a very edematous dermis with splayed collagen bundles, significant epidermal spongiosis, and occasionally subepidermal bullae.[14,27]

Treatment
Usually resolves with resolution of edema and, generally, no additional treatment is necessary.[14,27]

Porphyria Cutanea Tarda

Background
Porphyrias are a group of disorders resulting from acquired or inherited defects in the enzymes responsible for heme synthesis. Porphyria cutanea tarda results from decreased activity of uroporphyrinogen decarboxylase[6,10] and is the most common porphyria presenting in an adult population. Iron overload plays an integral part in its pathogenesis.

History
The initial symptoms include photosensitivity along with skin breakdown, and are usually precipitated by a variety of risk factors, such as alcohol consumption, increased estrogen levels, increased iron levels (as seen in hemochromatosis), hepatitis C, and human immunodeficiency virus (HIV).[6,10] Lesions are typically very slow to heal.

Physical examination
Minimal trauma leads to blistering and erosions with overlying crust symmetrically distributed on photoexposed skin (especially the face and dorsal hands). These areas heal with postinflammatory pigmentary alterations. Milia and waxy, yellow, plaquelike scarring may develop. In rare cases, contractures of the digits may occur. Patients may also have a unique finding of increased hair on the bitemporal and malar cheeks. In some cases, permanent loss of scalp hair and fingernails can be seen. Urine is usually slightly brown or discolored.[6,10]

Differential diagnosis
Drug-induced bullae, pseudoporphyria (**Table 3**), and ABDs (BP, epidermolysis bullosa acquisita, bullous lupus) (see **Table 2**).

Diagnostic study/biopsy
Diagnosis is confirmed with laboratory abnormalities showing increased serum and urine uroporphyrin, urine coproporphyrin, and fecal isocoproporphyrin. Further evaluation should include tests for hepatitis C, HIV, hemochromatosis, hemoglobin/hematocrit, liver function, and iron studies (particularly ferritin). Biopsy is not always necessary because the condition is fairly recognizable based on clinical appearance and laboratory testing.[6,10]

Treatment/further work-up
Initially consider serial phlebotomies every 2–4 weeks with monitoring of hemoglobin, hematocrit, and iron levels with the goal to reach a hemoglobin level of 10 to 11 g/dL and the lower limits of normal range of serum ferritin concentration without induction of iron deficiency anemia. Low-dose antimalarials (ie, hydroxychloroquine 100 mg twice weekly) have also been successful. Erythropoietin has been reported to be helpful in patients with renal failure. Photoprotection, avoidance of triggers such as alcohol, and treatment of associated conditions are also recommended. It is important to monitor for the development of hepatocellular carcinoma given the increased long-term risk in these patients.[6,10]

Bullous Neutrophilic Dermatoses

Background
Bullous neutrophilic dermatoses are inflammatory dermatoses with 2 major subtypes: bullous Sweet syndrome (BSS) and bullous pyoderma gangrenosum (BPG). There has been a suggestion that BSS and BPG are variants of the same disease process.[28]

History
BPG presents with painful blisters that are acute in onset and rapidly progressive. BPG has been seen in association with systemic diseases, including hematologic malignancies and inflammatory bowel disease.[28] Sweet syndrome usually presents with fever, an increased neutrophil count, and joint involvement, and may be associated with myelogenous leukemia, medications, autoimmune disorders, and infections.[29]

Physical examination
BPG presents as flaccid hemorrhagic bullae sometimes overlying an erythematous plaque, and progresses to superficial ulcerations most commonly on the face and

Table 3
Bullous drug eruptions

Disease	Examination Findings	Time Interval	Notes	Notable Responsible Drugs	Treatment
Fixed drug eruption	• Sharply circumscribed erythematous to dusky violaceous patches • Central blisters or erosions may appear • Often resolves with postinflammatory hyperpigmentation • Recurrence at same locations following drug reexposure • Can involve mucosa and genitalia	• First exposure, 1–2 wk • Reexposure, <48 h, usually within 24 h	• May have mucosal, acral, and genital involvement	Sulfonamides, TMP-SMX, NSAIDs, aspirin, acetaminophen (paracetamol), barbiturates, phenolphthalein, tetracyclines, metronidazole, pseudoephedrine	—

SJS
TEN
	• Prodromal symptoms: fever and painful skin
	• Dusky macules with or without epidermal detachment
	• Macular atypical targets
	• Flaccid bullous lesions, confluence, wide erosions + Nikolsky sign
	• Involves mucosa, face, trunk
	• Systemic symptoms: fever, lymphadenopathy, hepatitis, and cytopenias
		7–21 d	• Mucosal, acral, and genital involvement
			• Percentage detachment of BSA
			  ○ SJS <10%
			  ○ SJS-TEN overlap 10%–30%
			  ○ TEN >30%
				Sulfonamides, TMP-SMX, allopurinol, β-lactam Abx, NSAIDs, piroxicam, anticonvulsants (aromatic), lamotrigine, phenytoin, barbiturates	• Critical = early withdrawal of responsible drug
					• No definitive therapy
					• Supportive care with burn team
					• Corticosteroids controversial
					• IVIg, cyclosporine, cyclophosphamide, plasmapheresis, N-acetylcysteine, TNF-α antagonists

(continued on next page)

Table 3
(continued)

Disease	Examination Findings	Time Interval	Notes	Notable Responsible Drugs	Treatment
EM	• Rarely drug induced, ~90% from infections (HSV-1/2, *Mycoplasma pneumoniae*, VZV, EBV, CMV, *Histoplasma capsulatum*, dermatophytes, and so forth) • Targetoid lesions on extremities/face • EM minor: target lesions, papular atypical targets, possible mucosal involvement. No systemic symptoms • EM major: as above + severe mucosal involvement, systemic symptoms, may have bullous lesions	—	• Rarely drug induced • Mostly from infections • No progression to TEN	NSAIDs, sulfonamides, anticonvulsants, aminopenicillins, allopurinol	• Consider prophylaxis for recurrent disease (acyclovir/valacyclovir/famciclovir) • Early systemic corticosteroids or pulse methylprednisolone may help • Refractory disease: azathioprine, thalidomide, dapsone, cyclosporine, mycophenolate mofetil, PUVA
AGEP	• Acute onset with high fever • Usually occurs within 2 d of drug exposure • Areas of erythema studded with pustules and occasionally vesicles • Lesions begin on face or intertriginous areas	<4 d	• High fever • Malaise, leukocytosis • >90% of cases drug induced	β-Lactams, macrolides, pristinamycin, terbinafine, hydroxychloroquine, calcium channel blockers (diltiazem), carbamazepine, acetaminophen, metronidazole	• Withdrawal of responsible drug • Topical corticosteroids • Antipyretics
Phototoxic drug eruption	• Limited to sun-exposed areas • Resembles exaggerated sunburn	—	—	Tetracyclines (especially doxycycline), quinolones, psoralens, NSAIDs, diuretics	—

	Clinical features		Causative drugs	Treatment
Drug-induced linear IgA bullous dermatosis	• Circumferential and linear vesicles and bullae • Annular and herpetiform vesicopustules and plaques	—	Vancomycin most common, β-lactam Abx, captopril, NSAIDs	• Topical steroids and withdrawal of drug usually lead to improvement • Systemic steroids and SSTs can be considered for patients with chronic disease
Drug-induced PV	• Most develop painful oral erosions • Flaccid blisters • Widespread cutaneous erosions • Associated pruritus uncommon (unlike bullous pemphigoid)	—	• 80% caused by drugs with a thiol group: penicillamine, ACE inhibitors (captopril), gold sodium thiomalate, pyritinol • Nonthiol drugs: antibiotics (especially β-lactams), pyrazolone derivatives, nifedipine, propranolol, piroxicam, and phenobarbital	• Mainstay = systemic corticosteroids • Topical = corticosteroids, antibiotics, immunomodulators (eg, tacrolimus) • If unresolved after medication withdrawal and corticosteroids, similar to pemphigus (see **Table 2**)
Drug-induced bullous pemphigoid	• Most common autoimmune subepidermal blistering disease • Associated with severe pruritus • Tense bullae on normal and erythematous skin • Concomitant erythematous or urticarial plaques • May have mucosal, acral, and genital involvement • Predominantly elderly • May be preceded by a pruritic urticarial or exanthematous phase	—	Furosemide, penicillin and other β-lactams, sulfasalazine	• Mainstay = systemic corticosteroids • Topical = corticosteroids, antibiotics, immunomodulators (eg, tacrolimus) • If unresolved after medication withdrawal and corticosteroids, consider SSTs (see **Table 2**)
Drug-induced pseudoporphyria	• Resembles PCT • Porphyrins are within normal limits	—	NSAIDs (naproxen), nalidixic acid, thiazides, furosemide, tetracyclines	Withdrawal of responsible drug

Abbreviations: Abx, antibiotics; ACE, angiotensin-converting enzyme; AGEP, acute generalized exanthematous pustulosis; BSA, body surface area; CMV, cytomegalovirus; d, days; EBV, Epstein-Barr virus; h, hours; EM, erythema multiforme; HSV, herpes simplex virus; IVIG, intravenous immunoglobulins; NSAID, nonsteroidal antiinflammatory drug; PCT, porphyria cutanea tarda; PUVA, psoralen (P) and ultraviolet A (UVA) therapy; PV, pemphigus vulgaris; SJS, stevens johnson syndrome; SSTs, steroid-sparing treatments; TEN, toxic epidermis necrolysis wk, week(s); TMP-SMX trimethoprim-sulfamethoxazole; TNF-α, tumor necrosis factor alpha; VZV, varicella zoster Virus.

Adapted from Bolognia JL, Jorizzo JL, Schaeffer JV, editors. Dermatology. London: Saunders; 2012.

upper extremities.[28] The typical lesions of Sweet syndrome are edematous, translucent, and erythematous papules and plaques that tend to localize to the head, neck, trunk, and upper extremities, but can also be widespread. Oral involvement may be seen in cases associated with hematologic malignancies. In BSS, vesicles containing viscous fluid can occasionally proceed to ulceration.[29]

Differential diagnosis

V vulnificus, leishmaniasis, and exaggerated bite reactions.

Diagnostic study/biopsy

Biopsies of both processes show a neutrophilic dermal infiltrate. Papillary dermal edema is prominent in BSS, and a subepidermal split is seen in BPG. A thorough history, review of medications, and evaluation for an underlying malignancy are important, and both diseases have shown a strong association with myelogenous leukemia. These diagnoses are of exclusion, and infectious causes of blisters and ulcerations should be excluded with a tissue culture.[28,29]

Treatment/further work-up

Systemic corticosteroids can be initiated when infection has been excluded. These disorders may require a longer course of therapy with corticosteroids or steroid-sparing agents such as dapsone, potassium iodide, and colchicine. Work-up to determine an underlying cause is critical.[28,29]

Small Vessel Vasculitis

Background

Small vessel vasculitis may occasionally present with blisters, and can have multiple causes, including medications and autoimmune, infections, paraneoplastic, and idiopathic causes.[14] Because the pathogenesis involves immune complex deposition on small vessel endothelium, the subsequent vascular destruction and erythrocyte extravasation lead to focal skin necrosis, with hemorrhagic blistering as a consequence.

History

Patients can present with a variety of symptoms based on cause. Pruritus can be associated with drug-induced vasculitis, and systemic symptoms can occur with connective tissue diseases, infections, and with paraneoplastic causes.[14]

Physical examination

Palpable purpura can precede hemorrhagic vesicles typically on the lower extremities. These lesions then progress to ulceration.[14]

Diagnostic study/biopsy

Biopsy shows small vessel leukocytoclastic vasculitis.[14] Further testing is based on suspicion for underlying causes.

Treatment

If the cause is idiopathic and removal of a possible underlying cause fails to resolve the vasculitis, systemic corticosteroids are the mainstay of treatment. Dapsone, colchicine, and immunosuppressive medications can be considered as steroid-sparing therapy.[14]

INFECTIOUS VESICULOBULLOUS DERMATOSES

Several bacterial, viral, and fungal infections can present with vesicles and bullae (**Table 4**).[3,11,12,30–32] Herpes infections usually present as localized or dermatomal

Table 4
Infectious bullous diseases

Form of Infection	Clinical Characteristics	Diagnosis and Management
HSV	• HSV-1 and HSV-2 (most prevalent serotypes) • Predominantly orolabial (vermillion border) and genital. Occasionally, also seen on buttocks, finger (herpetic whitlow), face, and other sites of contact (herpes gladiatorum) • Vesicles and erosions in a cluster preceded by burning and pain • Primary infection: occurs within a week after exposure. Usually accompanied by symptoms of fatigue, lymphadenopathy, and occasional fevers. Takes 2–6 wk to resolve • Recurrent HSV infections: spontaneous or secondary to stress, UV light, or immunosuppression. Usually takes 7–10 d to resolve and are mild compared with primary HSV • Immunocompromised: tend to have disseminated vesicles and are at risk for systemic involvement. Cutaneous findings: atypical with persistent enlarging ulcerations, as well as verrucous lesions oddly distributed in some cases on the tongue, esophagus, and gastro-intestinal mucosa • Disseminated form: also seen in patients with extensive skin barrier breakdown such as eczema	• Diagnostic tests: Tzanck smear, DFA, viral culture, serology and VZV PCR. Biopsy shows viral cytopathologic changes • Recurrent genital herpes: oral acyclovir (800 mg PO bid × 5d), valacyclovir(1 g PO qd × 5 d), and famciclovir(1 g PO bid × 1 d) can be used in immunocompetent hosts. A protracted course is used in the setting of orolabial herpes flare • Immunocompromised: disseminated HSV requires IV acyclovir at 10 mg/kg every 8 h in most cases or 1 g PO bid valacyclovir until all cutaneous lesions have resolved. Foscarnet may be used in resistant cases • >6 episodes a year: chronic suppressive therapy with acyclovir (400–800 mg PO bid to tid), or valacyclovir (500 mg qd to 1 g qd PO bid), or famciclovir (250 mg PO bid) is recommended

(continued on next page)

Table 4
(continued)

Form of Infection	Clinical Characteristics	Diagnosis and Management
VZV	• Primary varicella infection (chicken pox): prodromal systemic symptoms such as fevers and malaise with subsequent erythematous papulopustular eruption that then progress to vesicles on an erythematous base predominantly on the trunk with significant pruritus. Lesions at a given time can be at any stage of development. The lesions crust over within 10 d. Adults may have systemic complications such as pneumonia • Herpes zoster: prodromal burning pain or itching with subsequent development of clustered vesicles on an erythematous base in a dermatomal distribution usually on the trunk. They seldom cross the midline. Occasionally they can progress to bullae. Elderly or immunocompromised patients may develop postherpetic neuralgia with burning pain in the affected distribution. Pneumonitis and hepatitis occasionally develop • Immunocompromised: can have a more disseminated presentation with more than 20 vesicles outside of the dermatome along with occasional internal organ involvement	• Diagnostic tests: Tzanck smear, DFA, viral culture, serology, and VZV PCR • Biopsy shows viral cytopathologic changes • Varicella zoster immunoglobulin within 4 d of exposure can be considered in immunocompromised and pregnant women along with neonates without previous immunity • Primary varicella infection: acyclovir (20 mg/kg PO qid × 5 d) or Valacyclovir (20 mg/kg PO tid × 5 d) is the treatment of choice • Reactivation: valacyclovir 1 g tid × 7 d with optimal results if treatment is initiated within 3 d of presentation. Oral acyclovir and famciclovir can also be used • Immunocompromised: IV acyclovir 10 mg/kg every 8 h for 7-10 days or until lesions healed in some cases • In patients with postherpetic neuralgia, treatment with gabapentin or tricyclic antidepressants should be considered. Topical options include lidocaine creams, and 8% capsaicin patch • VZV live viral vaccine is effective in children • VZV vaccine is recommended for patients older than 60 y to prevent development of zoster and decrease the incidence of postherpetic neuralgia
Bullous impetigo	• Results from *Staphylococcus aureus*–derived local exfoliative toxin, which binds to a desmosomal protein leading to a blister formation. It is the same exfoliative toxin that mediates staphylococcal skin syndrome • It is usually seen in newborns and presents as small vesicles that progress to flaccid blisters that easily rupture leaving a collaret of scale predominantly on the trunk, axillae, face, buttock, and extremities • This is more localized, in contrast with staphylococcal scalded skin syndrome(also seen in children), which presents with diffuse erythema, flaccid bulla with positive Nikolsky sign, positive Asboe-Hansen sign, peeling, and erosions with accentuation in the intertriginous folds and perioral furrowing • Adult patients SSSS are typically more ill and complain of severe generalized skin tenderness. They have a prodrome of conjunctivitis, pharyngitis, and fever	• Culture: blister fluid usually grows *S aureus*. Biopsy shows acantholysis in the granular layer of the skin • Treatment: it usually resolves on its own by 6 wk. Topical antibiotic creams such as mupirocin, retapamulin, or fusidic acid can be used as first line and IV ceftriaxone can be used for complicated cases such as concomitant cellulitis or in patients with poor immunity • In adults, the mortality for SSSS is high and is seen most commonly in immunosuppressed individuals with HIV and renal failure. Isolation of exotoxin A and B may be difficult • Biopsy usually shows intraepidermal split. Blood cultures are positive in adults more often than in children • Toxic shock syndrome and TEN are on the differential • Pneumonia is the most frequent complication

Bullous cellulitis	• Severe cases of cellulitis can actually present with vesicles and bullae overlying the erythematous, swollen, very painful, and poorly defined areas of involvement (usually unilateral) • Systemic symptoms of fatigue and fever typically precede the skin presentation • Most common causes: S aureus and GAS • Immunocompromised: mixed flora • Long-term monitoring: renal function for acute glomerulonephritis in the setting of GAS cellulitis	• Mostly a clinical diagnosis • Differential diagnosis: deep venous thrombosis, superficial thrombophlebitis, and stasis dermatitis • Treatment: oral antibiotics in most cases. IV antibiotics (usually reserved for patients with complicated cellulitis) • Recurrent cellulitis: most common in patients with stasis dermatitis. These patients should also be evaluated for interdigital macerations and tinea pedis
V vulnificus	• Vibrio skin infection usually presents with violaceous purpuric macules that progress to hemorrhagic bullae and vesicles that can ulcerate • Severe complications: sepsis and necrotizing fasciitis • It is mostly seen in men more than 40 y of age with exposure of open wounds to warm coastal seawater and/or raw seafood (shellfish) • Risk factors: diabetes, hemochromatosis, cirrhosis, antacid use, renal disease, as well as immunosuppression	• Wound culture: confirms the diagnosis • Pseudomonas infection should be considered on the differential diagnosis • Treatment: combination of doxycycline and IV ceftriaxone. Other alternatives are cefotaxime or ciprofloxacin • Given high mortality from sepsis, prompt empiric treatment within 24 h is indicated • Surgical debridement and occasionally amputation may be needed in severe cases with rapidly expanding bullae
Bullous tinea	• Inflammatory variant of tinea pedis can present with vesicles and bullae, especially on the medial foot • Severe cases may present with a concomitant id reaction/dermatophytid response with poorly demarcated symmetric eczematous patches in distant sites such as the face and extremities	• Fungal culture: Trichophyton mentagrophytes (most common) • Treatment: topical antifungal such as econazole or terbinafine cream is usually sufficient. In severe cases especially with id reaction and/or onychomycosis, consider oral antifungals (fluconazole and terbinafine). We recommend avoidance of oral ketoconazole because of inherent greater hepatic risks

Abbreviations: bid, twice a day; d, days; DFA, direct fluorescent antibody; GAS, group A *Streptococcus*; h, hours; HSV, herpes simplex virus; IV, intravenous; Kg, kilogram; mg, milligram; PO, orally; qd, every day; qid; S aureus, staphylococcus aureus; SSSS, staphylococcal scalded skin syndrome; TEN, toxic epidermal necrolysis; 4 times a day; tid, 3 times a day; UV, ultraviolet; VZV, varicella zoster virus; wk, weeks; y, years.

vesicles, but are occasionally disseminated or form bullae in immunocompromised hosts.[3] Tinea pedis (especially zoophilic species such as *Trichophyton mentagrophytes*) can present as vesicles and bullae on the bilateral feet, which can often be confused with ACD from footwear.[32] *Staphylococcus aureus* produces exotoxins against desmoglein-1 that result in bullous impetigo when localized and SSSS when systemic.[31] *V vulnificus* presents acutely with hemorrhagic blisters and sepsis.[11] Treatment and management depend on the type of infection and extent of involvement. Immunocompromised hosts tend to have more extensive involvement and generally require more aggressive therapy.[3]

BULLOUS DRUG ERUPTIONS

This entity consists of different vesiculobullous eruptions seen in the setting of medications, as detailed in **Table 3**.[14,33] Note that although some drug-induced reactions result in cytotoxic or cytokine-induced necrosis of keratinocytes (eg, fixed drug eruption or Stevens-Johnson syndrome [SJS]/TEN), others can result in drug-induced autoantibody-mediated bullous diseases, such as vancomycin-induced linear IgA bullous dermatosis. Management includes discontinuation of the medication along with management of symptoms. Some acute severe reactions, such as SJS/TEN, require an urgent multidisciplinary approach along with ophthalmology and a burn team.[12]

ACKNOWLEDGMENT

The authors would like to thank Samuel Kwak for his help with the images.

REFERENCES

1. Fine J-D, Mellerio JE. Epidermolysis Bullosa. In: Bolognia JL, Jorizzo JL, Schaffer JV, editors. Dermatology. 3rd edition. London: Saunders; 2012. p. 501–13.
2. Kneisel A, Hertl M. Autoimmune bullous skin diseases. Part 1: clinical manifestations. J Dtsch Dermatol Ges 2011;9(10):844–56 [quiz: 857].
3. Mendoza N, Madkan V, Sra K, et al. Human Herpes Viruses. In: Bolognia JL, Jorizzo JL, Schaffer JV, editors. Dermatology. 3rd edition. London: Saunders; 2012. p. 1321–43.
4. Johnston GA. Treatment of bullous impetigo and the staphylococcal scalded skin syndrome in infants. Expert Rev Anti Infect Ther 2004;2(3):439–46.
5. Contestable JJ, Edhegard KD, Meyerle JH. Bullous systemic lupus erythematosus: a review and update to diagnosis and treatment. Am J Clin Dermatol 2014;15(6):517–24.
6. Schulenburg-Brand D, Katugampola R, Anstey AV, et al. The cutaneous porphyrias. Dermatol Clin 2014;32(3):369–84, ix.
7. Vereecken P, Tas S, Verraes S, et al. Phototoxic contact phytodermatitis: clinical and biological aspects. Rev Médicale Brux 1998;19(3):131–4 [in French].
8. Almahameed A, Pinto DS. Pernio (chilblains). Curr Treat Options Cardiovasc Med 2008;10(2):128–35.
9. Mota ANC de M, Nery NS, Barcaui CB. Case for diagnosis: bullosis diabeticorum. An Bras Dermatol 2013;88(4):652–4.
10. Frank J, Poblete-Gutierrez P. Porphyria. In: Bolognia JL, Jorizzo JL, Schaffer JV, editors. Dermatology. 3rd edition. London: Saunders; 2012. p. 717–27.

11. Hsiao C-T, Lin L-J, Shiao C-J, et al. Hemorrhagic bullae are not only skin deep. Am J Emerg Med 2008;26(3):316–9.
12. Levitt J, Markoff B. Vesiculobullous skin disease. Hosp Med Clin 2014;3(4): 582–96.
13. Hull CM, Zone JJ. Dermatitis Herpetiformis and Linear IgA Bullous Dermatosis. In: Bolognia JL, Jorizzo JL, Schaffer JV, editors. Dermatology. 3rd edition. London: Saunders; 2012. p. 491–500.
14. Mascaro Jr. J. Other Vesiculobullous diseases. In: Bolognia JL, Jorizzo JL, Schaffer JV, editors. Dermatology. 3rd edition. London: Saunders; 2012. p. 515–22.
15. Amagai M. Pemphigus. In: Bolognia JL, Jorizzo JL, Schaffer JV, editors. Dermatology. 3rd edition. London: Saunders; 2012. p. 461–74.
16. Bernard P, Borradoria L. Pemphigoid Group. In: Bolognia JL, Jorizzo JL, Schaffer JV, editors. Dermatology. 3rd edition. London: Saunders; 2012. p. 475–90.
17. Nosbaum A, Vocanson M, Rozieres A, et al. Allergic and irritant contact dermatitis. Eur J Dermatol 2009;19(4):325–32.
18. Usatine RP, Riojas M. Diagnosis and management of contact dermatitis. Am Fam Physician 2010;82(3):249–55.
19. Cohen D, Souza AD. Irritant Contact dermatitis. In: Bolognia JL, Jorizzo JL, Schaffer JV, editors. Dermatology. 3rd edition. London: Saunders; 2012. p. 249–59.
20. Reider N, Fritsch PO. Other Eczematous Eruptions. In: Bolognia JL, Jorizzo JL, Schaffer JV, editors. Dermatology. 3rd edition. London: Saunders; 2012. p. 219–31.
21. McGovern TW. Dermatoses due to plants. In: Bolognia JL, Jorizzo JL, Schaffer JV, editors. Dermatology. 3rd edition. London: Saunders; 2012. p. 279–81.
22. Bottoni U, Mauro FR, Cozzani E, et al. Bullous lesions in chronic lymphocytic leukaemia: pemphigoid or insect bites? Acta Derm Venereol 2006;86(1):74–6.
23. Baum S, Sakka N, Artsi O, et al. Diagnosis and classification of autoimmune blistering diseases. Autoimmun Rev 2014;13(4–5):482–9.
24. Otten JV, Hashimoto T, Hertl M, et al. Molecular diagnosis in autoimmune skin blistering conditions. Curr Mol Med 2014;14(1):69–95.
25. Huilaja L, Mäkikallio K, Tasanen K. Gestational pemphigoid. Orphanet J Rare Dis 2014;9:136.
26. Cole MB, Smith ML. Environment and Sports-Related Skin Diseases. In: Bolognia JL, Jorizzo JL, Schaffer JV, editors. Dermatology. 3rd edition. London: Saunders; 2012. p. 1492–4.
27. Chacon AH, Farooq U, Choudhary S, et al. Coma blisters in two postoperative patients. Am J Dermatopathol 2013;35(3):381–4.
28. Sakiyama M, Kobayashi T, Nagata Y, et al. Bullous pyoderma gangrenosum: A case report and review of the published work. J Dermatol 2012;39(12):1010–5.
29. Voelter-Mahlknecht S, Bauer J, Metzler G, et al. Bullous variant of Sweet's syndrome. Int J Dermatol 2005;44(11):946–7.
30. Millett CR, Halpern AV, Reboli AC, et al. Bacterial diseases. In: Bolognia JL, Jorizzo JL, Schaffer JV, editors. Dermatology. 3rd edition. London: Saunders; 2012. p. 1187–220.
31. Patel GK, Finlay AY. Staphylococcal scalded skin syndrome: diagnosis and management. Am J Clin Dermatol 2003;4(3):165–75.
32. El-Segini Y, Schill W-B, Weyers W. Case Report. Bullous tinea pedis in an elderly man. Mycoses 2002;45(9–10):428–30.
33. Revuz J, Laurence V-A. Drug Reactions. In: Bolognia JL, Jorizzo JL, Schaffer JV, editors. Dermatology. 3rd edition. London: Saunders; 2012. p. 335–56.

Atopic Dermatitis

A Common Pediatric Condition and Its Evolution in Adulthood

Deepti Gupta, MD

KEYWORDS

- Atopic dermatitis • Eczema • Pruritus • Atopy • Corticosteroids • Phototherapy
- Bleach bath

KEY POINTS

- Clinical presentation of atopic dermatitis varies from infancy to adulthood, and it is important for the clinician to recognize these different presentations.
- Atopic dermatitis has a significant effect on an individual's quality of life.
- Atopic dermatitis is associated with multiple comorbidities.
- Treatment of atopic dermatitis is multifactorial and targeted at the various components of pathogenesis.
- The treatment and management of atopic dermatitis is similar across age groups.

PATIENT HISTORY/SYMPTOMS

Atopic dermatitis (AD), which is also more commonly referred to as eczema, is a common chronic and pruritic inflammatory skin disorder with a relapsing course that can affect any age group.[1] The term *atopic* or *atopy* refers to a tendency to develop an increased sensitivity to common environmental antigens. AD affects approximately 25% of children and 2% to 3% of adults. AD has a predilection for presenting in early childhood, with 60% of patients presenting within the first year of life and 90% present by 5 years of age.[2,3] A small percentage of individuals do have adult-onset AD, often presenting by 30 years of age; approximately 10% to 30% of individuals continue to have persistent AD into adulthood. Increased rates of adult-onset AD are seen in individuals who move from a more humid, tropical climate to a more temperate one located at higher latitude.

Disclosure statement: The author has no disclosures or financial relationships.
Division of Dermatology, Department of Pediatrics, Seattle Children's Hospital, 4800 Sand Point Way Northeast OC 9.834, Seattle, WA 98105, USA
E-mail address: Deepti.Gupta@seattlechildrens.org

Med Clin N Am 99 (2015) 1269–1285
http://dx.doi.org/10.1016/j.mcna.2015.07.006

Historically, AD has been referred to as the itch that rashes. Pruritus is a hallmark symptom of this disease and causes a significant effect on quality of life. Seventy percent of patients with AD have a positive family history of atopic disease, including other conditions, such as allergic rhinitis/rhinoconjunctivitis, food allergies, asthma, and environmental allergies. The odds of developing AD are 2 to 3 fold higher in a child with one atopic parent and 3 to 5 fold higher with 2 atopic parents.[4]

The atopic march describes the observation that patients with AD commonly go on to develop other allergic conditions, such as asthma and allergic rhinitis. Some estimates suggest one-third of children go on to develop asthma and two-thirds go on to develop allergic rhinitis.[5] More recent studies have also linked AD to other nonallergic conditions, the most compelling being attention-deficit/hyperactivity disorder.[6] Patients with AD have more irregular and altered sleep patterns at baseline as compared with individuals without AD. During flares of AD, rates of sleep disturbance are significantly increased and can affect entire families. Increased rates of depression and anxiety have also been noted in both teenagers and adults with AD.[7] Patients with AD are also more at risk for secondary complications, such as skin infections.

PATHOPHYSIOLOGY

The pathogenesis of AD is multifactorial and results from dysfunction of the skin barrier, dysregulation of the immune system, and environmental triggers. The dysfunction of the skin barrier can be genetically based with mutations in filaggrin (FLG gene).[8] Filaggrin plays a key role in epidermal differentiation and formation of the skin barrier, including the stratum corneum. The stratum corneum plays an important role in preventing transepidermal water loss and prevention of skin infections. Filaggrin also breaks down to the skin natural moisturizing factor, which aids in skin barrier function and hydration. In addition to a dysfunctional skin barrier, patients with AD also have dysregulation of their immune system. This dysregulation causes an upregulation of the T helper type 2 (Th2) pathway, impaired innate immunity, and increased allergic sensitization.

The hygiene hypothesis explains the increasing prevalence of AD and other allergic conditions. This theory postulates that improved hygiene decreases early life exposure to infectious agents. These infections exert their effect through the Th1 pathway. There is thought to be an inverse relationship between Th1 and Th2 pathways. Therefore, decreased infectious exposures leads to decreased Th1 activation and increased Th2 pathway activity. This shift to the Th2 arm of the pathway leads to increased allergic sensitization. Finally, environmental triggers also play a role in the development and propagation of AD. It has been shown that, in climates with higher humidity, increased mean temperatures, lower precipitation, decreased indoor heating, and higher ultraviolet light index, there are lower incidences of AD.[9]

PHYSICAL EXAMINATION

AD presents acutely as an erythematous and pruritic rash typically with ill-defined xerotic papules and plaques with scattered erosions and often with oozing and crusting. In more chronic cases, one can see lichenified and hyperpigmented plaques (**Fig. 1**). AD has an age-specific morphology and distribution that can change over time. In infants and young children (<2 years of age), we see a predilection for face (**Fig. 2**), neck, scalp, wrists, and extensor extremities (**Fig. 3**) and a higher incidence of exudative rash. These areas correlate with infants' activities (eg, crawling) and are areas that they are able to rub or scratch. This infantile pattern often disappears by 2 years of age. Classic flexural involvement of the antecubital and popliteal fossa

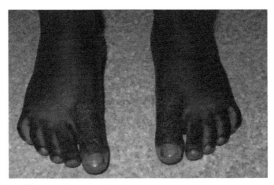

Fig. 1. Lichenified and hyperpigmented plaques.

(**Fig. 4**) can be seen at any age but tends to more often occur after 2 years of age. The rash during childhood tends to be less exudative and can also show predilection for the neck circumferentially, eyelids, and flexural wrists. In adolescents, there is classic flexural involvement but also common involvement of the forehead, periocular area (**Fig. 5**), and neck. In adults, AD localizes to specific areas of involvement, mainly the hands, feet, nipple, and eyelids with occasional generalized involvement in classic flexural areas. Lichenification and prurigo nodule development are more commonly seen in adolescent and adult patients with AD. Specific clinic findings to AD are nipple involvement and upper lip cheilitis (**Fig. 6**). Other clues to AD that help distinguish it from other conditions are the relative sparing of the groin, axilla, nasal tip, and diaper area. This distinction is largely caused by retention of moisture in these areas, presence of a protective covering, and the oily nature of the nasal tip. Xerosis and pruritus are universally present. Patients with AD may also have an impaired ability to sweat and may complain of increased pruritus related to exercise or heat. Other associated clinical features that can be seen in patients with AD are listed in **Box 1**.

DIAGNOSTIC TESTS/IMAGING STUDIES

AD is a clinical diagnosis that is made based on morphology, distribution of skin rash, historical features, physical examination, and clinical findings. Diagnostic criteria for AD have been proposed by Hanifin and Rajka[10] in 1980 but are difficult to use in clinical practice with 4 major criteria and 23 minor criteria. The American Academy of

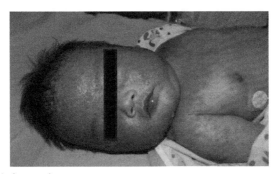

Fig. 2. Infant with face rash.

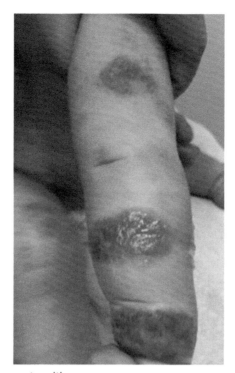

Fig. 3. Rash on extensor extremities.

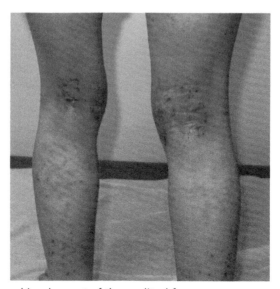

Fig. 4. Classic flexural involvement of the popliteal fossa.

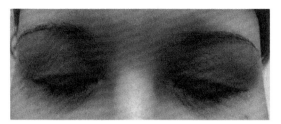

Fig. 5. Rash on the forehead, periocular area.

Dermatology Consensus group and UK working group have revised the criteria making them more applicable to clinical practice. **Table 1** identifies the revised criteria.

Skin biopsy and other laboratory evaluations are used to rule out other diagnoses or confirm other associated skin disorders. There is currently no biomarker that is completely specific to AD. If serum testing is done, one can find AD associated with an elevation of total immunoglobulin E level or elevation of peripheral eosinophilia; but this is not uniformly present in every case. These laboratory findings do not correlate with disease severity and are not sensitive or specific to AD.

DIFFERENTIAL DIAGNOSIS

The differential diagnosis of AD is broad (**Box 2**). There are a variety of nutritional and immunodeficiency disorders that present with eczema as a hallmark feature. There may be subtle morphologic clues in these cases, but in general a high level of suspicion is needed. Scabies can often be mistaken for AD. Scabies can be distinguished by evidence of burrows, which are thin tortuous gray lines often with a pustule or papule housing the mite at the end. In adults, the head and neck are often spared; there is a high predilection of rash in the interdigital web spaces, genital region, and umbilicus. In infants and children, the rash of scabies is polymorphic and widespread, with a predilection often for the palms and soles (**Figs. 7** and **8**); but the rash can be present anywhere. There are often other family members with a pruritic rash given that scabies is spread by close contacts. Psoriasis is an inflammatory skin disorder that is characterized by well-defined, often symmetric pink papules and plaques with overlying micaceous scale (**Fig. 9**). Psoriasis has a predilection for the scalp, nails, extensor surfaces of the limbs, umbilicus, and sacrum. It can often be distinguished from AD by its morphology. Psoriasis also tends to be less exudative and is not prone to superinfection. Seborrheic dermatitis can be distinguished from AD as it has a predilection for more oily and warm areas (eg, scalp, eyebrows, nasolabial folds, groin,

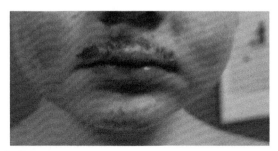

Fig. 6. Upper lip cheilitis.

Box 1
Other associated clinical features

Atypical vascular responses: facial pallor, white dermatographism, delayed blanch response

Keratosis pilaris

Hyperlinear palms

Ichthyosis vulgaris

Ocular and periorbital hyperpigmentation

Dennie-Morgan lines (prominent groove or line of the lower eyelid)

Perifollicular accentuation and lichenification (seen more in darker skinned individuals)

Lichenification

Prurigo nodules

Table 1
Diagnostic criteria for AD

Essential Features (Must Be Present)	Important Features (Seen in Most Cases, Adding Support to the Diagnosis)	Associated Features (These Clinical Features Help to Suggest the Diagnosis of AD but Are Too Nonspecific to Be Used to Define or Detect AD for Research or Epidemiologic Studies)	Exclusion of Other Conditions

1. Pruritus
2. Eczema (acute, subacute, chronic)
  a. Typical morphology and age-specific patterns
    i. Flexural lichenification in adults
    ii. Facial and extensor involvement in infancy
  b. Chronic and relapsing course
	1. Early age of onset
	2. Atopy
	  a. Personal and/or family history
	  b. Immunoglobulin E reactivity
	3. Xerosis
		1. Atypical vascular responses (ie, facial pallor, white dermatographism, delayed blanch response)
		2. Keratosis pilaris/ hyperlinear palms/ ichthyosis
		3. Ocular/periocular changes
		4. Other regional findings (ie, perioral changes, periauricular lesions)
		5. Perifollicular accentuation/lichenification/prurigo lesions
			1. Scabies
			2. Seborrheic dermatitis
			3. Contact dermatitis (irritant or allergic dermatitis)
			4. Ichthyoses
			5. Cutaneous T-cell lymphomas
			6. Psoriasis
			7. Immune deficiency disorders
			8. Tinea corporis

Data from Eicheifield LF, Hanifin JM, Luger TA, et al. Consensus conference on pediatric atopic dermatitis. J Am Aacd Dermatol 2003;49:1088–95.

Box 2
Differential diagnosis of AD

- Scabies
- Ichthyosis
- Seborrheic dermatitis
- Psoriasis
- Contact dermatitis
- Cutaneous T-cell lymphoma
- Nutritional deficiencies
  - Acrodermatitis enteropathica
  - Zinc deficiency (prematurity, deficient breast milk zinc, cystic fibrosis)
  - Gluten-sensitive enteropathy
  - Other nutritional deficiencies (biotin, essential fatty acids)
- Immune deficiency disorders
  - Hyper–immunoglobulin E syndrome
  - Severe combined immunodeficiency
  - Wiskott-Aldrich syndrome
  - Agammaglobulinemia
  - Netherton syndrome
  - Ataxia-telangiectasia
- Tinea corporis
- Langerhans cell histiocytosis

---

gluteal crease, umbilicus) because of its pathogenesis being linked to lipophilic yeast, *Pityrosporum ovale*. Seborrheic dermatitis has a yellow, greasy appearance on an erythematous base. The distribution and appearance can help distinguish this condition from AD. In infants, there is often overlap of these two conditions; therefore, it can be more difficult to distinguish them, but treatment in this age group is often similar for both conditions.

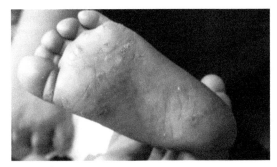

Fig. 7. Rash of scabies on the sole.

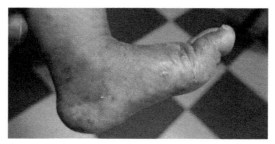

Fig. 8. Rash of scabies on the foot.

DIAGNOSTIC DILEMMAS

The diagnosis of AD is often made based on history and physical examination, but there can be some overlap with the conditions mentioned earlier. If there is diagnostic uncertainty, further testing can be done, such as skin biopsy, patch testing for allergic contact dermatitis, scabies scrapings, and laboratory evaluation to rule out other disorders. Skin biopsy or repeat skin biopsy should be considered when the rash is recalcitrant to adequate and appropriate therapy, progressing despite treatment, or patients have other positive review of systems or physical examination findings that are concerning.

TREATMENT

Treatment of AD often includes multiple modalities of therapy being used together, some of them being nonpharmacologic, to target different aspects of AD pathogenesis. Treatment and management of AD is to control symptoms of an acute flare but then to be proactive and minimize future relapses of the disease.

When treating an individual with AD, all of the following concerns should be assessed and addressed for optimal treatment and management:

1. Restore and maintain the skin barrier function
2. Minimize inflammation
3. Control pruritus
4. Consider and manage external environmental triggers
5. Treat infection

Restoring the Skin Barrier

Patients with AD have a defect in their skin barrier leading to greater transepidermal water loss and xerosis. There is very strong evidence that use of moisturizers is very beneficial to patients with AD.[11] Moisturizing decreases the amount of medication

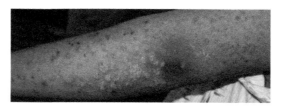

Fig. 9. Psoriasis papules and plaques with overlying micaceous scale.

used and symptoms of AD (ie, erythema, pruritus, skin fissuring). Moisturizers should be fragrance and dye free to limit possible irritants, and liberal and frequent application is recommended to prevent xerosis. Application of the moisturizers immediately after bathing can further improve skin hydration in patients with AD by sealing in moisturize from the bath. Moisturizing alone can be a treatment of mild disease and is a very important part of maintenance therapy and prevention of flares. The various formulations of emollients are listed in **Table 2**.

Antiinflammatories

Topical corticosteroids

Topical corticosteroids (TCSs) are the first-line treatment of AD and are a mainstay of therapy. They are grouped in 7 classes from very low potency (class 7) to high potency (class 1) and come in various strengths and formulations (**Table 3**). The choice of TCS is guided by location applied, severity of disease, extent of disease, availability, patient preference, and cost. A guide to the adequate amount of medication to be applied is approximately 0.5 g or an adult fingertip (from distal interphalangeal joint to distal fingertip) to 2 palms of rash (approximately 2% body surface area).

When choosing a TCS, the general principles to consider are thickness of the skin the medication will be applied to, body surface area affected, and if there will be occlusion of the medication. Lower-potency TCSs are recommended in thin skin areas (eg, face, neck, and genital area) and areas of occlusion (eg, skin folds and intertriginous areas) where there is increased absorption of medication and higher risk of skin thinning. Higher-potency TCSs should be used in thick-skin areas (eg, palms and soles) to penetrate the stratum corneum. When applying TCS to a larger body surface, higher-potency steroids should be avoided to prevent significant systemic absorption. Application of TCS is recommended twice a day and should be used until inflammatory lesions are significantly improved, which could be for several weeks at a time. There has been recent evidence suggesting that individuals who have frequent flares of disease in the same site can use a more proactive approach of applying TCS once to twice weekly to these areas as maintenance therapy to reduce rates of relapse and increase time between flares. This use of intermittent TCS has been shown to be more effective than moisturizers alone.[12]

Table 2
Emollient vehicles

Vehicle	Pros	Cons
Ointment	• Greatest moisturizing effect • Highest proportion of lipid • Free of preservatives, does not sting when applied	Greasy

Cream	• An emulsion of water in lipid
	  ○ More hydrating than lotions
	  ○ Less greasy
		Contains preservatives, can sting or burn with application

Lotion	• Emulsion of a higher proportion of water to lipid than creams • Well tolerated • Not greasy	May need increased applications to keep skin hydrated
Oil	• Easy to spread over a large surface area	Can contain some preservatives and fragrances that could be irritating
Gel	• Not appropriate for AD	Drying

Table 3
TCS formulations by class

Class	Medication	Strength (%)	Form
I. Superpotent	Augmented betamethasone dipropionate	0.05	Ointment
	Clobetasol propionate	0.05	Ointment, cream, solution, foam
	Diflorasone diacetate	0.05	Ointment
	Fluocinonide	0.1	Cream
	Halobetasol propionate	0.05	Ointment, cream
II. High potency	Betamethasone dipropionate	0.05	Ointment, cream, foam, solution
	Budesonide	0.025	Cream
	Desoximetasone	0.25	Ointment, cream
	Diflorasone diacetate	0.05	Cream
	Fluocinonide	0.05	Ointment, cream, and gel
	Halcinonide	0.1	Ointment, cream
	Mometasone furoate	0.1	Ointment
	Triamcinolone acetonide	0.5	Ointment, cream
III–IV. Medium potency	Betamethasone valerate	0.1	Ointment, foam
	Clocortolone pivalate	0.1	Cream
	Desoximetasone	0.05	Cream
	Fluocinolone acetonide	0.025	Ointment, cream
	Flurandrenolide	0.05	Cream
	Fluticasone propionate	0.005	Ointment
	Mometasone furoate	0.1	Cream
	Triamcinolone acetonide	0.1	Ointment, cream
V. Lower-medium potency	Hydrocortisone butyrate	0.1	Ointment, cream, solution
	Hydrocortisone probutate	0.1	Cream
	Hydrocortisone valerate	0.2	Ointment, cream
	Triamcinolone acetonide	0.25	Ointment, cream
VI. Low potency	Alclometasone dipropionate	0.05	Ointment, cream
	Desonide	0.05	Ointment, cream
	Fluocinolone acetonide	0.01	Cream, oil, solution
	Flurandrenolide	0.025	Cream
VII. Lowest potency	Dexamethasone	0.1	Cream
	Hydrocortisone	2.5	Ointment, cream, lotion
	Hydrocortisone acetate (over the counter)	0.5 and 1.0	Cream, ointment

Overall, TCSs have a good safety profile with low adverse effects reported.[13] Most of the side effects reported are cutaneous but are uncommon with proper use. The cutaneous side effects include purpura, telangiectasias, striae, focal hypertrichosis, and acneiform and rosacealike eruptions. The highest risk of developing adverse cutaneous effects are with application of TCS in sites of occlusion and thinner-skin areas, use of higher potency TCS, and use of TCS in older patients with thinner skin. Most cutaneous side effects are reversible after stopping TCS but may take months to resolve. Patients can also develop an allergic contact dermatitis or type 4 hypersensitivity reactions to TCS themselves or to the ingredients within the formulation. It is important to consider this if a rash worsens or fails to respond to TCS and perform patch testing to determine the exact allergen.

Systemic side effects with TCS use, such as hypothalamic-pituitary-adrenal (HPA) suppression, are extremely low.[14] The risk of HPA suppression increases in children who have a high body surface area to weight ratio, individuals receiving other forms of corticosteroids (eg, inhaled, oral, and intranasal), and with prolonged and continued use of high-potency TCS. If there is a concern for HPA axis suppression, a cortisol stimulation test should be performed to assess adrenal response. Other systemic side effects, such as hyperglycemia and hypertension, have been rarely reported.[15] The risk of development of cataracts and glaucoma with TCS use has been unclear with current studies. One reason for this is about 10% of patient with AD develop cataracts as a secondary manifestation of their disease, and these cataracts are indistinguishable from cataracts induced by corticosteroids. Given this uncertainty, it is recommended to limit long-term periocular use of TCS and switch to a topical calcineurin inhibitor (TCI) if a long-term antiinflammatory is needed.

Some patients or parents of patients have a phobia of using corticosteroids, which can significantly interfere with the treatment of AD. These concerns should be addressed directly with patients and families to address any misunderstanding about the medications.[16]

Topical calcineurin inhibitors

TCIs are steroid-sparing agents that can be used in conjunction with TCS or by themselves. They are derived from the *Streptomyces* bacteria and inhibit T-cell activation, thereby blocking proinflammatory cytokines and mast cell activation. The various formulations of TCI are listed in **Table 4**. TCIs do not have the cutaneous adverse side effects that TCS have. Their use is indicated when there is evidence of steroid-induced atrophy, in areas at high risk for skin thinning, and when TCSs have been used continuously long-term. Like TCSs, TCIs can also be used as a maintenance therapy 1 to 3 times per week to prevent flares at recurrent sites of disease. Side effects of TCI include local reactions of burning and stinging. These side effects are more widely reported with TCIs than TCSs. These reactions tend to decrease over time. Use of TCSs before TCIs can also decrease sensations of burning and stinging. TCIs are not to be used when there is active infection according to the package insert; but no consistent increase in viral infections have been noted, and there has been some evidence to show a decrease in staphylococcal aureus colonization. There is also a black box warning for TCI regarding a theoretic risk of malignancy (ie, skin cancer and lymphoma). This warning is based on animal studies and is not directly

Table 4 TCSs			
Medication	**Pimecrolimus 1%**	**Tacrolimus 0.3%**	**Tacrolimus 0.1%**
Vehicle	Cream	Ointment	Ointment
FDA approved	• Mild to moderate AD • >2 y of age[a]	• Moderate and severe AD • >2 y of age[a]	• Moderate and severe AD • >15 y of age
TCS equivalent	No direct comparison study done; thought to be low–mid potency	Low–mid potency	Midpotency

Abbreviation: FDA, Food and Drug Administration.

[a] Studies have shown effective and safe use in children less than 2 years of age.

Data from Breuer K, Werfel T, Kapp S. Safety and efficacy of topical calcineurin inhibitors in the treatment of childhood atopic dermatitis. Am J Clin Dermatol 2005;6:65–77.

translatable to humans. There is currently no evidence for a causal relationship between TCI use and malignancy.[17]

Phototherapy
When patients fail optimal topical therapy, then the next step in treatment can be phototherapy or system medications. Phototherapy is the use of light waves for the treatment of medical conditions. There are various types of phototherapy including narrowband UVB (NBUVB), broadband UVB, UVA, topical and systemic psoralen plus UVA (PUVA), UVA and UVB, and Goeckerman therapy, which uses crude coal tar in combination with phototherapy. NBUVB is the most widely used and available form of phototherapy. Treatment protocols are in place for the treatment of AD with each specific type of phototherapy that are based on the minimal erythema dose and Fitzpatrick skin type. Phototherapy can be used as a monotherapy or in conjunction with emollients and TCS, but the use of phototherapy with calcineurin inhibitors is cautioned. Patients' personal and family history of skin cancer should be taken into account when determining if phototherapy is the best modality of treatment of an individual because of the increased actinic damage and potential risk of developing a skin cancer, though this risk is low. Also, patients should be counseled regarding the use of topical or systemic photosensitizing medications with use of phototherapy. The side effects of phototherapy that are more common include actinic damage, local erythema, tenderness, burning, pruritus, and stinging. Less commonly nonmelanoma and melanoma skin cancers can develop, but this is seen more with the use of PUVA or UVA.[18] The main barriers to phototherapy are cost, availability, time, and the logistical challenge of treatments 2 to 3 times per week. Home phototherapy units are also available and can be used under practitioner guidance but can be costly and difficult to obtain.

Systemic immunosuppressants
The most commonly used systemic immune-modulating medications used for AD are azathioprine, cyclosporine, mycophenolate mofetil, and methotrexate.[19] These medications have been recommended for the treatment of refractory AD when optimal topical treatments and/or phototherapy has been ineffective (**Table 5**). These agents are all steroid-sparing agents, and their use is off label for AD. The use of oral corticosteroids in AD should be avoided if possible. Oral corticosteroids only temporarily suppress disease, and short courses often lead to flares of the AD once medication is withdrawn. Corticosteroid use should be reserved for acute and severe flares of AD where a short course of corticosteroids can act as a bridge to a steroid-sparing systemic medications or phototherapy that may take a longer time to take effect.

Management of pruritus
Patients with AD have a significant component of pruritus that significantly affects their quality of life. Pruritus in AD is driven by the release of histamine from basophils and mast cells. Pruritus causes significant sleep disturbance as well as difficulty in concentration during the day in school or work for patients. Various topical and oral medications have been suggested to address pruritus. Topical antihistamines are not recommended, as they are not effective at controlling pruritus or inflammation and may cause burning and stinging. Use of intermittent sedating oral antihistamines is more effective at controlling pruritus related to AD and should be used in conjunction with other antiinflammatory treatments for AD and emollients. The intermittent use of a sedating antihistamine at night can be beneficial in decreasing pruritus and helping improve sleep patterns; but its effect on routine activities and school and work performance should be considered when dosing and scheduling medications. The use of

Table 5
Systemic medications for AD

Medication	Pros/Cons	Contraindications	Management Guidelines
Azathioprine	Pro: • May be more favorable long-term based on side-effect profile Cons: • Slower onset of action than CSA • Weeks to 2 mo until treatment effect noted • Risk of bone marrow suppression	Absolute: • Allergy to azathioprine • Pregnancy or attempting pregnancy • Active infection Relative: • Concurrent use of allopurinol • Live vaccines may be contraindicated	• Requires baseline TPMT activity to determine dosing • TPMT is an inducible enzyme, levels of azathioprine can be altered over time • Pregnancy category D
Cyclosporine	Pros: • Rapid onset of action • Significant decrease in disease activity noted within 2–6 wk of initiation • Shown to be effective in inducing remission of disease Cons: • Risk of malignancies (eg, cutaneous and lymphoproliferative) • Potential long-term adverse effects of renal dysfunction and hypertension	Absolute: • Abnormal renal function • Malignancy • Uncontrolled hypertension • Hypersensitivity to cyclosporine • Live vaccines contraindicated; killed vaccines may have decreased efficacy Relative: • Poorly controlled diabetes • Major infection • Concomitant use of PUVA, UVB, MTX, other immunosuppressant agents, coal tar	• FDA approved for use up to 1 y • Therapeutic in both 1-y continuous dosing and 3–6 mo intermittent courses • High rates of potential medication interactions (CYP3A4) • Quicker onset of action with microemulsion formulation • Should be administered in BID dosing • Pregnancy category C
Methotrexate	Pros: • Easily available • Can be given weekly • Well-known side-effect profile Cons: • Slower onset of action than CSA • Risk of malignancies (cutaneous and lymphoproliferative)	Absolute: • Pregnancy • Nursing mothers • Alcoholism • Alcoholic liver disease • Chronic liver disease • Immunodeficiency • Bone marrow hypoplasia, leukopenia, thrombocytopenia, or significant anemia • Hypersensitivity to MTX Relative • Abnormalities in renal or liver function • Active infection • Obesity • Diabetes mellitus • Live vaccines may be contraindicated	• Possible liver biopsy at 3.5–4.0 g cumulative dose, but studies lacking if this is needed in patients with AD • Folic acid supplementation may skip on day taking MTX • Pregnancy category X

(continued on next page)

Table 5
(*continued*)

Medication	Pros/Cons	Contraindications	Management Guidelines
Mycophenolate mofetil	Pros: • Favorable side-effect profile • Well tolerated • Longer clinical remission in some studies once medication was discontinued Cons: • Delayed onset of action • Insufficient data exist in regard to MMF and AD • Risk of malignancies (cutaneous and lymphoproliferative)	• Hypersensitivity to MMF and mycophenolic acid • Pregnancy or attempting pregnancy • Live vaccines may be contraindicated	• Pregnancy category D

Abbreviations: CSA, cyclosporine; FDA, Food and Drug Administration; MMF, Mycophenolate Mofetil; MTX, Methotrexate; TPMT, thiopurine methyl-transferase enzyme.

nonsedating antihistamines has not routinely shown to cause significant improvement in pruritus related to AD at standard doses. Rather, nonsedating histamines are more beneficial when urticaria is present on examination, when there is an identified environmental allergen trigger, or with a concomitant allergic condition (ie, allergic rhinitis, seasonal allergies.)

External environmental factors

Patients with AD have higher rates of sensitization to house dust mites, pollens, animal dander, and fungi. The relationship between AD and food allergies is cause for many questions and concern from patients. Patients with AD have increased rates of food allergies, but true food allergy-induced AD is rare. Food allergies as a cause of AD are most common in children less than 5 years of age. The National Institute of Allergy and Infectious Disease Food Allergy Expert Panel recommends consideration of allergy testing in individuals less than 5 years of age when (1) AD continues to be persistent despite optimized and appropriate treatment of AD, (2) reliable history of immediate allergic reaction after ingestion of a specific food, or (3) both. In older children and adults, food allergies tend to be less common. In these groups, allergy testing should be pursued if there is a reproducible history of a certain allergen causing AD flares. Testing should be dictated by a reproducible allergen or allergens that are most prevalent in a given population based on age. In children less than 5 years of age, common allergens include cow's milk, eggs, wheat, soy, and peanuts. In this age group, allergens should be retested over time as individuals can build tolerance and outgrow these allergies. In older children, tree nuts, shellfish, and fish are more common allergens. In adolescents and adults, pollen-related food allergies are more common, so individuals experience symptoms when eating certain foods if they are allergic to certain types of pollen. When performing allergy testing, either food-specific immunoglobulin E serum testing or skin prick testing, it is important to know that both tests have a high negative predictive value of greater than 95% and low positive predictive value of 40% to 60%. Negative test results are helpful to rule out food allergies, but positive tests signify sensitization and not always true allergy. Therefore, clinical correlation and history are very important to help confirm the true presence of an allergy. Another environmental trigger for AD is the house dust mite, *Dermatophagoides pteronyssinus*. Dust mite covers for pillows and mattresses can be used to decrease exposure, but evidence is limited supporting their overall effectiveness. Seasonal allergies can sometimes exacerbate AD; in these cases, the use of nonsedating antihistamines can be helpful in conjunction with AD management.

Skin infection

Patients with AD are more prone to skin infections because of impaired skin barrier, diminished immune recognition, and impaired antimicrobial peptide production. Patient with AD also have increased amounts of *Staphylococcus aureus* colonized on their skin: 76% to 100% in patients with AD compared with 2% to 25% in healthy controls. This colonization can be a driving force for increased inflammation and pruritus.[20] In addition to increased susceptibility to bacterial infections, patients with AD can also be prone to superinfection with viral pathogens, such as herpes simplex virus (eczema herpeticum), varicella, and recently a new strain of the Coxsackie virus A6 (eczema coxsackium).[21] Patients with AD may also develop extensive molluscum contagiosum and flat warts, which can be difficult to clear. These infections can spread quite rapidly and be severe because of the disrupted skin barrier.

The approach to combating bacterial superinfection in AD has 2 prongs: one aimed at treating current infection and second with decreasing bacterial colonization to prevent future infection. Application of topical antimicrobials to treat infection has not shown to have a clear benefit and can cause contact dermatitis and promote antimicrobial resistance. Therefore, they are not recommended in treatment of AD. Systemic antibiotics can be used when there is clinical evidence of bacterial infection and can be used in conjunction with TCS. It is recommended to document infection by culture and antibiotic sensitivity testing, confirming the type of bacteria present and any resistance patterns and serving as a helpful to guide to direct therapy. Application of mupirocin 2% ointment twice daily intranasally for the first 5 days of every month for 3 months has shown some effect in decreasing *Staphylococcus aureus* colonization when used in conjunction with dilute bleach baths. Dilute bleach baths (sodium hypochlorite) also solely have been effective for decreasing *Staphylococcus aureus* colonization.[22] Studies have also shown sodium hypochlorite to have antiinflammatory properties regulated through the inhibition of 2 important genes of nuclear factor-kB, which regulates the inflammatory response in the skin.[23] The concentration of sodium hypochlorite is 0.25 to 0.5 cups of 6% sodium hypochlorite to a bathtub of water (40 gallons) = 0.005%. Bleach baths can be used for maintenance therapy for individuals with recurrent bacterial infections. There is no optimal guideline for frequency of baths, but some recommendations are from 1 to 3 times per week. Dilute bleach baths are overall well tolerated; but if patients have numerous eroded areas, they can experience some stinging; therefore, it may be best to start bleach baths a few weeks after the acute flare of AD has subsided. If taking a bath is not possible or patients do not have a bathtub, other possible options to decrease bacterial colonization are using a spray bottle of dilute bleach in the shower or using chlorhexidine soap 4%. Chlorhexidine does have antimicrobial properties but does not have the antiinflammatory effects of sodium hypochlorite. It can also potentially be an irritant dermatitis.

Eczema herpeticum is more frequently seen in children and is secondary to transmission of herpes simplex virus (HSV)-1 often by a parent or caregiver. Once infected with HSV, patients with AD can have recurrent episodes of eczema herpeticum that presents with the appearance of sudden crusted, vesicular, eroded, and punched out papules in previous areas of AD. If there is periorbital involvement, an ophthalmologic evaluation is recommended to rule out the possibility of herpetic keratoconjunctivitis. Secondary bacterial infection in the setting of eczema herpeticum is common, so treatment with oral antivirals and oral antibiotics is warranted in this scenario. This treatment is in conjunction with use of TCS and optimal skin-directed management of AD. If an individual has recurrent episodes of eczema herpeticum, antiviral prophylaxis can be considered.

OTHER MANAGEMENT CONSIDERATIONS

In addition to the various treatments outlined earlier, there are other nonpharmacologic interventions that practitioners taking care of patients with AD should understand. Bathing is an important component to address in patients with AD. Once-a-day bathing for a maximum of 5 to 10 minutes in warm (not hot) water, with use of fragrance- and dye-free nonsoap cleansers, and application of an emollient immediately afterward to prevent drying out of the skin are recommended. Soap use can be harmful to the stratum corneum and can cause further irritation and damage to the skin barrier. Bath additives and water-softening devices have not shown any benefit to AD. Wet wraps are also an important therapeutic intervention that can be used in recalcitrant disease or during a severe flare of AD to improve penetration of topical medications, help heal the skin by providing a barrier from repeating traumatization, and decrease transepidermal water loss. Wet wraps consist of applying a topical agent (emollient +/- medication) to the skin and applying a wet first layer (eg, gauze, tubular bandages, cotton suit) that is damp and wrung out followed by a dry second layer. Use of TCS rather than just emollients has shown to be a more effective therapy. The easiest method for patients to do this is to apply 2 layers of nonirritating cotton clothing, one as the wet layer and the second as the dry layer. Wet wraps can be used for a few days up to 2 weeks and can be worn from a few hours to 24 hours. Often they are best tolerated and easiest for patients when worn overnight. Strength of TCS being used and the body surface area that it is being applied to should be considered carefully to prevent skin atrophy or increased systemic absorption. The risk of HPA suppression is very low with short courses of wet wrap therapy, once-a-day use, and use of lower to midpotency TCS for larger body surface areas.

REFERENCES

1. Mancini AJ, Kaulback K, Chamlin SL. The socioeconomic impact of atopic dermatitis in the United States: a systemic review. Pediatr Dermatol 2008; 25(1):1–6.
2. Kay J, Gawkrodger DJ, Mortimer MJ, et al. The prevalence of childhood atopic eczema in a general population. J Am Acad Dermatol 1994;30:35–9.
3. Garg N, Silverberg JI. Epidemiology of childhood atopic dermatitis. Clin Dermatol 2015;33:281–8.
4. Wen HJ, Chen PC, Chiang TL, et al. Predicting risk of early infantile atopic dermatitis by hereditary and environmental factors. Br J Dermatol 2009;161:1166–72.
5. Bantz SK, Zhou Z, Zheng T. The atopic march: progression from atopic dermatitis to allergic rhinitis and asthma. J Clin Cell Immunol 2014;5(2):1–16.
6. Romanos M, Gerlach M, Warnke A, et al. Association of attention-deficit hyperactivity disorder and atopic eczema modified by sleep disturbance in a large population based sample. J Epidemiol Community Health 2010;64:269–73.

7. Schmitt J, Romanos M, Pfennig A, et al. Psychiatric comorbidity in adult eczema. Br J Dermatol 2009;161:878–83.
8. Van den Oord R, Sheikh A. Filaggrin gene defects and risk of developing allergic sensitization and allergic disorders: systemic review and meta-analysis. BMJ 2009;339:1–12.
9. Silverberg JI, Hanifin J, Simpson EL. Climatic factors associated with childhood eczema prevalence in the United States. J Invest Dermatol 2013;133:1752–9.
10. Hanifin JM, Rajka G. Diagnostic features of atopic-dermatitis. Acta Dermatol Venereol 1980;92:44–7.
11. Eichenfield LF, Tom WL, Berger TG, et al. Guidelines of care for the management of atopic dermatitis. Section 2: management and treatment of atopic dermatitis with topical therapies. J Am Acad Dermatol 2014;71:116–32.
12. Schmitt J, von Kobyletzki L, Svensson A, et al. Efficacy and tolerability of proactive treatment with topical corticosteroids and calcineurin inhibitors for atopic eczema: systemic review and meta-analysis of randomized control trials. Br J Dermatol 2011;164:415–28.
13. Callen J, Chamlin S, Eichenfield LF, et al. A systematic review of the safety of topical therapies for atopic dermatitis. Br J Dermatol 2007;156:203–21.
14. Ellison JA, Patel L, Ray DW, et al. Hypothalamic-pituitary-adrenal function and glucocorticoid sensitivity in atopic dermatitis. Pediatrics 2000;105:794–9.
15. Hengge UR, Ruzicka T, Schwartz RA, et al. Adverse effects of topical glucocorticoids. J Am Acad Dermatol 2006;54:1–15.
16. Charman CR, Morris AD, Williams HC. Topical corticosteroid phobia in patients with atopic eczema. Br J Dermatol 2000;142:931–6.
17. Breuer K, Werfel T, Kapp S. Safety and efficacy of topical calcineurin inhibitors in the treatment of childhood atopic dermatitis. Am J Clin Dermatol 2005;6:65–77.
18. Sidbury R, Davis DM, Cohen DE, et al. Guidelines of care for the management of atopic dermatitis. Section 3: management and treatment with phototherapy and systemic agents. J Am Acad Dermatol 2014;71:327–49.
19. Slater NA, Morrell DS. Systemic therapy of childhood atopic dermatitis. Clin Dermatol 2015;33:289–99.
20. Huang JT, Abrams M, Tlougan B, et al. Treatment of Staphylococcus aureus colonization in atopic dermatitis decreases disease severity. Pediatrics 2009;123:808–14.
21. Mathes EF, Oza V, Frieden IJF, et al. "Eczema coxsackium" and unusual cutaneous findings in an enterovirus outbreak. Pediatrics 2013;132(1):e149–57.
22. Tollefson MM, Bruckner AL. Atopic dermatitis: skin directed management. Pediatrics 2014;134:1735–44.
23. Leung TH, Zhang LF, Wang J, et al. Topical hypochlorite ameliorates NF-kB medicated skin diseases in mice. J Clin Invest 2013;123(12):5361–70.

FURTHER READINGS

Sidbury R, Tom WL, Bergman JN, et al. Guidelines of care for the management of atopic dermatitis. Section 4: prevention of disease flares and use of adjunctive therapies and approaches. J Am Acad Dermatol 2014;71:1218–33.
Totri CR, Diaz L, Eichenfield LF. 2014 update on atopic dermatitis in children. Curr Opin Pediatr 2014;26:466–71.
Eichenfield LF, Tom WL, Chamlin S, et al. Guidelines of care for the management of atopic dermatitis. Section 1: diagnosis and assessment of atopic dermatitis. J Am Acad Dermatol 2014;70:338–51.

Rheumatologic Skin Disease

Andrea Kalus, MD

KEYWORDS

- Rheumatology • Dermatology • Skin • Lupus • Dermatomyositis • Morphea

KEY POINTS

- The cutaneous presentation of lupus is variable and attention to the clinical features assists in defining the chances of systemic disease.
- In dermatomyositis serologic studies help identify the associated conditions of lung disease and malignancy.
- Photoprotection and topical therapy are important therapeutic interventions in lupus and dermatomyositis.
- Clinical findings can differentiate morphea from systemic sclerosis. An important association with morphea is the common co-occurrence of genital lichen sclerosus.

LUPUS ERYTHEMATOSUS

Lupus is a chronic autoimmune disease with the potential for multiorgan disorder and prominent involvement of the skin. There is great variety in the clinical features and severity from one patient to the next. There are several distinct and recognizable patterns of skin involvement that are specific for lupus.

Patient History

Lupus preferentially affects young women but can occur at any age. The most common clinical presentation involves skin rashes and constitutional symptoms, with fatigue and musculoskeletal complaints predominating.[1,2] The skin manifestations of lupus are classified as acute cutaneous lupus, subacute cutaneous lupus, and chronic cutaneous lupus. Chronic cutaneous lupus includes several subtypes, the most common being discoid lupus.[3] Less common forms of chronic cutaneous lupus are lupus panniculitis, chilblain lupus, and tumid lupus. Some controversy exists about the relationship of tumid lupus to the rest of the lupus spectrum.[3]

Disclosure: The author has nothing to disclose.
Dermatology Division, Department of Medicine, University of Washington School of Medicine, 1959 NE Pacific St., Seattle, WA 98115, USA
E-mail address: akalus@uw.edu

Med Clin N Am 99 (2015) 1287–1303
http://dx.doi.org/10.1016/j.mcna.2015.07.007
medical.theclinics.com

Lupus is characterized by relapses and remissions. It is expected that the clinical pattern that develops early in the disease will predominate over the course of the illness. Recognition of the type of skin disease can help predict systemic disease because the subsets of cutaneous lupus relate to systemic disease differently (**Fig. 1**). Patients with lupus also present with skin findings that are not specific to lupus, and these include pernio, vasculitis, photosensitivity, alopecia, livedo, and bullous lesions.

It is important to carefully consider medications, because they can be a trigger for lupus. Subacute cutaneous lupus erythematosus (SCLE) is a form of lupus commonly attributed to medicines. More than 40 medications are reported to cause SCLE; of these, the most common are hydrochlorothiazide, diltiazem, angiotensin-converting enzyme inhibitors, and terbinafine.[4] In recent years it has been recognized that the tumor necrosis factor (TNF) inhibitors cause multiple presentations of autoimmunity, including lupus.[5,6] Patients often have systemic and cutaneous findings, although the systemic findings may be more prominent. In contrast with drug-induced lupus caused by procainamide, hydralazine, and minocycline, antihistone antibodies may not be present. Drug-induced forms often resolve when the offending medications have been stopped, although it may take months.

Clinical Findings

Acute cutaneous lupus
This condition presents as classic malar erythema, known as a butterfly rash (**Fig. 2**). It is present in about 40% to 50% of patients at the diagnosis of systemic lupus.[2] Erythema spreading over the cheeks and nose, sparing the sun-protected areas like the nasolabial fold, is characteristic. There can be extension onto the forehead and chest. In a few patients a more generalized eruption accompanies this rash, involving the extensor arms and hands and often localized to the interphalangeal skin and sparing the skin over the knuckles. Erythema and small papules tending toward confluence are present. Small amounts of scale may be found. The clinical course of the rash can worsen with sun exposure or reappear with systemic disease flares.

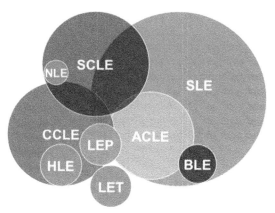

Fig. 1. Relationship of lupus subsets to systemic disease. ACLE, acute cutaneous lupus erythematosus; BLE, bullous lupus erythematosus; CCLE, chronic cutaneous lupus erythematosus; HLE, hypertrophic lupus erythematosus; LEP, lupus erythematosus profundus; LET, lupus erythematosus tumidus; NLE, neonatal lupus erythematosus; SCLE, subacute cutaneous lupus erythematosus; SLE, systemic lupus erythematosus. (*Courtesy of* J. Callen, MD, Louisville, KY.)

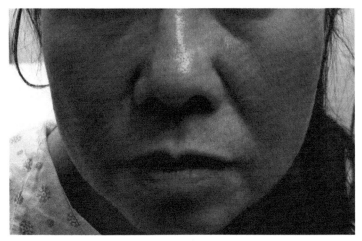

Fig. 2. Facial erythema in lupus, with redness over both cheeks, slightly over the nose. Rash does not extend over the nasolabial fold.

Many of these patients have systemic lupus and this is reflected in their serologies. Positive antinuclear antibodies (ANA) are common and titers are generally greater than or equal to 1:160. Anti–double-stranded DNA and anti-Smith antibodies are both specific for systemic lupus, with anti-Smith being seen less frequently. Multiple other antibodies can be found that are beyond the scope of this article. This rash resolves in days to weeks without scarring, although marked postinflammatory hyper-pigmentation is common.

Subacute cutaneous lupus

These patients have marked photosensitivity. The rash is characterized by erythema-tous, scaly, and polycyclic or ring-shaped macules and papules predominantly on the upper chest and back (**Fig. 3**). The rash can extend down the arms but rarely involves the legs. The central face is characteristically spared, although peripheral lesions do occur on the face. Up to 70% of patients have SSA (anti-Ro) antibodies, and although

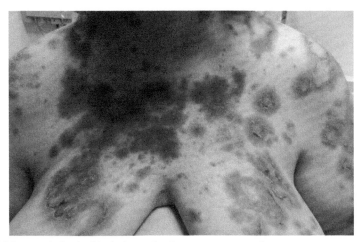

Fig. 3. Widespread classic skin lesions of subacute cutaneous lupus.

they may meet criteria for systemic disease they can be reassured that they are more likely to have a benign course.[4] Again, postinflammatory pigment changes are common but scarring is usually avoided. Careful scrutiny for a causative medication is important.

Discoid cutaneous lupus

Discoid lupus starts out as a papule that gradually expands into an indurated round plaque. As it enlarges the center develops a depressed scar that is hypopigmented (**Fig. 4**). There is often scale, and follicular plugging may be visible. When the scalp is involved the follicular changes result in scarring and irreversible alopecia. The lesions can be triggered by sun exposure and also by trauma (Koebner effect). The most common areas involved are the head and neck, and, when only here, the disease is deemed localized. When it extends below the neck, it is described as generalized. When the presentation is predominantly discoid lesions, the patients have minimal risk for systemic involvement. However, up to 20% of patients with systemic lupus have discoid lesions at some point in the course of their disease.[2]

Variations of lupus skin findings

There are several additional skin findings or variations that are less common but associated specifically with lupus. Overlaps occur between lichen planus and lupus, as well as lupus and erythema multiforme, known as Rowell syndrome. Patients can present

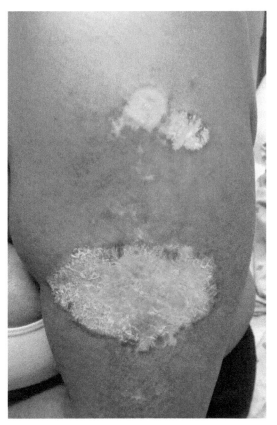

Fig. 4. Discoid lupus.

with lupus panniculitis, in which deep nodules are found in the skin, often with overlying discoid changes, most commonly on the head, neck, chest, and proximal arms. This condition is called lupus profundus. In addition to the mucosal ulcers often seen early in diagnosis, about 10% of patients with lupus have other mucosal findings.[7] These mucosal findings are more common in patients with discoid type skin disease. Any mucosa can be affected. In the mouth it is most likely to involve the lips and buccal mucosa. The appearance may resemble oral lichen planus.

Tumid lupus presents with erythematous, almost urticarial, plaques. On skin biopsy, it is characterized by prominent mucin deposition. Usually there is little of the interface dermatitis that is characteristic of other lupus skin presentations. These patients are typically ANA negative and do not progress to develop systemic lupus. Tumid lupus is marked by extreme photosensitivity with prominent involvement in photoexposed areas, including the face. Extension to photoprotected sites only rarely occurs. Because of its various nonlupus features, experts debate whether tumid lupus should be considered part of the lupus spectrum.[3]

Treatment

Treatment of cutaneous lupus is based initially on severity, with attention later to clinical response and escalation of therapy for resistant disease (**Fig. 5**). Large clinical trials evaluating therapies for skin disease are lacking, so treatment recommendations are often based on case reports, case series, and expert opinion. Topical therapy is a useful starting point[8] and may have additive benefit even in patients on systemic treatment. For the treatment of skin disease, systemic therapy beyond hydroxychloroquine is reserved for patients with widespread skin lesions, disfiguring or scarring lesions, and refractory disease.

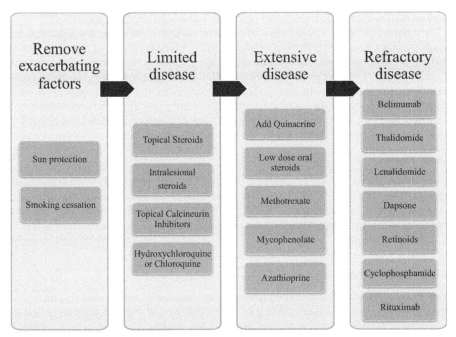

Fig. 5. Therapeutic considerations in cutaneous lupus.

Hydroxychloroquine is an important therapy for lupus. This therapy is effective for treating musculoskeletal complaints, skin findings, and constitutional symptoms. It also prevents flares of disease, reduces thrombotic complications of lupus, and improves survival.[9] It should be continued even when other therapy is added. Dosing is usually 200 to 400 mg per day up to a maximum of 6 mg/kg. Regular monitoring for eye toxicity is recommended. Patients may also develop blue-gray to brown pigment changes in the skin. When this occurs it is often subtle and can take years to develop. An alternative is chloroquine and in refractory cases quinacrine may be added.

Topical steroids of medium (ie, triamcinolone 0.1%) to high potency (ie, clobetasol 0.05%) are used up to 2 times per day. High-potency steroids are more effective and the risk of atrophy from therapy is often outweighed by the potential for disfiguring scars if left untreated. To minimize the risk of skin atrophy, use of steroids for 1 to 2 weeks then a 1-week break can be recommended. Alternating topical steroids with topical calcineurin inhibitors may avoid steroid-induced skin atrophy without interruption in therapy.[8]

If skin disease remains uncontrolled after initiating the treatment described earlier, then consideration for treatment with additional systemic agents is reasonable. Initial choices include methotrexate, mycophenolate, and azathioprine.[10] For SCLE and discoid lesions, thalidomide and lenalidomide are considered effective.[11–13] The historical context for these therapies and the demonstrated severe risk of birth defects have resulted in a required monitoring program for providers and patients to comply with in order for these medications to be prescribed. In 2011, belimumab, an infusion therapy that modulates B cells, was approved for the treatment of lupus and results show improvement in skin disease.[14] Rituximab has shown effect in case reports, but relapses are common and the role in lupus therapy is still being determined.[15] Oral retinoids (isotretinoin and acitretin) are used for hyperkeratotic lesions or lesions on the palms and soles. Dapsone has been recommended for bullous lesions, urticarial vasculitis, and oral ulcers. Overall response rates with dapsone are low.[3,10]

The inherent photosensitive nature of lupus along with routine recommendation for sun protection results in vitamin D deficiency,[16–18] which has been documented in multiple studies and ongoing investigations are underway to examine the complex interplay of the immune system and vitamin D. Clinical monitoring and supplementation when necessary are recommended. In addition to sun protection with broad-spectrum sunscreens (recommended ingredients are titanium, zinc, and Mexoryl),[19] it is also important to encourage smoking cessation. Smoking reduces the effectiveness of therapy and can be a risk factor for more severe disease.

Future Therapy

Future directions of therapy for lupus include anti-interferon therapies and clinical trials are currently underway.[20] Although photoprovocation of lupus is well documented there is interest in modulation of lupus and clinical improvement with specific wavelengths of light (ultraviolet [UV] A1, 340–400 nm).[21] The exact role in therapy is yet to be determined.

DERMATOMYOSITIS

Dermatomyositis is an autoimmune disease that classically affects skin and muscles. Vigilance for important associations with lung disease and malignancy can be aided by serology testing. Distinctive skin findings are readily identifiable and assist in diagnosis.

Patient History

Patients with dermatomyositis usually present in midlife and women are 2 times more often affected than men.[22] The incidence of dermatomyositis is increasing worldwide, although this is attributed to better diagnosis. It is associated with geographic latitude, and regions with higher surface UV exposure have higher incidences.[23] Photosensitivity is an important clinical feature of dermatomyositis.

Symptoms may come on quickly or develop over several months. Skin findings may precede or follow characteristic symmetric muscle weakness of the proximal muscle groups (classic dermatomyositis). It is important to recognize that skin findings can occur without ever developing muscle weakness (amyopathic dermatomyositis). Other subtypes have been described. Postmyopathic dermatomyositis follows classic dermatomyositis with persistent skin disease despite resolution of muscle symptoms. Hypomyopathic dermatomyositis is also described and these patients have very mild subclinical muscle disease.[22]

Patients may report difficulty swallowing or changes to their voice caused by effects on muscles in the pharynx and upper esophagus. This condition may portend more severe disease. Interstitial lung disease can occur and can be rapidly progressive and fatal.[24] Swallowing difficulty has been associated with lung disease.

Clinical Findings

The distinctive skin findings of dermatomyositis are periorbital erythema and swelling described as a heliotrope rash. Redness and papules overlying the knuckles are called the papules of dermatomyositis (Gottron papules) and are often seen in conjunction with ragged cuticles, dilated nail fold capillaries, and cuticle hemorrhage (**Fig. 6**). A less common hand finding is hyperkeratosis along the sides of the fingers and on the palms, sometimes with surrounding erythema known as mechanic's hands (**Fig. 7**). Gottron sign is violaceous erythema over the elbows and knees (**Fig. 8**). The finding of erythema, hypopigmentation and hyperpigmentation, and telangiectasia extending over the shoulders (shawl sign; **Fig. 9**), in a V distribution of the neck, and lateral thighs (holster sign), is often described simply as poikiloderma associated with dermatomyositis. Scale is often present and the rash is difficult to distinguish from lupus or other papulosquamous disorders. Attention to the characteristic distribution and careful examination of the nail folds is helpful in these cases. Scalp involvement with erythema, scale, and often intense pruritus can persist even when other areas of skin involvement have come under control.

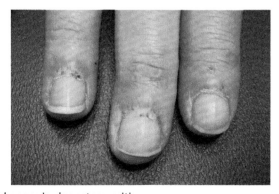

Fig. 6. Nail fold changes in dermatomyositis.

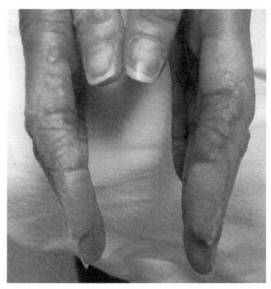

Fig. 7. Mechanics hands with dermatomyositis.

Cardiac involvement, with conduction abnormalities or arrhythmias, occurs infrequently.[25] Calcinosis of the muscles and skin, common in children but unusual in adults, is a challenging complication to treat.

Skin biopsy is not specific, but can support the diagnosis of dermatomyositis. It shows similar features to lupus, with interface dermatitis and perivascular lymphocytic inflammation. Clinical findings remain the most distinguishing feature. Along with strength testing, detection of increased muscle enzyme levels in serum can indicate muscle involvement. Levels of creatine kinase, lactate dehydrogenase, aldolase, aspartate aminotransferase, and alanine aminotransferase are all potentially increased in muscle disease, and checking several is reasonable. Although the complete evaluation of muscle disease is not discussed here it is important to remember that once dermatomyositis has caused extensive damage to the muscles and atrophy has occurred, the muscle enzyme levels may return to normal despite significant muscle disease.

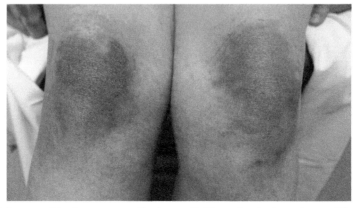

Fig. 8. Violaceous skin changes over the knees, Gottron sign in dermatomyositis.

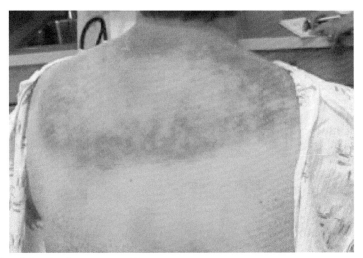

Fig. 9. Shawl sign in dermatomyositis.

A positive ANA test occurs in 80% to 90% of patients. In addition, multiple myositis autoantibodies can be detected, and increasing relevance and clinical implications are being recognized for these antibodies (**Table 1**).[22] Clinically important antibodies include Mi-2, MDA5, anti-p155/140, and antisynthetase antibodies. Mi-2 is most specific for dermatomyositis, but is not very sensitive. When present, it suggests treatment-responsive disease.

The constellation of rapidly progressive severe interstitial lung disease, myositis, arthritis, often mechanic's hands, and antisynthetase antibodies, sometimes with SSA antibodies, is referred to as the antisynthetase syndrome.[26,27] Fever and Raynaud phenomenon may be additional symptoms. There have been 8 distinct antisynthetase antibodies detected, and more are likely be to be found in the future. Of these, anti–Jo-1 is the most common. In some cases, lung disease is the initial presenting symptom and other features are less prominent.[24]

The presence of MDA5 antibodies is also associated with severe interstitial lung disease.[28] It is found in amyopathic forms of dermatomyositis and may be associated with punched-out–type ulcerations in the skin. In both of these scenarios the lung

Table 1
Frequency of antibodies in dermatomyositis (DM) and clinical associations

Antibody	Frequency in DM (%)	Clinical Association
Mi-2	20–30	Most specific antibody for DM. More responsive disease
MDA5	50	Associated with amyopathic DM. Increased ILD and skin ulcers, levels may decrease in response to therapy
P155/140	20–25 DM 40–75 cancer- associated DM	Cancer-associated myositis, severe skin disease, high negative predictive value for malignancy
Antisynthetase (Jo-1 and others)	5–10	Antisynthetase syndrome high frequency of ILD and arthritis

Abbreviation: ILD, interstitial lung disease.

disease is common, affecting more than 70% of patients, and mortality is significant as well (~30%).[29]

Overlaps exist between dermatomyositis and lupus, as well as systemic sclerosis. In these presentations, a variety of autoantibody patterns can be seen, including positive SSA, anti-RNP, anti-sm, and SCL.

An association between dermatomyositis and malignancy is well recognized. The clinical findings of dermatomyositis may precede, coincide with, or follow the cancer diagnosis. Recent analysis has suggested a 5-fold greater occurrence of cancer in these patients than would normally be expected.[30] The malignancies most represented in the setting of dermatomyositis are hematopoietic and lung. A variety of other cancers are also noted to be over-represented, including ovary, colon, bladder, breast, cervix, pancreas, and esophagus.[30,31] Cancer screening recommendations are not standardized. Consequently appropriate clinical decision making includes symptom-directed screening and the usual age-appropriate screening. It is reasonable to repeat the screening annually for 3 years, because this is when the risk of cancer-associated dermatomyositis tends to decrease. Because routine screening is not very effective for ovarian cancer, lung cancer, and pancreatic cancer, vaginal ultrasonography and a computed tomography scan of the chest, abdomen, and pelvis is ordered by some experts. The impact of anti-p155/140 antibodies on screening for malignancy remains to be determined. In light of the high negative predictive value (93%) for malignancy, in the setting of a negative anti-p155/140, it may be reasonable to consider cancer screening tests at diagnosis of dermatomyositis and then return to the usual recommended schedule for the patient's age.[32]

Treatment

Although treatment algorithms do not exist for dermatomyositis, a common approach is to start oral prednisone at doses around 1 mg/kg/d for patients with evidence of muscle disease. This dose is tapered slowly, often over months. With long courses of steroids, side effects are a predicted complication. Concurrent addition of a steroid-sparing immunosuppressive drug may shorten the need for high-dose steroids and prevent steroid-associated side effects. Commonly used therapies are methotrexate (10–20 mg per week), mycophenolate (1000–1500 mg twice daily), or azathioprine. Often these can be started at the same time as prednisone. In cases resistant to standard therapy, intravenous immunoglobulin or rituximab are reasonable choices. For interstitial lung disease, a more aggressive treatment regimen is usually required, and is not discussed here.

Once therapy has been initiated it seems that exercise, both resistance and aerobic, may benefit patients with myositis. It is reasonable to recommend an exercise program after about 4 weeks of systemic treatment.[33]

Skin disease in patients with dermatomyositis can be resistant and attention to skin-specific treatments is important. Photoprotection is recommended, with clothing and broad-spectrum sunscreen. Midpotency topical steroids and topical calcineurin inhibitors are also helpful for the rash and related itching. Addition of hydroxychloroquine or chloroquine can benefit patients significantly. Quinacrine can be added when patients do not respond to a single agent. In patients with amyopathic forms, escalation of therapy to other systemic agents, including methotrexate and mycophenolate, may be required to control symptoms.[34]

Future Therapy

Although TNF cytokines play a role in the pathogenesis of dermatomyositis, use of TNF blockers has not been uniformly successful. Note that dermatomyositis has been identified as an unusual autoimmune side effect of TNF blocker therapy.[35] Further research with new agents may identify effective treatments. In 1 patient, inhibition of the JAK pathway with ruxolitinib resulted in improvement of dermatomyositis.[36]

MORPHEA

Morphea is an idiopathic inflammatory skin disease that presents in a variety of ways, but ultimately causes skin hardening and in some cases loss of function. Although understanding of the pathophysiology is incomplete, it seems to share features with systemic sclerosis. Despite this common pathophysiology, morphea and systemic sclerosis are readily distinguished clinically and should be thought of separately. Morphea is largely confined to the skin and subcutaneous tissues, whereas systemic sclerosis is a multisystem disease. Distinctive findings on examination can help differentiate the two conditions and direct appropriate therapy.

Patient History

The onset of symptoms in morphea may be insidious, and studies have shown a delay in diagnosis of a year or longer.[37] Morphea is nearly 3 times more common in women than in men. It affects children and adults equally.[38] Patients may describe arthralgias, myalgias, and fatigue occurring along with morphea but the systemic symptoms of gastrointestinal reflux, pulmonary symptoms, and cardiac symptoms seen in systemic sclerosis are not characteristic of morphea.[39]

In addition to the skin findings, there are some special clinical considerations in patients with morphea. Morphea that involves the scalp or occurs around the eyes can be associated with symptoms of uveitis, headaches, or seizures.[40,41] Several reports show a strong association between morphea and genital lichen sclerosis. Frank discussion with patients about genital symptoms, including skin changes, itching, or burning, should be included in the history because patients may be reluctant to volunteer these concerns.[42]

The course of morphea is one of remission and relapse.[43] Ongoing monitoring is helpful to treat relapses early and avoid additional disability.

Clinical Findings

Plaque morphea
Several distinct patterns of morphea occur on the skin. Plaque-type morphea is the most common. The earliest lesions are often erythematous plaques with little induration; sometimes a lilac border is observed at the periphery of the lesion (**Fig. 10**). This condition progresses to central sclerosis with induration and smooth yellow to white scarring. There is often peripheral erythema or hyperpigmentation (**Fig. 11**). Over time, destruction of the hair and sweat glands occurs in the affected skin. The plaques can increase in size and number. Involvement in the inframammary area, the area around the hips, and on the low back together as a pattern is common.

Generalized plaque morphea
When the plaques are greater than 3 cm in size and there are more than 4 plaques involving 2 body areas it is classified as generalized plaque morphea. Patients can have superficial or deep involvement in the skin.

Pansclerotic morphea
In rare patients the course is rapid and progressive with multiple enlarging plaques that eventually result in widespread involvement of close to the entire skin, except

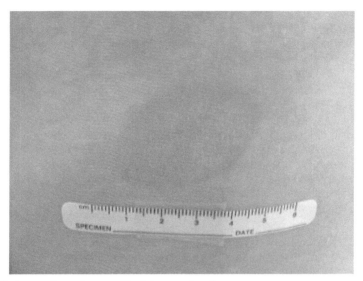

Fig. 10. Early morphea plaque with violaceous border.

for sparing of the hands and feet. This presentation is referred to as pansclerotic and requires aggressive treatment.

Linear morphea

The linear subtype of morphea occurs most commonly in children. In this type, plaques develop in a linear pattern, eventually coalescing into a single band of scarring that can extend the length of a limb. When it crosses joints it can cause loss of mobility

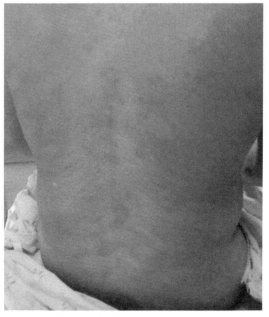

Fig. 11. Morphea plaques on the low back.

because of scarring. Linear morphea often involves deeper structures, including muscle and bone. When it involves the scalp and forehead it has been referred to as en coup de sabre (**Fig. 12**), which is a French term referring to the injuries sustained by soldiers hit on the head by a sword.

Patients often have a mixed presentation with both linear and plaque types. Several less common forms of morphea have been reported, including superficial morphea,[44] guttate morphea, bullous morphea,[45] and keloidal morphea.[46,47]

The diagnosis of morphea is made based on history and clinical examination of the skin. Differentiating from systemic sclerosis is an important first consideration. In contrast with systemic sclerosis, which begins with sclerodactyly, morphea usually does not involve the hands. Raynaud phenomenon is characteristic of systemic sclerosis and is absent in morphea. Nail fold and serologic findings of systemic sclerosis are not present in morphea. Examination of the genital skin is recommended to detect asymptomatic lichen sclerosus and to direct treatment if present. The most likely clinical differential diagnoses to consider are eosinophilic fasciitis, lipodermatosclerosis, graft-versus-host disease, and nephrogenic systemic fibrosis (**Box 1**).

Skin biopsy is usually not required. When performed it shows an inflammatory pattern of lymphocytes and plasma cells in the dermis and subcutis, and in late lesions thickened collagen bundles are present. The histologic findings may be indistinguishable from systemic sclerosis.

There are no specific laboratory tests to confirm the diagnosis of morphea. Patients with morphea, especially the linear and deep subtypes, often have a positive ANA test. The clinical utility of this test is yet to be determined and routine testing is not clinically useful.[48]

Treatment

For patients with early and limited skin involvement, topical therapy with high-potency steroids, topical calcineurin inhibitors, or calcipotriene is recommended. Patients with continued progression or generalized disease should be treated with either phototherapy (nbUVB [narrow band ultraviolet B], bbUVA [broad band ultraviolet A], or UVA1) or systemic treatment with either methotrexate or methotrexate combined with pulsed-dose steroids (1 g of Solu-Medrol intravenously daily for 3 consecutive days, repeated

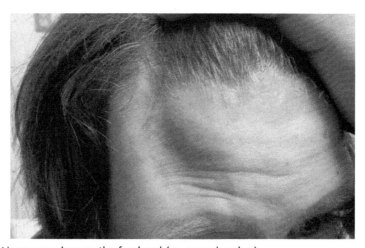

Fig. 12. Linear morphea on the forehead (en coup de sabre).

Box 1
Clinical differential diagnosis of morphea

Systemic sclerosis

Eosinophilic fasciitis

Lichen sclerosus

Lipodermatosclerosis

Graft-versus-host disease

Nephrogenic systemic fibrosis

Panniculitis

Chemical-induced skin hardening (taxane-induced scleroderma, silicone implant/injection complication, toxic oil syndrome)

Scleredema

Scleromyxedema

Myxedema

Dermatofibrosarcoma protuberans

Cutaneous T-cell lymphoma

Radiation-related skin changes

Carcinoma en cuirasse

Porphyria cutanea tarda

---

monthly for 3–6 months). Systemic therapy should be considered for linear morphea, which often is more aggressive and disabling. An alternative to methotrexate is mycophenolate using doses of 1000 to 1500 mg twice daily.[49]

Further progression after a period of quiescence is encountered. Treatment should be restarted in these cases. If the clinical findings are not clear and comparison photographs are not available a skin biopsy may be helpful. The finding of inflammation on the biopsy suggests clinical activity and may be compelling to restart therapy.

Future Therapy

Future therapeutic directions in morphea include studies to better understand the comparative effectiveness of systemic treatments and phototherapy. The timing of therapeutic intervention may also become an important part of treatment. As awareness increases it may be possible to treat early, when the disease is thought to be more responsive.

Ultrasonography and MRI studies have been able to detect the skin and deeper inflammatory and tissue changes associated with morphea. Ultrasonography or MRI may be useful for monitoring response to therapy, surveillance for recurrence, and to guide clinical decision making regarding the use of systemic therapy in this disease.[38]

REFERENCES

1. Rothfield N, Sontheimer RD, Bernstein M. Lupus erythematosus: systemic and cutaneous manifestations. Clin Dermatol 2006;24(5):348–62.
2. Walling HW, Sontheimer RD. Cutaneous lupus erythematosus: issues in diagnosis and treatment. Am J Clin Dermatol 2009;10(6):365–81.

3. Callen JP. Management of "refractory" skin disease in patients with lupus erythematosus. Best Pract Res Clin Rheumatol 2005;19(5):767–84.

4. Callen JP. Drug-induced subacute cutaneous lupus erythematosus. Lupus 2010; 19(9):1107–11.

5. Williams VL, Cohen PR. TNF alpha antagonist-induced lupus-like syndrome: report and review of the literature with implications for treatment with alternative TNF alpha antagonists. Int J Dermatol 2011;50(5):619–25.

6. Yanai H, Shuster D, Calabrese E, et al. The incidence and predictors of lupus-like reaction in patients with IBD treated with anti-TNF therapies. Inflamm Bowel Dis 2013;19(13):2778–86.

7. Lourenco SV, Nacagami Sotto M, Constantino Vilela MA, et al. Lupus erythematosus: clinical and histopathological study of oral manifestations and immunohistochemical profile of epithelial maturation. J Cutan Pathol 2006;33(10):657–62.

8. Kuhn A, Ruland V, Bonsmann G. Cutaneous lupus erythematosus: update of therapeutic options part I. J Am Acad Dermatol 2011;65(6):e179–93.

9. Croyle L, Morand EF. Optimizing the use of existing therapies in lupus. Int J Rheum Dis 2015;18(2):129–37.

10. Kuhn A, Ruland V, Bonsmann G. Cutaneous lupus erythematosus: update of therapeutic options part II. J Am Acad Dermatol 2011;65(6):e195–213.

11. Cortes-Hernandez J, Avila G, Vilardell-Tarres M, et al. Efficacy and safety of lenalidomide for refractory cutaneous lupus erythematosus. Arthritis Res Ther 2012; 14(6):R265.

12. Cortes-Hernandez J, Torres-Salido M, Castro-Marrero J, et al. Thalidomide in the treatment of refractory cutaneous lupus erythematosus: prognostic factors of clinical outcome. Br J Dermatol 2012;166(3):616–23.

13. Dalm VA, van Hagen PM. Efficacy of lenalidomide in refractory lupus pernio. JAMA Dermatol 2013;149(4):493–4.

14. Ginzler EM, Wallace DJ, Merrill JT, et al. Disease control and safety of belimumab plus standard therapy over 7 years in patients with systemic lupus erythematosus. J Rheumatol 2014;41(2):300–9.

15. Hofmann SC, Leandro MJ, Morris SD, et al. Effects of rituximab-based B-cell depletion therapy on skin manifestations of lupus erythematosus–report of 17 cases and review of the literature. Lupus 2013;22(9):932–9.

16. Schneider L, Colar da Silva AC, Werres Junior LC, et al. Vitamin D levels and cytokine profiles in patients with systemic lupus erythematosus. Lupus 2015; 24(11):1191–7.

17. Yap KS, Morand EF. Vitamin D and systemic lupus erythematosus: continued evolution. Int J Rheum Dis 2015;18(2):242–9.

18. Yap KS, Northcott M, Hoi AB, et al. Association of low vitamin D with high disease activity in an Australian systemic lupus erythematosus cohort. Lupus Sci Med 2015;2(1):e000064.

19. Kuhn A, Gensch K, Haust M, et al. Photoprotective effects of a broad-spectrum sunscreen in ultraviolet-induced cutaneous lupus erythematosus: a randomized, vehicle-controlled, double-blind study. J Am Acad Dermatol 2011;64(1):37–48.

20. Kirou KA, Gkrouzman E. Anti-interferon alpha treatment in SLE. Clin Immunol 2013;148(3):303–12.

21. Gambichler T, Terras S, Kreuter A. Treatment regimens, protocols, dosage, and indications for UVA1 phototherapy: facts and controversies. Clin Dermatol 2013;31(4):438–54.

22. Iaccarino L, Ghirardello A, Bettio S, et al. The clinical features, diagnosis and classification of dermatomyositis. J Autoimmun 2014;48-49:122–7.

23. Meyer A, Meyer N, Schaeffer M, et al. Incidence and prevalence of inflammatory myopathies: a systematic review. Rheumatology (Oxford) 2015;54(1):50–63.
24. Hallowell RW, Danoff SK. Interstitial lung disease associated with the idiopathic inflammatory myopathies and the antisynthetase syndrome: recent advances. Curr Opin Rheumatol 2014;26(6):684–9.
25. Zhang L, Wang GC, Ma L, et al. Cardiac involvement in adult polymyositis or dermatomyositis: a systematic review. Clin Cardiol 2012;35(11):686–91.
26. Katzap E, Barilla-LaBarca ML, Marder G. Antisynthetase syndrome. Curr Rheumatol Rep 2011;13(3):175–81.
27. Uribe L, Ronderos DM, Diaz MC, et al. Antisynthetase antibody syndrome: case report and review of the literature. Clin Rheumatol 2013;32(5):715–9.
28. Koichi Y, Aya Y, Megumi U, et al. A case of anti-MDA5-positive rapidly progressive interstitial lung disease in a patient with clinically amyopathic dermatomyositis ameliorated by rituximab, in addition to standard immunosuppressive treatment. Mod Rheumatol 2015;1–5 [Epub ahead of print].
29. Hozumi H, Enomoto N, Kono M, et al. Prognostic significance of anti-aminoacyl-tRNA synthetase antibodies in polymyositis/dermatomyositis-associated interstitial lung disease: a retrospective case control study. PLoS One 2015;10(3):e0120313.
30. Yang Z, Lin F, Qin B, et al. Polymyositis/dermatomyositis and malignancy risk: a metaanalysis study. J Rheumatol 2015;42(2):282–91.
31. Olazagasti JM, Baez PJ, Wetter DA, et al. Cancer risk in dermatomyositis: a meta-analysis of cohort studies. Am J Clin Dermatol 2015;16(2):89–98.
32. Selva-O'Callaghan A, Trallero-Araguas E, Grau-Junyent JM, et al. Malignancy and myositis: novel autoantibodies and new insights. Curr Opin Rheumatol 2010;22(6):627–32.
33. Alemo Munters L, Alexanderson H, Crofford LJ, et al. New insights into the benefits of exercise for muscle health in patients with idiopathic inflammatory myositis. Curr Rheumatol Rep 2014;16(7):429.
34. Callen JP, Wortmann RL. Dermatomyositis. Clin Dermatol 2006;24(5):363–73.
35. Lundberg IE, Vencovsky J, Alexanderson H. Therapy of myositis: biological and physical. Curr Opin Rheumatol 2014;26(6):704–11.
36. Hornung T, Janzen V, Heidgen FJ, et al. Remission of recalcitrant dermatomyositis treated with ruxolitinib. N Engl J Med 2014;371(26):2537–8.
37. Johnson W, Jacobe H. Morphea in adults and children cohort II: patients with morphea experience delay in diagnosis and large variation in treatment. J Am Acad Dermatol 2012;67(5):881–9.
38. Vasquez R, Sendejo C, Jacobe H. Morphea and other localized forms of scleroderma. Curr Opin Rheumatol 2012;24(6):685–93.
39. Nouri S, Jacobe H. Recent developments in diagnosis and assessment of morphea. Curr Rheumatol Rep 2013;15(2):308.
40. Chiu YE, Vora S, Kwon EK, et al. A significant proportion of children with morphea en coup de sabre and Parry-Romberg syndrome have neuroimaging findings. Pediatr Dermatol 2012;29(6):738–48.
41. Polcari I, Moon A, Mathes EF, et al. Headaches as a presenting symptom of linear morphea en coup de sabre. Pediatrics 2014;134(6):e1715–9.
42. Lis-Swiety A, Mierzwinska K, Wodok-Wieczorek K, et al. Co-existence of lichen sclerosus and localized scleroderma in female monozygotic twins. J Pediatr Adolesc Gynecol 2014;27(6):e133–6.
43. Saxton-Daniels S, Jacobe HT. An evaluation of long-term outcomes in adults with pediatric-onset morphea. Arch Dermatol 2010;146(9):1044–5.

44. McNiff JM, Glusac EJ, Lazova RZ, et al. Morphea limited to the superficial reticular dermis: an underrecognized histologic phenomenon. Am J Dermatopathol 1999;21(4):315–9.

45. Fernandez-Flores A, Gatica-Torres M, Tinoco-Fragoso F, et al. Three cases of bullous morphea: histopathologic findings with implications regarding pathogenesis. J Cutan Pathol 2015;42(2):144–9.

46. Chiu HY, Tsai TF. Images in clinical medicine. Keloidal morphea. N Engl J Med 2011;364(14):e28.

47. Wriston CC, Rubin AI, Elenitsas R, et al. Nodular scleroderma: a report of 2 cases. Am J Dermatopathol 2008;30(4):385–8.

48. Chiu YE. Practice gaps: evaluating the clinical utility of autoantibodies in morphea. JAMA Dermatol 2013;149(10):1166.

49. Fett N, Werth VP. Update on morphea: part II. Outcome measures and treatment. J Am Acad Dermatol 2011;64(2):231–42 [quiz: 243–4].

Common Dermatologic Procedures

Shelley Yang, MD, Jeremy Kampp, MD*

KEYWORDS

- Dermatologic procedures • Skin biopsy • Punch biopsy • Shave biopsy • Excision
- Curettage • Cryosurgery • Cryotherapy

KEY POINTS

- Performance of skin biopsies is a fundamental skill for all physicians who manage skin conditions.
- Esthetic procedures comprise a minority of most dermatologists' practices, although a wide array of procedures is available and growing.
- Choice of a biopsy technique is based on the type of skin lesion, anatomic site, and desired histologic information.
- Postoperative care and instructions minimize the risk of complications.

INTRODUCTION

Procedural training is an essential component of a dermatologist's education and practice. Procedures are performed in an outpatient setting and can range from the basic skin biopsy to advanced flaps and reconstructions. This article reviews common procedures performed by dermatologists, focusing on biopsies, which are also highly relevant and fundamental skills for all physicians who manage skin conditions.

PATIENT PREPARATION

A thorough preoperative evaluation is required before any procedure. Medical history should include information on drug allergies, current medications, presence of a pacemaker or implantable defibrillator, prosthetic devices, history of wound infections, or postoperative bleeding.

The risk of thrombotic events from discontinuing antithrombotic medications may outweigh the increased risk of bleeding.[1] Patients taking aspirin for primary prevention

The authors have nothing to disclose.
Division of Dermatology, University of Washington School of Medicine, Seattle, WA 98105, USA
* Corresponding author. UW Dermatology Center, 4225 Roosevelt Way Northeast, 4th floor, Seattle, WA 98105.
E-mail address: Jkampp@uw.edu

Med Clin N Am 99 (2015) 1305–1321
http://dx.doi.org/10.1016/j.mcna.2015.07.004
0025-7125/15/$ – see front matter © 2015 Elsevier Inc. All rights reserved.

medical.theclinics.com

may discontinue use 2 weeks before surgery, but this is not necessary for minor procedures such as biopsies. Some supplements, such as ginkgo and ginseng, can increase the risk of perioperative bleeding and should be discontinued several weeks before surgery.

Commonly used agents for antisepsis are addressed in **Table 1**.

SKIN ANESTHESIA

Lidocaine is the most commonly used local anesthetic in dermatologic surgery and has a rapid onset of action and intermediate duration. Longer-acting anesthetics, such as bupivacaine, have a delayed onset and may be used with lidocaine to maximize anesthesia duration.

Epinephrine is often added to local anesthetics to decrease bleeding through vasoconstriction, thereby prolonging anesthesia duration and decreasing systemic absorption of lidocaine. Vasoconstriction onset takes 15 minutes, thus adequate time must be allocated before starting the procedure. Epinephrine should be used cautiously in pregnancy and in patients with severe hypertension, peripheral vascular disease, or narrow-angle glaucoma. Multiple reviews have not identified evidence to support the dogma that epinephrine is contraindicated in the digits, ear, nose, and genitals due to risk of necrosis.[2–4]

Usually 1% lidocaine is used, but 0.5% lidocaine with 1:200,000 epinephrine has been shown to provide equivalent anesthesia to 1% lidocaine with 1:100,000 epinephrine. The maximum safe dosage is generally accepted as 5 mg/kg of 1% plain lidocaine and 7 mg/kg of 1% lidocaine with epinephrine. Refer to **Box 1** for strategies to minimize injection site pain and **Table 2** for potential injection side effects.

BIOPSIES

The skin biopsy is an essential procedure for clinical-histopathological correlation. Approaches include shave, saucerization, punch, and incisional biopsies.[5] It is always important to send any sampled specimens for pathologic evaluation.

Biopsies are indicated for suspected neoplastic lesions, for bullous disorders, and to help establish a diagnosis when the cutaneous disorder is unclear.[6] Although in most cases the purpose of a biopsy is to obtain a sample, in some situations the biopsy procedure itself may be curative. There are few absolute contraindications. Biopsies generally should not be performed at an infected site. Caution must be

Table 1 Commonly used agents for antisepsis		
Agent	**Advantages**	**Disadvantages**
Isopropyl alcohol	Inexpensive, commonly used for minor clean procedures, immediate effect	Weak antimicrobial activity, not recommended for extensive procedures, skin must remain wet for 2 min for maximum effect[5]
Chlorhexidine	Broad-spectrum activity against gram-positive and gram-negative organisms, rapid onset and prolonged activity	Should not be used near the ears or eyes due to risk of keratitis and ototoxicity
Povidone-iodine	Broad spectrum antimicrobial activity	Must dry and cannot be wiped off to be effective, skin irritant, leaves residual color

Box 1
Minimizing injection site pain
Use a small-gauge needle (30 gauge)
Add sodium bicarbonate (8.4%) at a 1:10 ratio to lidocaine
Apply ice, ethyl chloride, or vibratory distraction at the injection site
Inject slowly into the subcutaneous tissue rather than the dermis
Place subsequent injections in an already anesthetized location

exercised for patients with bleeding diatheses, including anticoagulant or platelet inhibitor use and thrombocytopenia. Even then, excessive bleeding is rarely a problem.

Appropriate site selection is critical to yielding accurate and relevant histologic information. Biopsy technique must take into consideration the anticipated depth of the lesion. For example, a pedunculated lesion may be biopsied via a superficial shave, but a deeper biopsy that includes subcutaneous tissue would be necessary for a suspected process such as panniculitis.

SHAVE BIOPSY

Shave and punch biopsies are the most commonly used biopsy techniques. Shave biopsies can be superficial or deep. Superficial shave biopsies are usually performed for raised lesions that are epidermal without suspected dermal extension, such as skin tags, seborrheic keratosis, actinic keratosis, and superficial basal cell carcinomas (BCC). They are not appropriate for pigmented, suspected melanocytic lesions. A superficial shave removes a thin disk of tissue across the skin surface, extending into the epidermis and a limited amount of superficial dermis. The goal is to create a shallow defect and obtain a single piece of unfragmented tissue with smooth edges. Anesthetic may be injected to create a wheal, thus raising the lesion to facilitate the shave. A slightly bent, double-edged razor blade, or number 15 blade on a scalpel held tangential to the surface may be used (**Fig. 1**).

The double-edged razor blade is flexible, and depth can be adjusted by increasing or decreasing the convexity of the blade. The blade is held with a slight bend and at a

Table 2	
Side effects of anesthesia	
Side Effect	**Comments**
Injection site pain	Please see **Box 1**
Vasovagal reactions	Lie patient flat during injection to reduce risk of vasovagal reaction. If vasovagal reaction occurs, apply cold compresses and place the patient in Trendelenburg position
Reported allergy	Obtain a thorough history of the reported allergy; most patients actually report a vasovagal reaction or epinephrine sensitivity rather than a true allergy. Most true allergies to local anesthetics have been reported with the ester class of anesthetics (eg, Procaine) due to the metabolite para-aminobenzoic acid, which does not cross-react with amides (eg, Lidocaine). True allergy to amides is very rare. If local anesthetic use is contraindicated, intradermal injection with diphenhydramine can be used

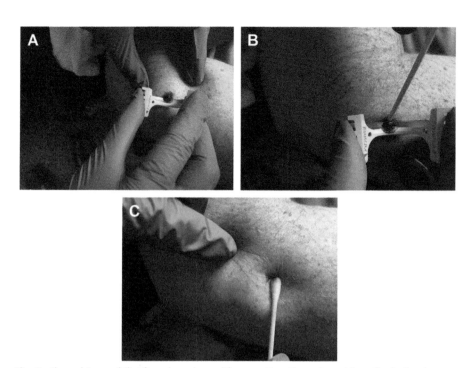

Fig. 1. Shave biopsy. (*A*) After cleansing with an antiseptic and marking, the lesion is anesthetized with lidocaine, usually with epinephrine and sodium bicarbonate. A slightly bent double-edged razor blade is held tangential to the surface, incising with a smooth back-and-forth motion, first only through the epidermis, before turning to a horizontal plane. (*B*) The shave biopsy specimen is removed by reversing the low angle to incise through the epidermis on the opposite side. To help stabilize the lesion, provide traction, and prevent tearing, forceps or the wooden end of a cotton-tipped applicator can be placed at the end of the lesion. (*C*) Aluminum chloride 20% solution is applied with firm pressure to achieve hemostasis.

low planing angle to the skin surface, incising with a smooth back and forth motion, first only through the epidermis, before turning to a horizontal plane. The shave biopsy specimen is removed by reversing the low angle to incise through the epidermis on the opposite side. To help stabilize the lesion, provide traction, and prevent tearing, forceps or the wooden end of a cotton-tipped applicator can be placed at the end of the lesion.

A deeper shave biopsy, also termed saucerization, allows more sampling of the dermis and is used for suspected BCC and squamous cell carcinomas (SCC), in which it is important to distinguish between in situ and invasive malignancy. The blade is bent further than for a superficial shave and then is moved forward in a smooth sawing motion, turning the blade up toward the surface to finish the biopsy.

Scissor or snip biopsy can be used for pedunculated lesions that are suspected to be benign growths, such as acrochordons (skin tags) and filiform warts. The lesion is first stabilized with toothed forceps and then cut at the base. The specimen is placed in the appropriate medium (**Table 3**).

Hemostasis for shave biopsies is usually obtained with aluminum chloride 20% solution. Aluminum chloride is more effective on a dry wound bed; thus, it is important to

Table 3	
Specimen processing	
Proposed Test	**Carrier Medium**
Routine light microscopy, immunohistochemistry, polymerase chain reaction	10% Buffered formalin
Direct immunofluorescence	Michel medium or fresh
Flow cytometry	Fresh
Culture for mycobacteria, fungi, bacteria	Fresh
Virus	Viral transport medium
Electron microscopy	Glutaraldehyde

Adapted from Olbricht S. Biopsy techniques and basic excisions. In: Bolognia J, Jorizzo JL, Schaffer JV, eds. Dermatology. Philadelphia: Elsevier Saunders; 2012.

blot away visible blood and then apply the aluminum chloride with firm pressure using gauze or a cotton-tipped applicator. **Box 2** lists common pitfalls in shave biopsies.

PUNCH BIOPSY

Punch biopsies yield full-thickness samples and can be used for lesions that require dermal or subcutaneous tissue for diagnosis. Sampling most of the lesion is desirable, but for large-sized suspected tumors, multiple "scouting" punch biopsies may be required.

A disposable instrument with a circular blade extends through the dermis to the subcutaneous fat to obtain a cylindrical specimen. The volume of tissue obtained varies depending on the diameter of the metal barrel. In general, punch biopsies smaller than 4 mm have a higher risk of yielding insufficient tissue for an accurate histologic diagnosis. For most punch biopsies, a 4-mm diameter is adequate. A larger diameter punch biopsy increases the likelihood of obtaining subcutaneous fat.

After marking, cleansing, and anesthetizing the skin, the lesion is stabilized with the thumb and forefinger and stretched slightly perpendicular to the relaxed skin tension lines (**Fig. 2**). This method helps create an oval, as opposed to a round, defect once the tissue is removed. The punch instrument is placed perpendicular to the skin. Gentle downward pressure is applied with a circular twisting motion. When the instrument reaches the subcutaneous fat, there is a sudden decrease in resistance. The punch instrument is removed and set aside. The core of the punched tissue is elevated gently at one superficial edge with forceps and detached at the base with small tissue scissors. Careful attention must be paid to avoid crushing the specimen with the forceps, which can distort histology.

After hemostasis is achieved with pressure, the wound is usually closed with 1 or 2 simple interrupted epidermal sutures, although healing by secondary intention is an option. Suture materials vary in elasticity, knot strength, memory, plasticity, tensile

Box 2
Common pitfalls: shave biopsies
The most common error when first performing shave biopsies is achieving insufficient depth, especially in areas with thick stratum corneum, such as the palms and soles. Careful attention must be paid to the angulation of the blade.

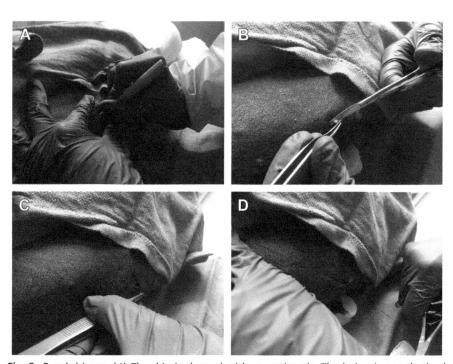

Fig. 2. Punch biopsy. (*A*) The skin is cleaned with an antiseptic. The lesion is anesthetized with lidocaine, usually with epinephrine and sodium bicarbonate. The punch biopsy instrument is held perpendicular to the surface of the lesion and rotated into the skin, usually down into the subcutaneous fat, and removed. (*B*) The specimen is gently lifted at the edge to avoid crush artifact and cut at the base. (*C, D*) The defect is closed with 1 to 2 simple interrupted epidermal sutures.

strength, tissue reactivity, infection potential, and cost (**Table 4**). Generally, 4-0 or 5-0 nylon or polypropylene monofilament suture can be used on the body and scalp, and 5-0 or 6-0 on the face, neck, or hands. Suture removal times vary depending on location (**Table 5**). Secondary intention healing has been shown to have similar cosmetic results as suturing for 1- to 4-mm punch biopsies.[7] However, healing by secondary intention healing takes longer and can result in a depressed or round scar. In sites with fragile skin, sutures may tear through the skin, and these wounds are best left to heal by secondary intention. An absorbable gelatin may be used to help achieve hemostasis by creating a matrix in which a clot can form while absorbing fluids.[8]

Special Considerations: Pigmented Lesions

Excisional biopsy, or entire removal of the lesion in question, is the preferred method for pigmented lesions suspicious for melanoma, although there are no consensus guidelines.[9] There is an increased risk of misdiagnosis and staging inaccuracy of nonexcisional biopsies compared with excisional biopsies. Up to 20% of initial partial biopsies underestimate the final Breslow depth.[10,11] The entire pigmented lesion should be removed down to the level of subcutaneous fat to allow for accurate staging. Small pigmented lesions may fit within a punch biopsy instrument; larger lesions should be excised completely using a scalpel.

Table 4 Sutures		
Classes	**Examples**	**Comments**
Absorbable	• Polyglactic acid (Vicryl) • Polydixanone (PDS) • Polyglycolic acid (Dexon) • Fast-absorbing gut	Fast-absorbing gut can be used for patients who are unable to return for suture removal
Nonabsorbable	• Nylon (Ethilon) • Polypropylene (Prolene) • Silk	• Braided sutures, including silk, have higher strength and knot security, but may harbor organisms between filaments and increase risk of infection • Silk and gut are natural materials and have high tissue reactivity

Postoperative Care

Proper wound care is important in optimizing cosmetic and functional results and helps minimize risk of complications.

Shave biopsy sites heal by second intention. The mature scar is flat or slightly depressed with slight hypopigmentation. The biopsy site should be kept moist with an occlusive ointment such as plain petrolatum, which has been shown to promote healing. Neomycin-containing ointments such as triple antibiotic ointments should be avoided in postoperative wound care because it is a common contact allergen. Bacitricin can also cause contact dermatitis, albeit at a lower frequency than neomycin. Similar rates of infection occur in patients who use petrolatum and bacitracin-containing ointment.[12–14] For deeper shave biopsies, electrodessication may be necessary to achieve hemostasis.

Antibiotic prophylaxis is generally not required for biopsies, but may be indicated for select patient populations undergoing procedures that breach the oral mucosa or on infected skin, such as with high-risk heart conditions or with recent prosthetic joint replacements.[15]

Bandaging may consist of an adhesive bandage with a central nonadherent dressing pad. For sutured wounds, a layered pressure dressing is applied. This dressing can consist of a nonadherent pad, followed by gauze, and dressing retention tape. Showering is permitted after 24 hours. The biopsy site may be cleansed gently with soap and water daily, followed by occlusive ointment and a bandage, until sutures are removed or the wound has re-epithelialized. In addition to verbal instructions, patients should receive written wound care instructions, including reasons to contact clinical staff if complications occur.

Complications

The complications of skin biopsies include bleeding, pain, infection, and scarring. The risk of postoperative hemorrhage was 0.1% for biopsies in one multicenter study.[16]

Table 5 Time to suture removal	
Location	**Days to Removal**
Face	5–7
Trunk, upper extremities, scalp	7–10
Back, lower extremities	12–14

Infection occurs rarely, in less than 1% of most procedures.[17] Biopsies on the lower limbs, lymphedematous or intertriginous areas, and ears are at higher risk of infections.

Pain is usually minimal. Paresthesias may occur rarely and can persist for months, especially on the forehead.[5] Wound dehiscence can occur and can be caused by infection, excessive tension, hematoma, or poor healing. Dehisced wounds may heal by secondary intention, and a delayed reconstruction can be attempted after inflammation resolves. Irritant or allergic reactions can occur, usually caused by topical antibiotics, tapes, and bandages. Tissue reactivity to suture material may also mimic a wound infection. Widened scars can occur in areas with higher skin tension, such as the back, shoulders, and breasts. Hypertrophic scars and keloids occur more commonly in the head and neck region, upper chest and back, and shoulders. The potential for keloid formation should be discussed in advance in those who are more susceptible (eg, African ethnicity) and having a procedure in the above-described locations.

Once the pathology report from the biopsy is received, the results should be discussed with the patient.

EXCISIONS

Excisional biopsy can be used to remove entire lesions for pathology and is the preferred technique for atypical pigmented lesions suspicious for melanoma. In this case, one is looking to acquire a narrowly clear margin (1–2 mm) for complete histologic analysis. Excisions are often the treatment for biopsy-proven cutaneous malignancies. Recommended margins depend on the clinical diagnosis. A small BCC or SCC is generally cured with a 4- to 5-mm visible surgical margin.[18] Moderately atypical nevi are excised with 3-mm margins, severely atypical nevi, or melanoma in situ with 5-mm margins, and thin invasive melanoma (Breslow depth ≤1.0 mm) with 1-cm margins.[19]

An excision is ideally designed as a fusiform shape, with a length-to-width ratio of 3 to 1 and the apical angles less than 30°. The line of closure is placed along relaxed skin tension lines, within skin folds or wrinkles, boundaries between cosmetic units, and following patterns of hair growth.[20] Precise, tension-free approximation of the skin edges allows for re-epithelialization and a barely visible scar.[21]

Intradermal interrupted buried stitches using absorbable sutures are placed after excision. The epidermis is then closed with superficial simple interrupted or running sutures.

Complications of excisions can include hematoma, infection, wound dehiscence, skin necrosis, suture reaction, excessive granulation tissue, contact dermatitis from tape adhesive or topical antibiotics, and hypertrophic scar or keloid. These risks, plus the possibility of recurrence of tumor, even with histologically negative surgical margins, must be discussed with the patient in advance as part of informed consent. An expanding hematoma may require removal of sutures for evacuation and electrocoagulation to stop bleeding arterioles. Skin necrosis can occur because of excessive tension and inadequate arterial supply. The superficial eschar acts as a biological dressing and should not be debrided. **Box 3** lists common pitfalls in suture reactions.

CURETTAGE

The curette is a round, semisharp device that is suitable for soft or friable lesions such as warts, skin tags, seborrheic keratosis, and molluscum contagiosum. It can be paired with electrodessication in the treatment of superficial BCC and SCC in situ.

> **Box 3**
> **Common pitfalls: suture reactions**
>
> Suture reaction may be mistaken for infection. Suture spitting results from deep sutures placed too high in the dermis and can occur weeks to several months after surgery. Suture granulomas present 1 to 3 months postoperatively as a pink papule or pustule along suture lines; they may resolve spontaneously or can be treated with intralesional steroid injections, or lancing the papule followed by suture removal.

Curettage for carcinoma is not an appropriate modality for infiltrative and micronodular types of BCC or invasive SCC. It is also not recommended on hair-bearing sites, because of possible extension down follicular units. It is not appropriate for treating recurrent tumors, lesions larger than 2 cm in diameter, tumors extending into the fat, lesions at sites of high risk for recurrence such as the face, or lesions with poorly defined borders.[22,23] A disadvantage is the lack of histologic confirmation of surgical margins.

Curette sizes vary from 0.5 to 10 mm, and typically a 3- to 5-mm curette is used, with smaller curettes used for smaller lesions. Multiple passes should be performed in several directions to ensure complete destruction of the tumor. A larger curette can be used for debulking, followed by a smaller curette to remove residual foci. Cancer cells are soft and less cohesive. When complete, the firm sensation of normal dermis can be felt, and punctate dermal bleeding occurs. If the subcutis is reached, excision should be performed, because the ability to reliably distinguish residual tumor from the more firm and curettage-resistant dermis is lost.

CRYOSURGERY

Cryosurgery is the localized application of liquid nitrogen to achieve destruction of skin lesions. It is a rapid and simple technique used for the treatment of benign lesions, such as small skin tags, warts, and seborrheic keratoses, and premalignant lesions, such as actinic keratoses. Liquid nitrogen exists at a temperature of $-195°C$ and induces tissue temperatures ranging from $-50°C$ to $-60°C$, which are adequate for tissue destruction.[24] Cell destruction results from intracellular and extracellular ice crystal formation, cellular dehydration, and protein and enzymatic denaturization.[25] Tissue damage is maximized with a slow thaw time. Multiple freeze–thaw cycles can further increase damage to the target.

Local anesthesia is usually not necessary, but may be recommended if large areas are being treated. Cryotherapy techniques include intralesional, direct-contact, and open-spray. The open-spray technique uses a hand-held device that permits insulated storage of liquid nitrogen attached to a nozzle that allows a constant rate of nitrogen vapor spray. The nozzle is adjustable to alter the size of the stream. A cone or disposable otoscope speculum can be used to help focus the delivery, resulting in less damage to uninvolved skin. Frozen areas will turn white, creating a cup-shaped ball of ice with a radius similar to the depth. The spray is directed at a 90° angle at a distance of 1 to 2 cm from the targeted lesion (**Fig. 3**). Pulse, continuous, spiral, and paintbrush techniques can be used.[26] A cotton-tipped applicator dipped in liquid nitrogen can be applied directly to the lesion and may offer a less frightening method than the spray for younger children. The degree of the freeze can be controlled by adjusting cotton-tip applicator pressure applied and length of skin contact. There is no consensus on the number of freeze-thaw cycles, the amount of surrounding tissue that should be

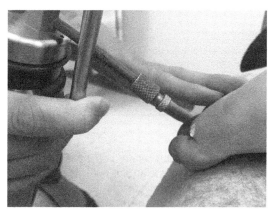

Fig. 3. Cryotherapy. The spray from the cryogun is directed at a 90° angle at a distance of 1 to 2 cm from the targeted lesion.

frozen, or the appropriate thaw time. In general, 2 freeze–thaw cycles with a freeze time of 10 to 15 seconds, and a complete thaw (30–60 seconds) in between is used.

Cryotherapy is effective in the treatment of actinic keratosis, with a cure rate of 99%.[27] Cryosurgery for genital warts and common warts has a cure rate of 60% to 86%.[28] Several treatment sessions may be necessary depending on the size and location of the warts, with plantar warts requiring the longest course of treatment. Paring down a hyperkeratotic wart before application of the cryogen may be beneficial.

There are few contraindications to cryosurgery but may include patients who are pain averse or for lesions with large areas involved. **Box 4** and **Table 6** summarize common reactions and possible complications of cryotherapy.

INTRALESIONAL STEROID INJECTIONS

Intralesional corticosteroid injections are a simple procedure used for a wide range of dermatologic conditions for their anti-inflammatory and atrophogenic properties. Common indications include hypertrophic scars, keloids, inflamed cysts, granuloma annulare, alopecia areata, lichen simplex chronicus, and prurigo nodularis. Intralesional therapy deposits the medication directly into a lesion with minimal systemic effects. The skin acts as a steroid reservoir, allowing the medication to be delivered over a period of time. Triamcinolone acetonide is the most widely used corticosteroid for intralesional injections. It is available as a micronized suspension with small corticosteroid particles that persist for extended periods of time after

---

Box 4
Reactions after cryotherapy

Immediate burning pain

Erythema

Edema

Blistering

Table 6	
Complications of cryotherapy	
Complication	**Comments**
Hypopigmentation	May be more prominent on darker skin. Melanocytes are sensitive to cold injury at −5°C, whereas malignant cells are damaged at −50°C
Nerve injury	Especially in locations with superficial nerves, such as the lateral sides of the digits. Tenting the skin up and away from the nerve may decrease the risk of nerve injury
Recurrence of the lesion	Some lesions, such as warts, may require multiple treatments before complete resolution
Alopecia	If hair follicles are destroyed
Paresthesias	—
Scarring	—

deposition, which is suitable for the treatment of chronic inflammatory dermatoses. Intralesional steroids decrease collagen synthesis and inhibit fibroblast proliferation, which can be desired in the setting of hypertrophic scars or keloids, but skin atrophy can be a side effect. There is a degree of systemic absorption associated with intralesional corticosteroids, especially with large amounts of corticosteroids or frequent injections.

Most intralesional therapy is administered with a syringe and needle. The corticosteroid is shaken to evenly suspend the drug and diluted to the desired strength with saline or 0.5% to 1% lidocaine without epinephrine. Typically, a small-bore, 30- or 27-gauge needle with a 1-mL syringe is used. Thirty-gauge needles produce less discomfort; however, there is a higher risk of blockage in the needle. The injection should target the dermis, where inflammation usually occurs, rather than the epidermis or subcutaneous layer. Only tenths of a milliliter may be necessary. For larger lesions, the needle should be partially withdrawn and redirected, or reinserted. Some resistance will be felt when injecting into the dermis. Avoid injecting into the subcutaneous layer, where the atrophic effect will be more prominent without the desired therapeutic effect. The patient may experience a burning sensation after injection. Hemostasis can be achieved with pressure.

The most common side effects of intralesional corticosteroid injections are atrophy and hypopigmentation. Atrophy and pigment changes usually resolve over time but can be permanent. Darkly pigmented skin is more susceptible to pigment changes. Complications can be minimized by using the lowest concentration and smallest quantity necessary and repeating the injections every 3 to 4 weeks.[29–31]

ADVANCED DERMATOLOGIC PROCEDURES

Procedural dermatology fellowships are available to board-eligible residents who have completed dermatology and are interested in advanced training in Mohs micrographic surgery, reconstruction of surgical defects, and cosmetic procedures. The next section covers Mohs surgery and selected common cosmetic procedures. Other procedures that are performed by dermatologists, but are beyond the scope of this article, include nail surgery, electrosurgery, sclerotherapy, skin resurfacing, and hair restoration.

MOHS MICROGRAPHIC SURGERY

Mohs micrographic surgery is a surgical technique allowing precise microscopic control of the margins by combining surgery with pathology. The technique was developed by Dr Frederic E. Mohs in the 1930s, who initially used zinc chloride paste to fix tissue in vivo before surgical procedures, and has evolved over the years to become the treatment of choice for most skin cancers on the head and neck, as well as for histologically aggressive or recurrent skin cancers (**Box 5**). It offers the highest cure rate for nonmelanoma skin cancer, with a 5-year cure rate of 99% for BCC, 94% for SCC.[32,33] It is also used to remove other skin malignancies, including lentigo maligna, extramammary Paget disease, microcystic adnexal carcinoma, and dermatofibrosarcoma protuberans.

The 4 major components are surgical excision, histopathologic examination, precise mapping, and wound management. Horizontal sections allow evaluation of peripheral and deep margins compared with the standard "bread loaf" vertical sectioning. Precise margin control allows maximal preservation of normal tissue. Reconstruction of the surgical defects is performed by the Mohs surgeon after removal of the skin cancer.

ESTHETIC PROCEDURES

The public's perception that dermatologists devote most of their time performing cosmetic procedures is unsubstantiated by dermatology workforce data. On average, dermatologists spend less than 10% of their total patient care time on cosmetic treatments, and many dermatologists choose not to incorporate cosmetics into their practice at all.[34] Preoperative consultation is paramount for all esthetic procedures. It is

---

Box 5
Indications for Mohs micrographic surgery

Tumor size >2 cm

Recurrent tumors

Poorly defined clinical borders

Positive margins on previous excision

High-risk histologic features (morpheaform, micronodular, infiltrative BCC, basosquamous, poorly differentiated and deeply infiltrative SCC, perineural invasion)

Chronic scar (Marjolin ulcer)

Immunocompromised patients

Prior radiated skin

Patients with genetic syndromes (eg, basal cell nevus syndrome, xeroderma pigmentosum)

Mask areas of face (central face, eyelids [including inner/outer canthi], eyebrows, nose, lips [cutaneous/mucosal/vermillion], chin, ear and periauricular skin/sulci, temple), genitalia (including perineal and perianal), hands, feet, nail units, ankles, and nipples/areola

Data from Ad Hoc Task Force, Connolly SM, Baker DR, et al. AAD/ACMS/ASDSA/ASMS 2012 appropriate use criteria for Mohs micrographic surgery: a report of the American Academy of Dermatology, American College of Mohs Surgery, American Society for Dermatologic Surgery Association, and the American Society for Mohs Surgery. J Am Acad Dermatol 2012;67;531–50.

important to evaluate patients carefully in order to determine if a procedure is indicated. Relative contraindications include unrealistic expectations or body dysmorphic disorder. The patient must be counseled on the potential benefits, limitations, and risks of the procedure.

Chemical Denervation

Botulinum toxin (BTX) is an injectable protein derived from neurotoxins produced by *Clostridium botulinum*. BTX weakens or paralyzes skeletal muscle through the inhibition of the release of acetylcholine from the presynaptic motor neuron, resulting in chemodenervation and paralysis of the treated muscle. The effects are transient; new nerve terminals form over time, creating new neuromuscular junctions and restoration of muscular function within a few months. BTX was initially used clinically in the treatment of strabismus,[35] and subsequently for numerous medical conditions such as cervical dystonia, blepharospasm, hemifacial spasm, migraine headaches, and hyperhidrosis.

Cosmetic use of BTX is predominantly for treatment of dynamic rhytids (wrinkles) on the upper third of the face. Results last from 3 to 6 months. When used appropriately, BTX has an excellent safety profile.[36] Side effects are usually temporary and mild and include injection site swelling or bruising, mild headache, or flulike symptoms.[37] Unintended muscle function impairment may occur, but is usually associated with poor technique. Although the risk of serious adverse effects is low, side effects such as dysphagia, aspiration, pneumonia, anaphylaxis, botulism, and death have been reported.[38]

Soft Tissue Augmentation

Facial aging results in progressive loss of tissue volume due to atrophy and displacement of subcutaneous fat. Soft tissue fillers may be used to replace lost volume on the face, such as within the glabellar lines and nasolabial folds, as well as other non-facial sites, such as the hands. Other therapeutic applications include HIV-associated lipoatrophy and facial scarring from acne. Numerous types of soft tissue fillers are available to correct contour abnormalities and provide cosmetic enhancement. Filler selection is determined by the defect type and desired effect duration (**Table 7**).

Lasers

Lasers are used for a variety of dermatologic conditions, including treatment of vascular lesions and pigmented lesions, hair removal, and ablative laser resurfacing. By definition, lasers are monochromatic, collimated, and coherent—that is, only one nondivergent wavelength is aligned in phase with peaks and troughs of the light.

Lasers are chosen by matching the particular wavelength with the absorption spectrum of the desired target. Longer wavelengths penetrate deeper into the skin. In selective photothermolysis, energy is absorbed and concentrated in the target by a light-absorbing structure called a chromophore (**Table 8**).[39] The target's thermal relaxation time should be greater than the pulse duration to confine heating and damage to the target.

Depending on the type of lesion treated, treatments every 4 to 6 weeks may be required, with gradual improvement after each session until the desired effect has been achieved. Most common side effects are pigment changes, hypertrophic scarring, infection, pain, and lack of efficacy.

Table 7
Injectable fillers

Type	Examples	Comments	Potential Side Effects
Temporary	• Collagen • Hyaluronic acid • Calcium hydroxylapatite • Poly-L-lactic acid	• Biodegradable • Most range in duration of 6–24 mo • Hyaluronic acid fillers are the most commonly used temporary fillers • Collagen and hyaluronic acids function through a volume-filling effect, whereas calcium hydroxylapatite provides scaffolding for endogenous collagen formation • Bovine collagen requires pretesting due to risk of allergy	• Bruising, hypersensitivity, granuloma formation, infection, and hematoma • Compression or obstruction of blood vessels can result in tissue necrosis, and aspiration before injection is important to prevent accidental infiltration into a vessel[42] • If the filler is placed improperly or excessively, hyaluronidase injections can be used to remove the agent[43]
Permanent	• Hydrogel polymers • Liquid injectable silicone • Autologous fat transfer	Aging results in structural changes over time, and temporary fillers offer the clinician flexibility to adjust placement	Permanent fillers persist indefinitely, but the effects, if undesired, are difficult to reverse and may require surgery

Chemical Peels

Chemical peels involve the application of chemical agents to produce controlled partial thickness injury. The subsequent regeneration results in an evening of pigmentation and improvement of skin texture. Peels are categorized by their intended depth of injury and are used in the treatment of photoaging, pigmentary dyschromias, rhytids, and actinic keratosis (**Table 9** lists indications per depth achieved). The main complications of peels are reactive hyperpigmentation and scarring. Reactive hyperpigmentation can occur after any depth of peel and occurs more frequently in skin with darker pigmentation. Patients with a history of herpes simplex infection are treated prophylactically with acyclovir or valacyclovir.[40,41]

Table 8
Lasers and target chromophores

Laser	Chromophore	Absorption Peaks (Nm)
Pulsed dye (PDL), potassium titanyl phosphate (KTP), copper vapor, argon	Hemoglobin	418, 542, 577
Neodymium-doped yttrium aluminum garnet (Nd:YAG), ruby, alexandrite, diode, PDL, KTP	Melanosome	300–1000 nm (Peak at 335)
CO_2, long-pulsed Nd:YAG, erbium, diode	Water	1450, 1950, 3000

Table 9
Chemical peels

Depth of Peel	Depth of Injury	Examples	Comments
Superficial	Epidermis, may reach papillary dermis	• Glycolic acid 70% • Salicylic acid 20%–30% • Trichloroacetic acid (TCA) 10%–25% • Jessner solution, a combination of resorcinol, salicylic acid, and lactic acid in ethanol	• May improve mild photoaging, pigmentary dyschromias • Often need multiple treatments to reach a desired result due to the superficial nature and limited wounding
Medium	Papillary dermis	Jessner solution or glycolic acid, followed by 35% TCA	Used for moderate photoaging, pigmentary dyschromia
Deep	Midreticular dermis	Baker–Gordon formula peel, consists of phenol, distilled water, septisol liquid soap, and croton oil	• May improve severe photodamage and advanced rhytides • Produce significant injury and patients have an extended period of post-treatment healing • Phenol can produce cardiac arrhythmias; thus full cardiopulmonary monitoring is required, and intravenous fluids are given preceding and after the peel to limit serum concentrations of phenol. Peeling slowly by cosmetic subunits over a total time of 60–90 min may reduce the risk[44]

SUMMARY

Dermatologists perform a wide variety of procedures on a daily basis. The skin biopsy is a fundamental technique that can be performed by all physicians who manage cutaneous conditions. Specimens should always be sent for pathologic evaluation, regardless of whether the sampled lesion appears benign. Postoperative care and education are critical for minimizing complications.

REFERENCES

1. Alcalay J, Alkalay R. Controversies in perioperative management of blood thinners in dermatologic surgery: continue or discontinue? Dermatol Surg 2004;30: 1091–4 [discussion: 1094].
2. Krunic AL, Wang LC, Soltani K, et al. Digital anesthesia with epinephrine: an old myth revisited. J Am Acad Dermatol 2004;51:755–9.
3. Häfner H-M, Röcken M, Breuninger H. Epinephrine-supplemented local anesthetics for ear and nose surgery: clinical use without complications in more than 10,000 surgical procedures. J Dtsch Dermatol Ges 2005;3:195–9.

4. Chowdhry S, Seidenstricker L, Cooney DS, et al. Do not use epinephrine in digital blocks: myth or truth? Part II. A retrospective review of 1111 cases. Plast Reconstr Surg 2010;126:2031–4.

5. Olbricht S. Biopsy techniques and basic excisions. In: Bolognia JL, editor. Dermatology. Philadelphia: Elsevier Saunders; 2012. p. 2381–97.

6. Alguire PC, Mathes BM. Skin biopsy techniques for the internist. J Gen Intern Med 1998;13:46–54.

7. Christenson LJ, Phillips PK, Weaver AL, et al. Primary closure vs second-intention treatment of skin punch biopsy sites: a randomized trial. Arch Dermatol 2005;141: 1093–9.

8. Howe N, Cherpelis B. Obtaining rapid and effective hemostasis: part I. Update and review of topical hemostatic agents. J Am Acad Dermatol 2013;69: 659.e1–17.

9. Sellheyer K, Nelson P, Bergfeld WF. Nonspecific histopathological diagnoses: the impact of partial biopsy and the need for a consensus guideline. JAMA Dermatol 2014;150:11–2.

10. Ng PC, Barzilai DA, Ismail SA, et al. Evaluating invasive cutaneous melanoma: is the initial biopsy representative of the final depth? J Am Acad Dermatol 2003;48: 420–4.

11. Ng JC, Swain S, Dowling JP, et al. The impact of partial biopsy on histopathologic diagnosis of cutaneous melanoma: experience of an Australian tertiary referral service. Arch Dermatol 2010;146:234–9.

12. Butler L, Mowad C. Allergic contact dermatitis in dermatologic surgery: review of common allergens. Dermatitis 2013;24:215–21.

13. Del Rosso JQ. Wound care in the dermatology office: where are we in 2011? J Am Acad Dermatol 2011;64:S1–7.

14. Nijhawan RI, Smith LA, Mariwalla K. Mohs surgeons' use of topical emollients in postoperative wound care. Dermatol Surg 2013;39:1260–3.

15. Wright TI, Baddour LM, Berbari EF, et al. Antibiotic prophylaxis in dermatologic surgery: advisory statement 2008. J Am Acad Dermatol 2008;59:464–73.

16. O'Neill JL, Taheri A, Solomon JA, et al. Postoperative hemorrhage risk after outpatient dermatologic surgery procedures. Dermatol Surg 2014;40:74–6.

17. O'Neill JL, Lee YS, Solomon JA, et al. Quantifying and characterizing adverse events in dermatologic surgery. Dermatol Surg 2013;39:872–8.

18. Miller SJ. The National Comprehensive Cancer Network (NCCN) guidelines of care for nonmelanoma skin cancers. Dermatol Surg 2000;26:289–92.

19. Bichakjian CK, Halpern AC, Johnson TM, et al. Guidelines of care for the management of primary cutaneous melanoma. American Academy of Dermatology. J Am Acad Dermatol 2011;65:1032–47.

20. Goldberg LH, Alam M. Elliptical excisions: variations and the eccentric parallelogram. Arch Dermatol 2004;140:176–80.

21. Ogawa R, Akaishi S, Huang C, et al. Clinical applications of basic research that shows reducing skin tension could prevent and treat abnormal scarring: the importance of fascial/subcutaneous tensile reduction sutures and flap surgery for keloid and hypertrophic scar reconstruction. J Nippon Med Sch 2011;78:68–76.

22. Neville JA, Welch E, Leffell DJ. Management of nonmelanoma skin cancer in 2007. Nat Clin Pract Oncol 2007;4:462–9.

23. Alam M, Ratner D. Cutaneous squamous-cell carcinoma. N Engl J Med 2001;344: 975–83.

24. Telfer NR, Colver GB, Morton CA, British Association of Dermatologists. Guidelines for the management of basal cell carcinoma. Br J Dermatol 2008;159:35–48.

25. Graham GF. Cryosurgery in the management of cutaneous malignancies. Clin Dermatol 2001;19:321–7.
26. Kuflik EG. Cryosurgery updated. J Am Acad Dermatol 1994;31:925–44 [quiz: 944–6].
27. Lubritz RR, Smolewski SA. Cryosurgery cure rate of actinic keratoses. J Am Acad Dermatol 1982;7:631–2.
28. Rivera A, Tyring SK. Therapy of cutaneous human Papillomavirus infections. Dermatol Ther 2004;17:441–8.
29. Jackson SM, Nesbitt LT. Glucocorticosteroids. In: Bolognia JL, editor. Dermatology. Philadelphia: Elsevier Saunders; 2012. p. 2075–88.
30. Firooz A, Tehranchi-Nia Z, Ahmed AR. Benefits and risks of intralesional corticosteroid injection in the treatment of dermatological diseases. Clin Exp Dermatol 1995;20:363–70.
31. Richards RN. Update on intralesional steroid: focus on dermatoses. J Cutan Med Surg 2010;14:19–23.
32. Mosterd K, Krekels GA, Nieman FH, et al. Surgical excision versus Mohs' micrographic surgery for primary and recurrent basal-cell carcinoma of the face: a prospective randomised controlled trial with 5-years' follow-up. Lancet Oncol 2008;9: 1149–56.
33. Pugliano-Mauro M, Goldman G. Mohs surgery is effective for high-risk cutaneous squamous cell carcinoma. Dermatol Surg 2010;36:1544–53.
34. Brezinski EA, Harskamp CT, Ledo L, et al. Public perception of dermatologists and comparison with other medical specialties: results from a national survey. J Am Acad Dermatol 2014;71:875–81.
35. Scott AB. Botulinum toxin injection into extraocular muscles as an alternative to strabismus surgery. Ophthalmology 1980;87:1044–9.
36. Naumann M, Jankovic J. Safety of botulinum toxin type A: a systematic review and meta-analysis. Curr Med Res Opin 2004;20:981–90.
37. Brin MF, Boodhoo TI, Pogoda JM, et al. Safety and tolerability of onabotulinumtoxinA in the treatment of facial lines: a meta-analysis of individual patient data from global clinical registration studies in 1678 participants. J Am Acad Dermatol 2009;61:961–70.e1–11.
38. Coté TR, Mohan AK, Polder JA, et al. Botulinum toxin type A injections: adverse events reported to the US Food and Drug Administration in therapeutic and cosmetic cases. J Am Acad Dermatol 2005;53:407–15.
39. Anderson RR, Parrish JA. Selective photothermolysis: precise microsurgery by selective absorption of pulsed radiation. Science 1983;220:524–7.
40. Nguyen T. Dermatology procedures: microdermabrasion and chemical peels. FP Essent 2014;426:16–23.
41. Jackson A. Chemical peels. Facial Plast Surg 2014;30:26–34.
42. Bachmann F, Erdmann R, Hartmann V, et al. The spectrum of adverse reactions after treatment with injectable fillers in the glabellar region: results from the Injectable Filler Safety Study. Dermatol Surg 2009;35(Suppl 2):1629–34.
43. Hirsch RJ, Brody HJ, Carruthers JDA. Hyaluronidase in the office: a necessity for every dermasurgeon that injects hyaluronic acid. J Cosmet Laser Ther 2007;9: 182–5.
44. Landau M. Cardiac complications in deep chemical peels. Dermatol Surg 2007; 33:190–3 [discussion: 193].

Skin Cancer Epidemiology, Detection, and Management

Sumul Ashok Gandhi, MD, Jeremy Kampp, MD*

KEYWORDS

- Basal cell carcinoma • Squamous cell carcinoma • Melanoma • Mohs surgery

KEY POINTS

- Multiple forms of cutaneous malignancy exist.
- Basal cell carcinoma is the most common skin malignancy in North America.
- Malignancy incidence rates are increasing.
- Preventive measures, screening, and early detection and treatment optimize outcomes.

INTRODUCTION

Skin cancer, when defined as a single entity, is the most common malignancy in the North America. Attention has often focused on melanoma, but the keratinocyte-based malignancies of basal cell carcinomas (BCCs) and squamous cell carcinomas (SCCs) also have a profound impact on the health of the public. Bickers and colleagues[1] estimated the aggregate US direct cost to treat skin cancer in 2004 to be $1.7 billion ($291 million for melanoma and $1.45 billion for nonmelanoma skin cancer [NMSC]), with an additional $3.8 billion ($2.85 billion for melanoma and $961 million for NMSC) in indirect costs from lost productivity. Although not as commonly referenced, other cutaneous malignancies, such as Kaposi sarcoma, cutaneous lymphoma, and Merkel cell carcinoma, need to be considered when patients present with new or changing lesions. Given the dramatic increase in psychosocial and economic burden of more advanced disease, knowledge about the prevention, early detection, and prompt treatment of skin cancer is an essential tool in the armamentarium of any physician.

Conflict of interest: There are no commercial or financial conflicts of interest and no sources of funding for this work.
Division of Dermatology, University of Washington School of Medicine, Seattle, WA 98105, USA
* Corresponding author. UW Dermatology Center, 4225 Roosevelt Way Northeast, 4th Floor, Seattle, WA 98105.
E-mail address: Jkampp@uw.edu

Med Clin N Am 99 (2015) 1323–1335
http://dx.doi.org/10.1016/j.mcna.2015.06.002
medical.theclinics.com

BASAL CELL CARCINOMA
Epidemiology

Of the 3.5 million cases of NMSC diagnosed each year, 80% are basal cell cancers, making it the most common cutaneous malignancy.[2] BCC is most prevalent in fair-skinned individuals, with a lifetime risk of 33% to 39% in white men and 23% to 28% in white women in the United States.[3] Given the known effects of ultraviolet (UV) light on the development of these lesions, there is a profound geographic variation in incidence, because states in proximity to the equator, like Hawaii (422 cases per 100,000 white residents living on the island of Kauai),[4] had twice the incidence that is seen in the Midwestern regions, like Rochester, Minnesota (146 cases per 100,000).[5]

Detection

Risk factors for BCC must be elicited during history. UV light, particularly intermittent, intense UVB light exposure, is the single most important environmental risk factor for BCC. Other well-established risk factors include radiation therapy, chronic arsenic exposure, and long-term immunosuppression. In patients with early-onset or numerous BCCs, a syndromic manifestation of a genetic cause (eg, basal cell nevus syndrome) should be considered.

BCCs are recognized on routine skin examination (**Box 1**, **Fig. 1**). They classically appear as pink, pearly papules, but in some cases look only slightly different from normal skin. Pigmented BCCs commonly appear brown or black-blue and must be distinguished from melanocytic lesions by histopathologic examination.

On physical examination, nodular BCC is the classic rodent-ulcer form that comprises half of all BCCs. As it grows in size, it often ulcerates centrally, leaving a peripherally raised, pearly border with vascular prominence. Superficial or multifocal BCC commonly presents as a flat, scaly pink or red macule and can mimic several inflammatory skin conditions. The morpheaform or sclerosing variant has an indurated texture, ivory color, with telangiectatic vessels. Its borders often blend with the surrounding skin, and it is known for subclinical extension and more frequent recurrence even after surgical treatment. Delay in diagnosis frequently occurs, because morpheaform BCCs can also mimic nonmalignant lesions such as scars.

Treatment

Tumor features (**Box 2**) as well as patient preference guide appropriate therapy. Although several treatment modalities exist (**Table 1**), Mohs micrographic surgery allows complete histologic margin evaluation to ensure full removal of cancerous tissue while limiting the resection of uninvolved tissue. Mohs surgery is the treatment choice of any BCC with high-risk characteristics as defined by the National Comprehensive Cancer Network (see **Box 2**).[6] When these criteria are not met, excision provides histologic margin evaluation, with a rapidly healing and optimal cosmetic outcome. With a 4-mm margin around lesional tissue of BCCs less than 2 cm in size, Wolf and Zitelli[7] found a 98% cure rate. Although BCC metastases are infrequent, rates approach

---

Box 1
Common BCC features

- Telangiectasia
- Nonhealing, oozing, or crusted ulcerative lesion on sun-exposed skin
- Scarlike lesion without prior injury (morpheaform pattern)

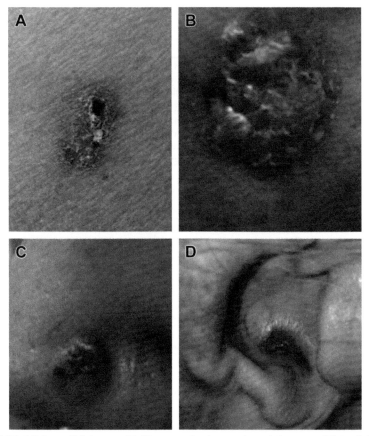

Fig. 1. BCC. (*A*) Superficial type. (*B*) Pigmented, ulcerated, nodular type. (*C*) Nodular type. (*D*) Pigmented, nodular type.

Box 2
BCC high-risk features

- Diameter greater than 20 mm on trunk and extremities
- Diameter greater than 10 mm on scalp, forehead, cheeks, or neck
- Diameter greater than 6 mm on genitals, hands, feet, or face (except as above)
- Poorly defined borders
- Recurrent tumor
- Patient immune suppression
- Prior radiation therapy to site
- Aggressive histology: morpheaform, sclerosing, infiltrative, micronodular features
- Perineural involvement

Data from Miller SJ, Alam M, Anderson J, et al. Basal cell and squamous cell skin cancers. J Natl Compr Canc Netw 2010;8:836–44.

Table 1 Common BCC treatment options	
Modality	**Description**
Mohs micrographic surgery	Complete histologic margin evaluation Maximizes tissue preservation during tumor eradication Treatment of choice for high-risk lesions May be time consuming and requires specialized training and equipment
Excision	Offers margin control but not 100% margin evaluation Margin control inferior to Mohs surgery in higher risk lesions Excision often requires larger margins and may sacrifice more normal tissue than in Mohs surgery
Electrodessication and curettage	Quick and easy No sample for histopathology: does not offer margin examination for high-risk lesions Lesion heals by secondary intent
Cryotherapy	In general reserved for smaller, lower risk lesions Quick and easy treatment No sample for histopathology: does not offer margin examination for high-risk lesions
Radiotherapy	Often used for lesions on nose, periocular area, and ear area Spares normal tissue High failure rate for lesions with aggressive histology Healing process after treatment may take weeks to months
Photodynamic therapy	Photoactivated medication results in tumor necrosis Reduced topical penetration limits utility to thin lesions
Topical agents	5-Fluorourcil Imiquimod
Oral agents	Vismodegib: competitive antagonist of smoothened receptor, a part of the sonic hedgehog pathway Systemic retinoids: isotretinoin, acitretin, etretinate

2% in lesions that are greater than 3 cm in diameter.[8] In such cases, prompt referral to a cutaneous oncology specialist is appropriate.

SQUAMOUS CELL CARCINOMA
Epidemiology

SCC is the second most common NMSC and is increasing in incidence worldwide. A study in Manitoba, Canada,[9] revealed a 266% increase in annual incidence in SCC rates in men from 1960 to 2000 and a 215% increase in the incidence rate in women during the same time. Studies estimated the number of new cases in the white population in the United States in 2012 to be between 186,000 and 419,000.[10] In the United States, lifetime risk of developing an SCC is 9% to 14% and 4% to 9% in men and women, respectively.[3] Although BCCs outnumber SCCs by a 4:1 ratio, cutaneous SCC causes more deaths and is responsible for approximately 2500 deaths in the United States each year.[11]

Detection

SCC has a multifactorial cause. The most important risk factor is cumulative sun exposure, with UVB light playing a greater role as tumor initiator and promoter than UVA. UV light produces mutations in the *p53* tumor suppressor gene, which subsequently results in proliferation of abnormal keratinocytes. Other factors in tumorigenesis include presence of scars and chronic dermatoses, exposure to several chemical compounds (arsenic, insecticides), prior radiation treatment, and human papillomavirus infection. Chronic immunosuppression, whether caused by diseases like human immunodeficiency virus (HIV)/AIDS or iatrogenic, has become increasingly important in increasing rates of SCC, with an SCC/BCC incidence ratio of 4:1, compared with the 1:4 ratio in the population at large. Patients with transplants have a mean onset to SCC development of 8 years after transplantation, with a 65-fold greater risk of immunosuppressed patients with heart and kidney transplants developing cutaneous SCC compared with the general population.[12,13] Many cases of transplant-associated SCC seem to be related to cutaneous HPV infection.

SCC can develop on any cutaneous surface but is most likely to arise in sun-exposed sites in fair-skinned individuals. SCC on nonexposed skin is more common in individuals with darker skin, in whom lesions tend to develop in areas of chronic scarring or inflammation.

Precursor lesions for SCC include actinic keratosis and SCC in situ (**Fig. 2**), which represent varying degrees of atypical keratinocyte proliferation limited to the epidermis. Classically these occur on sun-exposed skin of fair-skinned individuals as rough, scaly, red-brown, gritty papules and plaques with minimal erythema and scale.

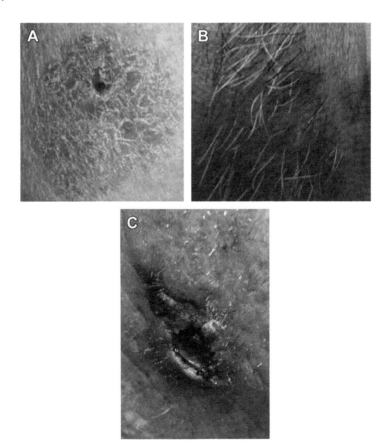

Fig. 2. SCC. (*A*) In situ. (*B*) Well-differentiated. (*C*) Moderately-differentiated.

Invasive SCC (see **Fig. 2**) can range in appearance from ill-defined, slightly elevated scaly papules and plaques to larger hyperkeratotic nodules that may show signs of ulceration. Lesions are often asymptomatic but local neurologic symptoms may indicate perineural spread. A biopsy is necessary to confirm the diagnosis.

Treatment

Treatment is intended to cure the tumor with preservation of function and cosmesis. Most patients have low-risk disease localized to the skin, which can be managed surgically in a manner similar to BCC (**Box 3**).

Mohs surgery is the preferred treatment of localized disease with high-risk features but is also indicated in lower risk tumors for which tissue-sparing is desired for cosmesis and functionality.

Standard surgical excision is also commonly used to effectively treat lower risk SCC. With 4-mm margins of grossly normal tissue excised around well-defined SCCs of less than 2 cm with no high-risk features, a cure rate of 92% was obtained for a previously untreated lesion whereas only a 77% cure rate was obtained for excision of recurrent SCCs.[14]

High-risk SCC (**Box 4**) should be treated more aggressively to maximize likelihood of cure after initial treatment. Although Mohs surgery or standard excision with margin examination may achieve local clearance, SCC treatment must further weigh the possibility of in transit, lymph node, and/or distant metastasis during the course of care. Treatment of NMSC involves long-term close follow-up to assess treatment-related complications, recurrence, and the development of new lesions. A full skin and lymph node examination should be performed every 3 to 6 months for the first 2 years, and then annually if no other signs of cancer are seen. Any suspicious lesions should be biopsied, because these patients have a much higher incidence of a second skin cancer compared with the general population, with an 18% 3-year cumulative risk of a second SCC within 3 years of detecting the first,[15] and a 50% chance of a second BCC or SCC in 5 years.[16]

MELANOMA
Epidemiology

Melanoma accounts for approximately 4.6% of all new cancers in the United States and was the fifth and sixth most common new cancer diagnosis in men and women, respectively. In 2014, approximately 76,100 Americans (43,890 men and 32,210 women) were diagnosed with melanoma. Melanoma is responsible for an estimated 9710 deaths, which represents 1.7% of all cancer-related deaths in the United States. Incidence rates for melanoma are gradually increasing, with an annual increase in

---

Box 3
SCC treatment options for localized, cutaneous disease

- Mohs micrographic surgery
- Standard surgical excision
- Electrodessication and curettage
- Cryotherapy
- Radiation therapy
- Photodynamic therapy

Box 4
SCC high-risk features

- Diameter greater than 2 cm on trunk or extremities
- Diameter greater than 1 cm on scalp, forehead, cheeks, or neck
- Diameter greater than 0.6 cm on genitals, hands, feet, or face (except as above)
- Poorly defined borders
- Recurrent tumor
- Rapid tumor growth
- Patient immune suppression
- Prior radiation therapy to site
- Moderately or poorly differentiated tumor
- Adenoid (acantholytic), adenosquamous, or desmoplastic histology
- Perineural or vascular involvement
- Depth greater than or equal to 2 mm

Data from Miller SJ, Alam M, Anderson J, et al. Basal cell and squamous cell skin cancers. J Natl Compr Canc Netw 2010;8:836–44.

---

incidence of 2.4% in men between the years 1992 and 2000; in women, an annual incidence increase of 3.9% from 1992 to 1997 was detected, with a 1.7% increase from 1997 to 2010. Although median age of diagnosis is 64 years, incidence steadily increases with age, reaching a peak of 91.2 cases per 100,000 between the ages of 80 and 84 years. Even though incidence rates have been steadily increasing, 5-year relative survival in melanoma has increased from 81.8% in 1975 to 92.8% in 2006, suggesting that patient education, early detection, and prompt treatment may play a role in increased survival rates.[17,18]

Detection

Several risk factors have been correlated with the development of melanoma. Although 10% of melanomas have a familial component, there is considerable heterogeneity in presentation, suggesting that the interaction of multiple genes with environmental factors plays a prominent role in patient presentation. Patients with 2 atypical nevi have roughly twice the risk and those with 5 atypical nevi possess more than 6 times the risk of melanoma development compared with those without any atypical moles.[19] In addition, Gandini and colleagues[19] found that patients with greater than 100 common nevi have a nearly 7-fold risk of melanoma development compared with those with fewer than 15. Evidence suggests that higher rates of melanoma are present in patients with extensive sunlight exposure, particularly in the setting of intermittent exposure with sunburn history.[20] Several studies[21] have also shown the link between indoor tanning and melanoma. Phenotypic characteristics that place patients at high risk include light skin, red or blonde hair, light eye color, and dense freckling pattern.

Melanoma can present in the eye, mucosa, and anywhere on the skin surface (**Fig. 3**). Examination should be performed with sources of bright light and magnification to view any difficult areas. The ABCDEs (asymmetry, border, color, diameter, evolving) of melanoma[22] recognition (**Table 2**) are essential to any examination, and

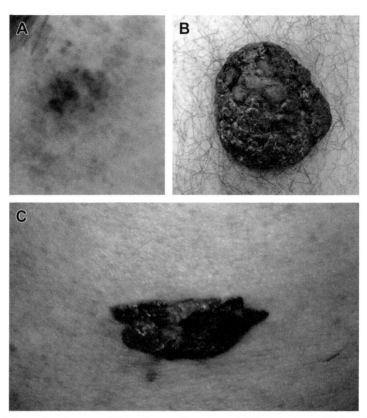

Fig. 3. Malignant melanoma. (*A*) Lentigo maligna type. (*B*) Nodular type. (*C*) Nodular type.

history should also be gathered regarding change in color, shape, and size along with irritation, redness, bleeding, or pain in any areas of concern.

Recommended screening intervals remain controversial. The American Academy of Dermatology recommends annual screening for higher risk patients, whereas the American Cancer Society recommends skin cancer examinations as part of a broader cancer-related checkup every 3 years for those between 20 and 39 years of age and

Table 2 ABCDEs of melanoma	
A = Asymmetry	One half is different from the other
B = Border	An irregular, poorly defined border
C = Color	Variegated color with shades of tan, brown, black. Occasionally has blue, white, or red features
D = Diameter	Usually >6 mm, or the size of a pencil eraser
E = Evolving	A lesion that looks different from other moles or one that is changing in size, shape, or color

Data from American Academy of Dermatology. What to look for: the ABCDEs of melanoma. Available at: https://www.aad.org/spot-skin-cancer/learn-about-skin-cancer/detect-skin-cancer/what-to-look-for. Accessed February 11, 2015.

annually after 40 years of age. Although screening can be conducted through self-examination or by any physician, the American College of Preventative Medicine recommends that health care professionals who screen patients have specific training to ensure high-quality skin examinations to increase detection and reduce unnecessary biopsies.[23]

Full excision with margins of 1 to 3 mm through the dermis to the subcutaneous fat to allow adequate measurement of depth is the preferred method of biopsy when the diagnosis of melanoma is under consideration. Full depth of lesion, and therefore avoidance of transection, is critical in prognosis (discussed later). Small biopsies can be prone to misdiagnosis and, when a larger, ill-defined melanocytic lesion is present, the most sensitive technique for definitive diagnosis may be a broad superficial shave biopsy. In this case, or any others when the nondermatologist is not comfortable managing a suspicious pigmented lesion, referral is appropriate.

Treatment

Treatment is based on clinical and histopathologic features of the tumor along with presence of lymph node involvement and local and distant metastasis as formulated

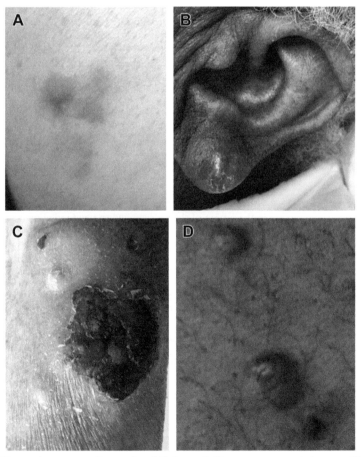

Fig. 4. Other cutaneous malignancies. (*A*) Dermatofibrosarcoma protuberans. (*B*) Merkel cell carcinoma. (*C*) Cutaneous T-cell lymphoma. (*D*) Kaposi sarcoma.

Table 3
Other cutaneous neoplasms

Neoplasm	Key Features
Merkel cell carcinoma	Rare, often lethal neuroendocrine skin cancer Risk factors: UV exposure, fair skin, immune suppression, Merkel cell polyomavirus infection Rapidly growing, firm, asymptomatic, skin-colored to red to violaceous dermal nodule Commonly on sun-exposed areas
Microcystic adnexal carcinoma	Typically located on face, with preference for upper lip Most commonly occurs in adults in their sixties, with female predominance Ill-defined indurated plaque or nodule with slow growth Prominent subclinical extension
Sebaceous carcinoma	Most commonly on the eyelid Slow-growing firm nodule, often ulcerated Strong association with Muir-Torre syndrome
Paget disease	Mammary and extramammary forms Extramammary form commonly affects vulva or scrotum, perineum, and/or axillae Mammary form commonly associated with breast mass or abnormal mammogram Appears as a nonresolving dermatitis; an erythematous scaly plaque that may become ulcerated, edematous, or macerated

Kaposi sarcoma	• Reactive, multifocal, vascular, neoplastic process thought to originate from endothelial cell infected with human herpes virus 8
	• Varying appearance: well-defined red to violaceous bruiselike patches to firm indurated subcutaneous nodules
	• Four types:
	  1. Epidemic: AIDS related
	  2. Iatrogenic: immune suppression related
	  3. Classic: in elderly of Mediterranean descent
	  4. Endemic: occurs in Africa, not HIV related

Angiosarcoma	Rare, aggressive tumor that occurs on head and neck in elderly and in the setting of chronic lymphedema and radiation Ill-defined nonhealing bruiselike lesions or facial edema with minimal erythema. Advanced lesions may form nodules. Often ulcerated Extensive subclinical spread is common
Dermatofibrosarcoma protuberans	Slow-growing flesh-colored to violaceous firm papule or plaque that progresses to a deep multinodular mass Often on trunk or extremities Rarely metastasizes
Atypical fibroxanthoma	Locally aggressive red plaque or nodule on sun-exposed skin. Often ulcerated Common seen in elderly Rare metastasis
Malignant fibrous histiocytoma	Also known as undifferentiated pleomorphic sarcoma Most common soft tissue sarcoma in adults

(continued on next page)

Table 3 (continued)	
Neoplasm	**Key Features**
	Deep subcutaneous mass, often occurring on extremities
	Aggressive tumor with potential for metastasis
Leiomyosarcoma	Pink dermal or subcutaneous nodule
	Most commonly found on extremities
Cutaneous lymphoma (mycosis fungoides)	Most commonly cutaneous T-cell lymphoma, of which mycosis fungoides is the most common variant
	Mycosis fungoides presents similarly to inflammatory dermatoses but is often recalcitrant to treatment and may indolently progress from patches to plaques and tumor nodules
	Classically affects breasts, buttocks, and intertriginous regions
	May progress to Sézary syndrome, an aggressive leukemic variant of cutaneous T-cell lymphoma that presents with erythroderma, edema, palmoplantar keratoderma, and fine scale

by the American Joint Committee on Cancer. Sentinel lymph node biopsy is widely used for the staging of clinically node-negative primary melanomas that have high-risk features with respect to tumor thickness, ulceration, and mitoses.

Early wide location excision based on Breslow thickness (thickness of tumor from the stratum granulosum) is the mainstay of treatment. However, in the lentigo maligna and acral lentiginous forms of melanoma, subclinical extension and asymmetric growth are often prominent. In these cases, Mohs micrographic surgery or staged excision with examination of permanent histologic sections may be considered. In patients who may not tolerate surgery, topical therapy with imiquimod and/or radiotherapy may be considered.

Adjuvant chemotherapy, immune therapy, or vaccine therapy should be considered in patients with high risk of tumor recurrence; most commonly those with positive nodes or in node-negative melanoma with greater than 4 mm Breslow depth. Treatment of metastatic disease varies based on extent of disease involvement.

Patients with history of melanoma need to be followed closely given the risk of recurrence and metastasis, as well as development of other forms of skin cancer. Individuals with prominent atypical and/or numerous nevi may benefit form having their cutaneous surface photographed to serve as a baseline with which future examinations can be compared. Patients with melanoma should initially be followed every 2 to 6 months depending on the characteristics of the lesion, but, even in the absence of tumor recurrence, every patient should be monitored annually.

OTHER CUTANEOUS NEOPLASMS

Any cell type in skin has the potential for disordered growth, and, as such, cutaneous neoplasia is broad in scope (**Fig. 4**, **Table 3**). Although the malignant potential of each neoplasm may vary, prompt biopsy and treatment are essential in each case.

SUMMARY

Although the signs and symptoms of the 3 most common skin malignancies are well known to physicians, any new or changing lesions should be monitored and worked up to rule out varying forms of cutaneous malignancy. Classic presenting features of each condition exist, but patients may present with overlapping or atypical features, and a biopsy is almost always required to definitively determine the true nature of each disorder. Given the intense psychosocial ramifications of skin cancer diagnosis and treatment, early detection remains the hallmark in producing favorable outcomes.

REFERENCES

1. Bickers DR, Lim HW, Margolis D, et al. The burden of skin diseases: 2004 a joint project of the American Academy of Dermatology Association and the Society for Investigative Dermatology. J Am Acad Dermatol 2006;55(3):490–500.
2. American Skin Cancer: Skin cancer– basal and squamous cell cancers. Available at: http://www.cancer.org/cancer. Accessed February 10, 2015.
3. Miller DL, Weinstock MA. Nonmelanoma skin cancer in the United States: incidence. J Am Acad Dermatol 1994;30(5 Pt 1):774–8.
4. Reizner GT, Chuang TY, Elpern DJ, et al. Basal cell carcinoma in Kauai, Hawaii: the highest documented incidence in the United States. J Am Acad Dermatol 1993;29(2 Pt 1):184.
5. Chuang TY, Popescu A, Su WP, et al. Basal cell carcinoma. A population based study in Rochester, Minnesota. J Am Acad Dermatol 1990;22(3):413.
6. Miller SJ, Alam M, Anderson J, et al. Basal cell and squamous cell skin cancers. J Natl Compr Canc Netw 2010;8(8):836–44.
7. Wolf DJ, Zitelli JA. Surgical margins for basal cell carcinoma. Arch Dermatol 1987;123(3):340–4.
8. Snow SN, Sahl W, Lo JS, et al. Metastatic basal cell carcinoma. Report of five cases. Cancer 1994;73(2):328–35.
9. Demers AA, Nugent Z, Michalcioiu C, et al. Trends of nonmelanoma skin cancer from 1960 through 2000 in a Canadian population. J Am Acad Dermatol 2005; 53(2):320–8.
10. Karia PS, Han J, Schmults CD. Cutaneous squamous cell carcinoma: estimated incidence of disease, nodal metastasis, and deaths from disease in the United States, 2012. J Am Acad Dermatol 2013;68(6):957.
11. Johnson T, Rowe DE, Nelson BR, et al. Squamous cell carcinoma of the skin. J Am Acad Dermatol 1992;26:467–84.
12. Ramsey HM, Fryer AA, Reece S, et al. Clinical risk factors associated with nonmelanoma skin cancer in renal transplant patients. Am J Kidney Dis 2000; 36(1):167–76.
13. Jensen P, Hansen S, Moller B, et al. Skin cancer in kidney and heart transplant recipients and different long-term immunosuppressive therapy. J Am Acad Dermatol 1999;40:177–86.
14. Rowe DE, Carroll RJ, Day CL. Prognostic factor for local recurrence, metastasis, and survival rates in squamous cell carcinomas of the skin, ear, and lip. J Am Acad Dermatol 1992;26:976–90.
15. Marcil I, Stern RS. Risk of developing a subsequent nonmelanoma skin cancer in patients with a history of nonmelanoma skin cancer: a critical review of the literature and meta-analysis. Arch Dermatol 2000;136(12):1524–30.
16. Karagas MR, Stukel TA, Greenberg ER, et al. Risk of subsequent basal cell carcinoma and squamous cell carcinoma of the skin among patients with prior skin cancer. Skin Cancer Prevention Study Group. JAMA 1992;267(24):3305–10.
17. Siegel R, Mah J, Zou Z, et al. Cancer statistics, 2014. Ca Cancer J Clin 2014; 64(1):9–29.
18. SEER program. Available at: http://seer.cancer.gov/registries/data.html. Accessed February 10, 2015.

19. Gandini S, Sera F, Cattaruzza MS, et al. Meta-analysis of risk factors for cutaneous melanoma: common and atypical nevi. Eur J Cancer 2005;41(1):28–44.
20. Elwood JM, Jopson J. Melanoma and sun exposure: an overview of published studies. Int J Cancer 1997;73(2):198.
21. International Agency for Research on Cancer Working Group on Artificial Ultraviolet Light and Skin Cancer. The association of use of sunbeds with cutaneous malignant melanoma and other skin cancers: a systematic review. Int J Cancer 2007; 120(11):2526.
22. American Academy of Dermatology. What to look for: the ABCDEs of melanoma. Available at: http://www.aad.org. Accessed November 2, 2015.
23. Ferrini RL, Perlman M, Hill L. American College of Preventive Medicine policy statement: screening for skin cancer. Am J Prev Med 1998;14(1):80–2.

Approach to the Patient with a Suspected Cutaneous Adverse Drug Reaction

Laura Swanson, MD, Roy M. Colven, MD*

KEYWORDS

- Urticaria • Exanthematous eruption • SJS/TEN
- Drug-induced hypersensitivity syndrome

KEY POINTS

- Adverse drug reactions are common and the skin is the most common site of manifestation.
- Most cutaneous adverse drug reactions are benign and self-limited, and typically present as exanthematous (morbilliform) eruptions or urticaria.
- A small subset of cutaneous adverse drug reactions is more severe, carries a risk of morbidity and mortality, and requires intervention.
- The single most important first step in any cutaneous adverse drug reaction is identifying and withdrawing the culprit medications.

INTRODUCTION

An adverse drug reaction (ADR) is defined by the World Health Organization as "a response to a drug which is noxious and unintended, and which occurs at doses normally used in man for the prophylaxis, diagnosis, or therapy of disease, or for the modifications of physiologic function." ADRs are common, occurring in up to 15% of hospitalized patients.[1] These events cause significant morbidity and mortality and financial burden, costing up to $2500 per adverse event.[2] The skin is among the most common organs of manifestation for adverse reactions and accounts for at least 15% of all ADRs. Recent epidemiologic data estimate 636,000 cutaneous adverse drug eruption-related health care visits in the United States annually.[1]

Cutaneous ADRs (CADRs) present in a variety of ways and have a spectrum of complication rates and prognoses ranging from no long-term sequelae to significant

Harborview Medical Center, Dermatology Section, Box 359763, 325 9th Avenue, Seattle, WA 98115, USA
* Corresponding author. Harborview Medical Center, Dermatology Section, Box 359763, 325 9th Avenue, Seattle, WA 98115, USA.
E-mail address: rcolven@uw.edu

Med Clin N Am 99 (2015) 1337–1348
http://dx.doi.org/10.1016/j.mcna.2015.06.003
0025-7125/15/$ – see front matter © 2015 Elsevier Inc. All rights reserved.

morbidity and mortality. For this reason, it is essential that the clinician be able to distinguish the signs and symptoms that suggest a more serious or severe CADR. This article describes a systematic approach to evaluating a patient with a suspected CADR, and the characteristics and management of different types of CADRs.

RECOGNIZING COMPLICATED VERSUS UNCOMPLICATED CUTANEOUS ADVERSE DRUG REACTIONS

The two most common forms of CADRs are urticarial and exanthematous eruptions, together accounting for 90% to 95% of all CADRs.[3] These two types of eruptions carry few to no long-term consequences. On the other end of the spectrum are the severe cutaneous adverse reactions (SCARs), which include, but are not limited to, acute generalized exanthematous pustulosis (AGEP), Stevens-Johnson syndrome/toxic epidermal necrolysis (SJS/TEN), and drug reaction with eosinophilia and systemic symptoms/drug-induced hypersensitivity syndrome (DRESS/DIHS). The percentage of CADRs that are considered to be severe or serious varies but most data suggest around 2%.[3,4] SCARs are associated with high rates of morbidity and mortality, and therefore, rapid recognition of the reaction, withdrawal of the offending agent, and appropriate triage, work-up, and treatment are critical.

Taking into account this spectrum of severity of CADRs, it is helpful for the clinician to think in terms of "complicated versus uncomplicated" reactions when evaluating a suspected CADR (**Fig. 1**). When patients exhibit features of a complicated CADR (discussed later and listed in **Box 1**), the clinician should have a low threshold to admit the patient to the hospital, perform a thorough work-up, including obtaining consultation from specialty services, and initiate therapy when indicated. However, most uncomplicated CADR can be managed in the outpatient setting with withdrawal of the offending agent and supportive therapy.

The first step in making this distinction between complicated and uncomplicated reactions is taking a detailed history. The history should include a complete medication exposure list with accurate dates of all drug exposures. It is important to ask not only about prescription medications, but also over-the-counter medications, such as

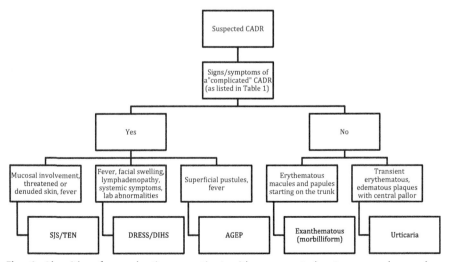

Fig. 1. Algorithm for evaluating a patient with a suspected cutaneous adverse drug reaction.

Box 1
Features suggestive of a "complicated" cutaneous adverse drug reaction

- Fever
- Facial swelling
- Lymphadenopathy
- Bullous or pustular lesions
- Threatened skin or a positive Nikolsky sign
- Mucosal involvement
- Systemic symptoms
- Laboratory abnormalities including but not limited to peripheral eosinophilia, circulating atypical lymphocytes, elevated liver function tests, elevated creatinine

---

nonsteroidal anti-inflammatory drugs (NSAIDs), which are common CADR-causing culprits. Time from medication initiation to development of a cutaneous reaction varies depending on the subtype of CADR (**Fig. 2**). Often patients have been exposed to multiple medications and creating a "drug chart" that details the dates of all medications taken is helpful in narrowing down the most likely culprits. The history should also include details of the rash onset and evolution. Prodrome symptoms, such as skin pain, new fever, and malaise, should be asked about, because visible rash may not be the earliest sign of a CADR. Completing a review of systems to determine if there are any associated symptoms, such as abdominal pain, ocular discomfort, or dysuria, is also key in differentiating a complicated versus uncomplicated reaction.

The examination should include vital signs, a full skin examination including groin and genitalia, evaluation of the eyes and oropharynx, and abdominal and lymph node palpation. The clinician should pay particular attention to whether or not there is mucosal involvement, abdominal tenderness, facial swelling, or lymphadenopathy because these signs are particularly suggestive of a complicated reaction. Additionally, the clinician should determine if there are pustular or bullous lesions, or areas of "threatened" or denuded epithelium, including mucosae and skin. To evaluate for threatened skin, the clinician should check for a positive Nikolsky sign by placing a gloved finger tangentially on several erythematous areas. The sign is considered positive if the epidermis detaches or sloughs with frictional traction. A positive Nikolsky sign indicates poor attachment of the epidermis to the dermis, which is the case in SJS/TEN because of confluent necrosis of keratinocytes.

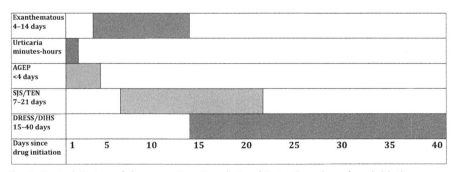

Fig. 2. Typical timing of drug eruptions in relationship to time since drug initiation.

Additional work-up should include basic laboratory studies, including complete blood count with differential and smear, a complete metabolic panel including creatinine and hepatic transaminases, and a urinalysis. If the patient is febrile, cultures of blood and other sites as directed by symptoms and signs should be taken. If eye signs or symptoms are present a detailed ophthalmologic examination is necessary. Often a skin biopsy, although not always diagnostic, is helpful. Occasionally additional specialty consultation and/or imaging studies are warranted.

If the work-up reveals a nonbullous, nonpustular rash with no fever, associated signs or symptoms, or laboratory abnormalities (excluding isolated eosinophilia), the reaction can be considered "uncomplicated" and usually falls into the category of urticarial or exanthematous eruptions. Exanthematous (also called morbilliform) eruptions are the most common CADR. Although the pathogenesis is not fully understood, they are thought to be cell-mediated hypersensitivity reactions.[4] Cutaneous features typically appear 7 to 14 days after drug exposure and are characterized by erythematous macules and papules (although lesions can be polymorphous) that begin on the trunk and spread outward (**Fig. 3**). Mucous membranes are usually spared, although a nonerosive enanthem can be observed in some. The eruption typically fades over 1 to 2 weeks without complications or long-term sequelae.

Acute drug-induced urticaria often occurs within minutes to hours of drug exposure and is considered an IgE-dependent immunologically mediated reaction. Clinically, urticaria is characterized by transient erythematous, edematous, pruritic papules and plaques that often have central pallor and no surface change otherwise (**Fig. 4**). These lesions can occur anywhere on the body. A key diagnostic feature is that individual lesions last less than 24 hours. Immunologic assays are available for some medications (mostly antibiotics) that can confirm the diagnosis. Treatment includes withdrawal of the medication and oral antihistamines. Most reactions resolve over days to weeks with no long-term sequelae.

If the work-up reveals any signs or symptoms concerning for a complicated reaction as discussed previously and as listed in **Box 1**, the next step is to determine what subset of complicated drug reaction is most likely, because each subset has different management strategies and prognoses. The three complicated reactions (all considered SCARs) covered in this article include AGEP, SJS/TEN, and DRESS/DIHS. Although it is helpful and important to differentiate among these three entities because of their differing treatments and prognoses, it should be noted that it is not uncommon for these entities to have overlapping features. Also of note, other reaction patterns considered by some to be SCARs that are not covered in this article include anaphylaxis, anticoagulant-induced skin necrosis, drug-induced vasculitis, and generalized fixed drug eruption.

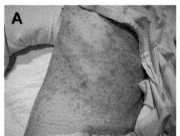 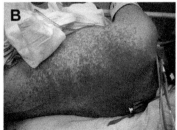

Fig. 3. (*A, B*) Exanthematous (morbilliform) eruption. Multiple erythematous macules and papules are present on the trunk. (*Courtesy of* J. Vary, MD, Seattle, WA.)

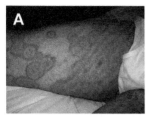
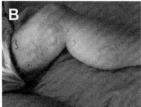
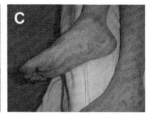

Fig. 4. (*A–C*) Urticaria. Multiple erythematous, edematous plaques with central pallor are present. (*Courtesy of* [A] M. Shinohara, MD, Seattle, WA; and [C] A. Kalus, MD, Seattle, WA.)

ACUTE GENERALIZED EXANTHEMATOUS PUSTULOSIS

In patients who present with recent drug exposure, fever, and a pustular eruption, AGEP should be considered. AGEP is a rare CADR with an estimated incidence of one to five cases per million per year.[5,6] Males and females seem to be affected equally. The pathogenesis of AGEP is incompletely understood and there is still controversy regarding a link to a personal or family history of psoriasis.[5,7] Although the genetics are less well studied in AGEP than in the other SCARs, early data suggest HLA-B5, Dr11, and DQ3 are more common in patients with AGEP.[4,5] There are some data to support an immunologic recall phenomenon where memory T cells are activated and produce neutrophil-promoting cytokines, such as interleukin-3 and -8.[6]

AGEP usually occurs within 1 to 4 days of drug initiation, which is a shorter time interval than most drug eruptions and is possibly explained by the recall reaction theory mentioned previously. Antibiotics, specifically β-lactam antibiotics, are among the most common culprit agents but the list of reported culprits is long and includes antimalarials, antihypertensives, and antiepilectics.[4,6]

Clinically, AGEP presents as diffuse superficial, nonfollicular, sterile pustules often on a background of erythematous, edematous skin (**Fig. 5**). The pustular eruption typically begins in the intertriginous zones and spreads rapidly. Patients often complain of burning or itching. The skin findings are usually accompanied by fever and sometimes by peripheral neutrophil-predominant leukocytosis. A peripheral eosinophilia has also been reported.[6] The pustules typically last 1 to 2 weeks and resolve with desquamation. Histologically, subcorneal spongiform neutrophil collections are seen.

In managing patients with AGEP, discontinuation of the causative agent is the most important intervention. Systemic treatment is usually not required because AGEP is

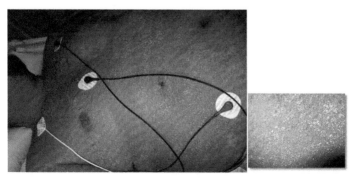

Fig. 5. AGEP. Superficial, nonfollicular, pustules are present on a background of erythematous skin. (*Courtesy of* M. Shinohara, MD, Seattle, WA.)

generally benign and self-limited.[8] The mortality rate is thought to be less than 5% and probably closer to 1% to 2%.[4,5]

STEVENS-JOHNSON SYNDROME/TOXIC EPIDERMAL NECROLYSIS

Mucosal involvement, flaccid vesicles and bullae, a positive Nikolsky sign, skin pain, and fever are features highly suggestive of SJS/TEN, a mucocutaneous disease with significant morbidity and mortality. SJS and TEN exist on a spectrum of severity described next. SJS/TEN is rare, with incidence estimates of 1.2 to 6 and 0.4 to 1.2 per million person-years, respectively.[9] Although rare, this disease affects all ages, all races, and both sexes, but certain populations including the elderly and HIV-infected patients have been shown to be at higher risk for TEN.[9,10]

Most cases of SJS/TEN are drug-induced. Clinical manifestations usually begin 7 to 21 days after drug exposure. Drugs with the highest risk include antibiotics, anticonvulsants, NSAIDs, and allopurinol.[11] Evidence suggests that SJS/TEN is associated with an impaired capacity to detoxify reactive intermediate drug metabolites.[12] The reaction is thought to be an immune response to an antigentic complex formed by the reaction of these metabolites with certain host tissues.[12] As with other SCARs, there seems to be a genetic susceptibility in patients with particular HLA subtypes, including HLA-B*1502 in Asians and East Indians exposed to carbamazepine, HLA-B*5801 in Han Chinese and some Europeans exposed to allopurinol, HLA-A*3101 in Japanese and Europeans exposed to carbamazepine, and HLA-B*5701 in whites and African Americans exposed to abacavir.[5] The US Food and Drug Administration recommends genotyping of all Asians before treatment with carbamazepine and of all patients before treatment with abacavir. Lastly, it has been noted that white patients with HLA-DQB1*0601 allele are at a particularly increased risk for SJS with ocular complications.[12]

The tissue damage in SJS/TEN is a reflection of massive keratinocyte apoptosis that starts as scattered individual-cell necrosis and progresses to confluent full-thickness necrosis. Epidermal necrosis is thought to be mediated by drug-specific cytotoxic T cells and increased expression of the cytolytic molecule FasL on keratinocytes and granulysin secretion from cytotoxic T cells. This leads to FasL and granulysin-mediated apoptosis of keratinocytes and subsequent epidermal necrosis and detachment.[12]

Initial clinical features of SJS/TEN include fever, ocular pain, and oral pain. Skin manifestations, particularly erythema and pain, follow shortly after. Skin lesions often begin as erythematous, dusky, or sometimes purpuric macules and patches. These lesions progress over hours to days to form flaccid bullae with a positive Absoe-Hansen sign (slight pressure on the blister extends the bullae laterally) and areas of denuded skin (**Fig. 6**). SJS and TEN exist on a spectrum with the term SJS being used when less than 10% body surface area (BSA) of epidermis is detached or detachable and TEN being used for greater than 30% BSA detached or detachable. When 10% to 30% BSA is detached or detachable, this is considered SJS/TEN overlap. Of note, skin that is erythematous but not detached visibly or inducibly (negative Nikolsky sign) should not be included in the BSA calculation.

Oral involvement is reported in 71% to 100% of patients.[13] Ocular involvement is also common and is reported in up to 74% of patients. Ocular involvement can have significant long-term complications including decreased visual acuity, photophobia, chronic dry eye, eyelid malposition, and blindness.[12,14,15] Respiratory, gastrointestinal, gynecologic, otolaryngologic, and renal involvement have been reported with long-term complications including, but not limited to, vaginal scarring and stenosis, esophageal strictures, bronchiectasis, and glomerulonephritis.[13]

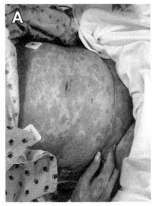
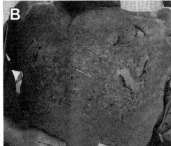
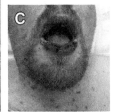

Fig. 6. SJS/TEN. (*A*) Erythematous and dusky patches are present in a patient with TEN. (*B*) Diffusely threatened skin with many denuded areas with exposed dermis are present in a patient with TEN. (*C*) Erosions and crusting of the vermillion lips is present in a patient with SJS.

The differential diagnosis of SJS/TEN includes erythema multiforme major, generalized bullous fixed drug eruption, staphylococcal scalded skin syndrome, autoimmune bullous disorders, and exfoliative dermatitis. Skin biopsy is helpful in confirming the diagnosis of SJS/TEN, because the histologic findings are definitively distinguishable from all of the previously listed disorders, with the exception of erythema multiforme major. In early lesions of SJS/TEN apoptotic keratinocytes are seen scattered in the epidermis. In later stage full-thickness epidermal necrosis is seen. Of note, a punch biopsy is often not needed to establish the diagnosis histologically. At our institution we frequently obtain a "skin roll" by placing a cotton swab at one edge of a ruptured bullae and rolling along the necrotic skin. This elevates the necrotic epidermis, which can then be sent in formalin for frozen or permanent sectioning. Alternatively, a pair of pick-ups and scissors can be used to gently elevate a piece of necrotic skin. These two methods are quick, do not cause any additional scarring, and do not require local anesthetic or sutures. Because the diagnostic pathology in SJS/TEN is solely in the epidermis, these methods are still able to confirm the diagnosis. Absence of keratinocyte necrosis should direct one to consider alternatives in the differential diagnosis, at which point a punch biopsy of lesional skin for routine histology and of perilesional skin for direct immunofluorescence should be considered.

Management of SJS/TEN involves identification and discontinuation of the correct culprit drug and providing intensive supportive care. There is significant controversy surrounding the use of systemic therapies in SJS/TEN. Supportive care is aimed at preventing common complications, which include hypovolemia, infection, electrolyte abnormalities, and renal impairment. Patients often require intensive care unit admission with some evidence to suggest better outcomes with admission to a burn intensive care unit.[16] Daily wound care includes covering denuded skin with paraffin gauze, porcine xenografts, human allografts, and/or other skin substitutes. Management of ocular involvement includes lubrication, topical antibiotics, lysis of adhesions, and in more severe cases amniotic membrane transplantation.[17]

Treatment with systemic therapies, such as systemic corticosteroids, IVIG, and cyclosporine, remains controversial and study outcomes of these interventions remain mixed. Early studies suggested increased infection rates and prolonged hospitalization with the use of systemic steroids,[18,19] although more recent studies suggest some benefit from systemic corticosteroids.[20] The data on IVIG are also mixed. Recently, the first meta-analysis on the efficacy of IVIG in TEN patients was performed and concluded that although IVIG exhibited a trend toward improved mortality, the evidence does not support a clinical benefit to IVIG and more randomized controlled trials are needed.[21] A recent retrospective review comparing IVIG with cyclosporine in patients with SJS/TEN demonstrated a mortality benefit with the use of cyclosporine over the use of IVIG.[22]

Mortality rates are less than 5% for SJS but 30% for TEN.[9] Infection is the leading cause of death in TEN.[16] Other causes of morbidity include but are not limited to myocardial infarction, gastrointestinal bleeding, pulmonary embolism, and pulmonary edema.[16] The Severity of Illness Score for Toxic Epidermal Necrolysis (**Box 2**) was developed to predict mortality in patients. Mortality ranges from 3.2% for 0 to 1 point to up to 90% for those with 5 points.[16]

DRUG REACTION WITH EOSINOPHILIA AND SYSTEMIC SYMPTOMS/DRUG-INDUCED HYPERSENSITIVITY SYNDROME

Fever, lymphadenopathy, facial swelling, a morbilliform to polymorphous rash, peripheral eosinophilia, atypical circulating lymphocytes, internal organ involvement (particularly liver and/or renal), and a longer lag time between drug exposure and reaction development are features highly suggestive of DRESS/DIHS. The incidence of DRESS/DIHS is estimated to be between 1 in 1000 and 1 in 10,000 for particular drugs, such as anticonvulsants and sulfonimides.[4] The incidence is thought to be higher in African American patients and the risk is significantly increased in Northern European populations with HLA-A*3101 allele in the setting of carbamazepine exposure, and in particular populations with HLA-B*5801 exposed to allopurinol.[23] Of note, HLA types have been extensively studied in the Han Chinese population and the following associations with CADRs have been found: carbamazepine-induced SJS/TEN, allopurinol-induced CADRs, methazolamide-induced SJS/TEN, and salazosulfapyridine-induced DRESS, which were respectively strongly associated with HLA-B*15:02, HLA-B*58:01, HLA-B*59:01, and HLA-B*13:01.[24] The American College of Rheumatology recommends screening for HLA-B*5801 in all Han Chinese, Thai, and Korean populations before initiation of allopurinol.[5]

Although the pathogenesis of DRESS/DIHS is not fully understood, it is thought to be related to alteration in the metabolism of certain drugs.[4] Polymorphisms of the epoxide hydroxylase and slow N-acetylator phenotypes confer an increased risk of DRESS.[5] Additionally, demonstration of reactivation of human herpesvirus-6

Box 2
The Severity of Illness Score for Toxic Epidermal Necrolysis (one point is given for each of the seven variables)

1. Age 40 years or older
2. Heart rate $\geq$120 beats per minute
3. Comorbid malignancy
4. Epidermal detachment of >10% BSA on Day 1
5. Blood urea nitrogen >28 mg/dL
6. Glucose >252 mg/dL
7. Bicarbonate >20 mEq/L

and -7 in patients with DRESS/DIHS has raised suspicion for a potential viral cause. There is some suggestion that human herpesvirus reactivation may contribute to severity, prolongation, or relapse of DRESS/DIHS.[25]

The list of culprit medications causing DRESS/DIHS is extensive and includes aromatic amine anticonvulsants, β-lactam antibiotics, allopurinol, NSAIDs, antiretrovirals, and sulfonamide antibiotics.[23] Multiple drug hypersensitivity (defined as drug allergies to two or more chemically different drugs) has been well documented in DRESS/DIHS.[26,27] It is hypothesized that costimulatory signals provided by viral reactivation and/or first-drug sensitization lead to an immune response to another drug-protein conjugate, resulting in allergy to a different drug class. This multiple drug hypersensitivity can be long lasting and have serious implications for future medication administration.[26]

In DRESS/DIHS, there is a longer lag time between drug exposure and development of the drug reaction, typically 15 to 40 days. Fever and rash are the most common manifestations. The rash can be polymorphous but typically begins as a morbilliform eruption involving the face, neck, upper extremities, and trunk (**Fig. 7**). The eruption can become edematous and include vesicles, bullae, pustules, and even purpuric lesions.[4] Additional clinical features include facial edema, lymphadenopathy, and occasionally arthralgias. Characteristic laboratory abnormalities include prominent peripheral eosinophilia, mononucleosis-like atypical lymphocytosis, and elevated hepatic enzymes.

Any internal organ can be affected in DRESS/DIHS, but the liver is the most common and often the most severe site of visceral involvement. Hepatitis can be fulminant and is responsible for most deaths in DRESS/DIHS.[4] Other potential systemic involvement can include myocarditis, interstitial pneumonitis, interstitial nephritis, and thyroiditis.[4]

Treatment includes prompt discontinuation of the offending agent and initiation of systemic steroids. Relapses with tapering of systemic steroids are common and long courses of systemic steroids with exceptionally slow tapers are often required.[4] Autoimmune disease as a long-term consequence of DRESS/DIHS is not uncommon,

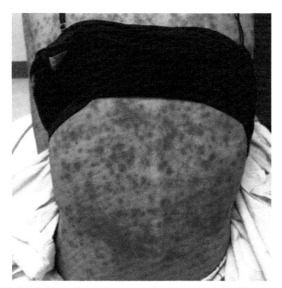

Fig. 7. DRESS/DIHS. Brightly erythematous papules are present diffusely on the trunk.

and can include autoimmune thyroid disease, insulin-dependent diabetes, scleroder-moid graft-versus-host disease–like lesions, and systemic lupus.[28] Estimates of mortality rates in DRESS/DIHS vary but are reported to be up to 10% with some anticonvulsant drugs.[5]

ADDITIONAL MANAGEMENT CONSIDERATIONS

The most important piece of managing any CADR, and particularly any SCAR, is correctly identifying and stopping the culprit drugs and preventing re-exposure. Unfor-tunately, identifying the culprit medication is difficult when patients are exposed to multiple medications and re-exposure challenges are dangerous. Creating a drug chart is a helpful tool. Additionally, patch tests are a low-risk method of testing that is helpful, although not universally successful. A recent multicenter study reported positive patch tests in 56.7% of 134 cases evaluated (58% of cases of AGEP, 64% of cases of DRESS/DIHS, but only 24% of cases of SJS/TEN). In only one of these cases was patch testing associated with recurrence of the rash.[26] The value of patch testing varies according to the type of SCAR and implicated drug. Patch testing yields more positives in AGEP and DRESS/DIHS than in SJS/TEN. Additionally, for unclear reasons, patch testing tends to be unhelpful in cases of SCAR induced by allopurinol among a few other common drug culprits.[26]

From a practical perspective, keys to preventing re-exposure include listing the allergy in the patient's medical chart and ensuring that the patient and family are aware of the allergy and are knowledgeable regarding the medication class and reaction type. Also, it is reasonable to suggest that patients wear medical alert bracelets and have the allergy listed in their wallets and on their refrigerators.

SUMMARY

CADRs are common and generally have a mild, self-resolving course with minimal associated morbidity and mortality. However, subsets of CARDs are more severe, require intervention, and have significant risk of associated morbidity and mortality. For this reason, it is crucial that the clinician recognize signs and symptoms worrisome for a more severe CARD so that appropriate triage, work-up, and treatment are initi-ated. In all CADRs the most important first step is identification and withdrawal of the culprit medications.

REFERENCES

1. Koelblinger P, Dabade TS, Gustafson CJ, et al. Skin manifestations of outpatient adverse drug events in the United States: a national analysis. J Cutan Med Surg 2013;17:269–75.
2. Bates DW, Spell N, Cullen DJ, et al. The costs of adverse drug events in hospi-talized patients. Adverse Drug Events Prevention Study Group. JAMA 1997; 277:307–11.
3. Bachot N, Roujeau JC. Differential diagnosis of severe cutaneous drug eruptions. Am J Clin Dermatol 2003;4:561–72.
4. Revuz J, Valeyrie-Allanore L. Drug reactions. In: Bolognia JL, Jorrizo JL, Schaffer JV, editors. Dermatology. London: Elsevier; 2012. p. 335–56.
5. Dodiuk-Gad RP, Laws PM, Shear NH. Epidemiology of severe drug hypersensi-tivity. Semin Cutan Med Surg 2014;33:2–9.
6. Sidoroff A, Halevy S, Bavinck JN, et al. Acute generalized exanthematous pustu-losis (AGEP)–a clinical reaction pattern. J Cutan Pathol 2001;28:113–9.

7. Sidoroff A, Dunant A, Viboud C, et al. Risk factors for acute generalized exanthematous pustulosis (AGEP)-results of a multinational case-control study (EuroSCAR). Br J Dermatol 2007;157:989–96.
8. Sidoroff A. Acute generalized exanthematous pustulosis. Chem Immunol Allergy 2012;97:139–48.
9. Roujeau JC, Stern RS. Severe adverse cutaneous reactions to drugs. N Engl J Med 1994;331:1272–85.
10. Bastuji-Garin S, Zahedi M, Guillaume JC, et al. Toxic epidermal necrolysis (Lyell syndrome) in 77 elderly patients. Age Ageing 1993;22:450–6.
11. Roujeau JC, Kelly JP, Naldi L, et al. Medication use and the risk of Stevens-Johnson syndrome or toxic epidermal necrolysis. N Engl J Med 1995;333:1600–7.
12. French LE, Prins C. Erythema multiforme, Stevens-Johnson syndrome and toxic epidermal necrolysis. In: Bolognia JL, Jorizzo JL, Schaffer JV, editors. Dermatology. London: Elsevier; 2012. p. 323–33.
13. Saeed H, Mantagos IS, Chodosh J. Complications of Stevens-Johnson syndrome beyond the eye and skin. Burns 2015. http://dx.doi.org/10.1016/j.burns.2015.03.012.
14. Mouafik SB, Hocar O, Akhdari N, et al. Ophthalmic manifestations after Lyell and Stevens-Johnson syndromes. Ann Dermatol Venereol 2015;142:393–8 [in French].
15. Gueudry J, Roujeau JC, Binaghi M, et al. Risk factors for the development of ocular complications of Stevens-Johnson syndrome and toxic epidermal necrolysis. Arch Dermatol 2009;145:157–62.
16. Schwartz RA, McDonough PH, Lee BW. Toxic epidermal necrolysis: part II. Prognosis, sequelae, diagnosis, differential diagnosis, prevention, and treatment. J Am Acad Dermatol 2013;69:187.e1–16 [quiz: 203–4].
17. Hsu M, Jayaram A, Verner R, et al. Indications and outcomes of amniotic membrane transplantation in the management of acute Stevens-Johnson syndrome and toxic epidermal necrolysis: a case-control study. Cornea 2012;31:1394–402.
18. Ruiz-Maldonado R. Acute disseminated epidermal necrosis types 1, 2, and 3: study of sixty cases. J Am Acad Dermatol 1985;13:623–35.
19. Halebian PH, Corder VJ, Madden MR, et al. Improved burn center survival of patients with toxic epidermal necrolysis managed without corticosteroids. Ann Surg 1986;204:503–12.
20. Kardaun SH, Jonkman MF. Dexamethasone pulse therapy for Stevens-Johnson syndrome/toxic epidermal necrolysis. Acta Derm Venereol 2007;87:144–8.
21. Huang YC, Li YC, Chen TJ. The efficacy of intravenous immunoglobulin for the treatment of toxic epidermal necrolysis: a systematic review and meta-analysis. Br J Dermatol 2012;167:424–32.
22. Kirchhof MG, Miliszewski MA, Sikora S, et al. Retrospective review of Stevens-Johnson syndrome/toxic epidermal necrolysis treatment comparing intravenous immunoglobulin with cyclosporine. J Am Acad Dermatol 2014;71:941–7.
23. Pavlos R, Mallal S, Ostrov D, et al. Fever, rash, and systemic symptoms: understanding the role of virus and HLA in severe cutaneous drug allergy. J Allergy Clin Immunol Pract 2014;2:21–33.
24. Yang F, Yang Y, Zhu Q, et al. Research on susceptible genes and immunological pathogenesis of cutaneous adverse drug reactions in Chinese Hans. J Investig Dermatol Symp Proc 2015;17:29–31.
25. Oskay T, Karademir A, Ertürk OI. Association of anticonvulsant hypersensitivity syndrome with herpesvirus 6, 7. Epilepsy Res 2006;70:27–40.

26. Barbaud A, Collet E, Milpied B, et al. A multicentre study to determine the value and safety of drug patch tests for the three main classes of severe cutaneous adverse drug reactions. Br J Dermatol 2013;168:555–62.
27. Gex-Collet C, Helbling A, Pichler WJ. Multiple drug hypersensitivity: proof of multiple drug hypersensitivity by patch and lymphocyte transformation tests. J Investig Allergol Clin Immunol 2005;15:293–6.
28. Kano Y, Tohyama M, Aihara M, et al. Sequelae in 145 patients with drug-induced hypersensitivity syndrome/drug reaction with eosinophilia and systemic symptoms: survey conducted by the Asian Research Committee on Severe Cutaneous Adverse Reactions (ASCAR). J Dermatol 2015;42:276–82.

Inpatient Consultative Dermatology

Lauren K. Biesbroeck, MD, Michi M. Shinohara, MD*

KEYWORDS

- Dermatology hospitalist • Inpatient dermatology • Consultative dermatology

KEY POINTS

- Dermatology consultation aids in diagnosis and management of inpatients, while allowing for increased teaching of consulting services and time for patient and family education.
- A broad range of skin disorders are seen by dermatologists in the inpatient setting, with overrepresentation by inflammatory and infectious dermatoses.
- Common cutaneous infections can present with atypical or severe morphologies in immunosuppressed patients, and opportunistic infections can disseminate rapidly.
- Calciphylaxis and pyoderma gangrenosum should be considered in unusual or recalcitrant wounds arising during hospitalization.

INTRODUCTION

Dermatologists play a vital role in the diagnosis and management of hospitalized patients. Skin problems in hospitalized patients are common, with approximately one-third demonstrating significant skin findings, and more than 10% with skin findings directly relevant to their hospitalization or otherwise indicative of a systemic disease.[1] Patients admitted for dermatology-related diagnoses accounted for nearly $900 million in Medicare reimbursements in 1 study.[2]

WHY INVOLVE DERMATOLOGY?

Dermatology consultation improves diagnostic accuracy. Dermatology consultation changes the diagnosis made by consulting teams frequently (45%–80% of patients), often leading to changes in treatment.[3–6] For example, when patients with suspected cellulitis were evaluated by dermatologists, cellulitis was confirmed in only 10%, potentially saving unnecessary antibiotic therapy and costly hospital stays.[7]

Disclosure Statement: The authors have nothing to disclose.

Division of Dermatology, University of Washington School of Medicine, 1959 Northeast Pacific Street BB-1353, Box 356524, Seattle, WA 98195-6524, USA

* Corresponding author.

E-mail address: mshinoha@uw.edu

One-third of those with suspected cellulitis had alternative dermatoses, including eczematous dermatitis, lymphedema, and lipodermatosclerosis, and one-quarter of those with confirmed cellulitis also had another dermatitis (eg, eczematous dermatitis or tinea), possibly predisposing them to cellulitis.[8]

Potential Cost Savings of Dermatology Involvement

Whether dermatology involvement leads to overall cost savings in the inpatient setting is not known presently, although it seems intuitive that with correct diagnosis, prompt initiation of appropriate therapy, and earlier discharge, cost savings follows. Helms and colleagues[9] comment that it is not unusual for patients to be discharged immediately after dermatology consultation, and our own experience reflects this. Dermatologists rely on physical examination alone the majority of the time, with potential costs savings with respect to laboratory testing and imaging.[4,6] Skin biopsy is an exception to this; when skin biopsies are performed in the inpatient setting, however, the yield can be high, with more than 80% of biopsies yielding a definitive diagnosis.[6]

The Dermatologist as Teacher

Dermatology inpatient consultation plays an important role in the education of consulting services (particularly trainees) as well as patients. Inpatient dermatology consultation offers an opportunity to fill a widening gap in dermatology medical education. Exposure to dermatology during medical training is limited, with a median dermatology exposure during medical school of only 10 hours (and decreasing).[10] Despite a significant number of visits for primary dermatology issues in the outpatient setting, family practice residents report only 1 to 4 weeks of dermatology training during their residency, and almost 20% report no exposure to dermatology.[11] Dermatology inpatient consultation can be an opportunity for in-depth, face-to-face discussion of a patient between the primary and consulting teams.

The inpatient setting also provides additional time for the often extensive patient and caregiver education needed to manage patients with complex skin disease. In erythroderma, for example, patients are sometimes admitted for intensive wet-wrap therapy, which entails full-body application of topical steroids followed by damp bandages or pajamas and an occlusive overlayer.[12] Hospitalization can provide a setting to educate patients and caregivers on skin care, better assess compliance with outpatient therapy, and get critical "buy in" about the effectiveness of topical therapies as they see their skin improve daily.

Barriers to Inpatient Consultation and the Dermatology Hospitalist Movement

Despite the benefits of dermatology involvement in the inpatient setting, access to dermatologists willing or able to consult on inpatients is limited, particularly in hospitals not affiliated with an academic or teaching institution. The majority of dermatology programs no longer admit directly to dedicated dermatology beds, instead acting solely as consultants.[13]

Solutions for providing inpatient dermatology coverage are being explored. Combined internal medicine–dermatology residencies have been introduced, and may provide a source of well-equipped trainees with a special interest in hospital consults. Teledermatology has been shown to be an effective tool for triaging inpatient consultations, improving the efficiency of inpatient consultation while still providing timely and reliable service.[14] Last, the "dermatology hospitalist" model was proposed in 2009 by Fox and colleagues[15]; in this model, specialized dermatologists are dedicated to inpatient care, with a goal of maximizing clinical expertise in the inpatient setting and maintaining a high standard of care.

COMMON CONSULTATIONS SEEN BY THE INPATIENT DERMATOLOGIST

The range of diagnoses that dermatologists see in the inpatient setting is broad, although in our experience inflammatory and infectious dermatoses are overrepresented, and series from other centers confirm this.[6]

Morbilliform Drug Eruptions

One of the most common inpatient consults to dermatology is evaluation of the patient with a suspected cutaneous drug eruption.[3,4,6] Skin rashes are among the most frequent manifestations of drug reactions, occurring in an estimated 2% of inpatients.[16] Uncomplicated morbilliform eruptions account for about 95% of skin manifestations of drug eruptions.[17] Dermatologist evaluation of these patients can help to confirm the diagnosis and identify a culprit medication, or at least narrow the list if a single agent cannot be identified.

Morbilliform eruptions present approximately 1 to 2 weeks after initial exposure, although can occur sooner on rechallenge. Skin examination shows morbilliform ("measleslike") morphology, with erythematous macules and papules starting centrally on the trunk and intertriginous areas, or in dependent areas (the back, posterior legs) of bedbound patients (**Fig. 1**). Mucosal involvement is typically absent. Moderate to severe pruritus is typical. The rash spreads peripherally, slowly resolving over 1 to 2 weeks.[18] The main differential diagnosis includes viral exanthems, which occur in increased frequency in immunosuppressed patients,[19] and early stages of severe cutaneous adverse drug reactions, including drug rash with eosinophilia and systemic symptoms, Stevens Johnson syndrome, and toxic epidermal necrolysis; severe cutaneous adverse drug reactions are covered in more detail elsewhere in this issue. In patients who have undergone stem cell transplantation (SCT), acute graft-versus-host disease (GVHD) and eruption of lymphocyte recovery also need to be considered. In those with bleeding diathesis, morbilliform eruptions may seem quite purpuric (**Fig. 2**), and may mimic vasculitis.

High fever or significant laboratory abnormalities not otherwise explainable (transaminitis, marked eosinophilia, neutrophilia, or renal insufficiency) should raise concern for a more serious drug eruption. Skin biopsies of morbilliform drug eruption are often nonspecific,[20] but can be useful in eliminating other diagnostic considerations.

Treatment of morbilliform drug eruption is supportive, with discontinuation of the offending drug, and midpotency topical steroids and oral antihistamines to control pruritus while awaiting resolution of the eruption.[21,22] We avoid the use of systemic

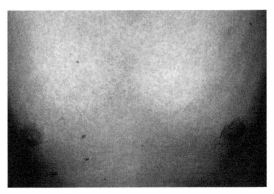

Fig. 1. Morbilliform drug eruption.

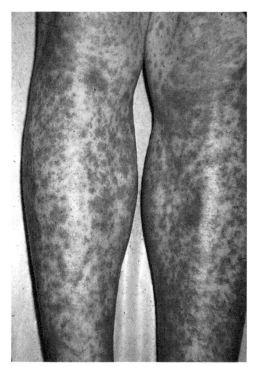

Fig. 2. Morbilliform drug eruption with a hemorrhagic appearance, which can simulate cutaneous vasculitis.

corticosteroids, because they can potentially further immunosuppress ill, hospitalized patients, and there is no evidence that systemic corticosteroids speed resolution of uncomplicated drug eruptions.

One of the most important tools when evaluating an inpatient with suspected drug eruption is construction of a drug chart that lists all of the medications a patient is exposed to within a 1- to 2-week window before the onset of the rash. Drug charting helps to eliminate medications as a cause of the eruption. For example, medications administered the day of or after a rash started are unlikely culprits. It is not unusual, in our experience, for inpatients to have multiple possible culprit medications identified by drug charting. In that case, we recommend discontinuing all unnecessary medications and changing critical medications to alternative medications in a different class. Drug charting minimizes unnecessary stopping and starting of medications; similarly, it is an excellent opportunity to reduce polypharmacy.[23]

Rash in the Hospitalized Immunosuppressed Patient

A common and challenging scenario for the inpatient dermatologist is evaluating the immunosuppressed patient with rash, including the neutropenic patient (owing to hematologic malignancy or chemotherapy associated neutropenia), solid organ transplant (SOT) patient, advanced human immunodeficiency virus infection/AIDS, malnutrition, and patients on immunosuppressive medications for other reasons, such as rheumatologic conditions. The decision to perform a skin biopsy in immunosuppressed patients is not taken lightly, particularly when patients are neutropenic and/or thrombocytopenic; 1 series found a generally higher rate of biopsy complications among inpatients, although this represents a single institution experience.[24]

Acute Graft-Versus-Host Disease

Acute GVHD (aGVHD) typically occurs within 2 to 6 weeks after SCT, but can occur at any point with alterations in immunosuppression regimens or donor lymphocyte infusion.[25] Differentiating aGVHD from drug eruption is particularly difficult, and may not be possible in some circumstances. The presentation can be identical, with morbilliform eruptions overlapping with mild (stage 1–2) aGVHD (**Fig. 3**) and toxic epidermal necrolysis overlapping with blistering or desquamating (stage 4) aGHV[26] (**Fig. 4**). GVHD may more frequently involve the face and acral surfaces compared with morbilliform eruptions[25] (**Fig. 5**). The presence of transaminitis or colitis may also favor aGVHD, but are not specific, because hepatitis can be seen in severe cutaneous adverse drug reactions.[27,28] Skin biopsy is of questionable utility, especially very early after SCT,[29] and dermatologists rely heavily on clinical examination and history in this setting.

Acute Graft-Versus-Host Disease in the Solid Organ Transplant Recipient

Recipients of SOT can also develop GVHD, and it is associated with high mortality (80%). The frequency of SOT GVHD varies depending on the organ transplanted, with the highest incidence (5.6%) in small intestine transplants, likely owing to periorgan lymphocyte transfer.[30,31] The incidence in liver transplant patients is 1% to 2%; few cases occur in other SOT. Early symptoms are nonspecific and easily mistaken for medication reactions or infections.[30,31] As with SCT patients, SOT GVHD initially presents with a morbilliform rash (**Fig. 6**). Diarrhea and fever are typical. The transplanted liver is often spared, but can be involved in other SOT settings.[31] Patients succumb to sepsis or gastrointestinal hemorrhage from bone marrow failure after infiltration by donor T cells. Diagnosis can be suggested by skin histology,[30,31] but is confirmed by demonstrating lymphocyte chimerism in peripheral blood or biopsies of affected tissues.

Cutaneous Infections in the Immunosuppressed Patient: Herpes Group Infections

Immunocompromised patients, including those with malignancy, advanced human immunodeficiency virus infection, malnutrition, and SOT or SCT patients, are at increased risk for cutaneous infections, oftentimes with atypical presentations. Herpes simplex virus (HSV) infection in the immunosuppressed, for example, may present as

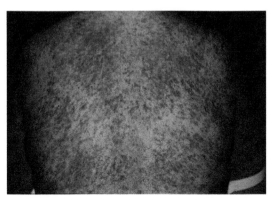

Fig. 3. Acute (morbilliform) graft-versus-host disease (GVHD). This patient also has evidence of early lichenoid changes suggestive of chronic GVHD.

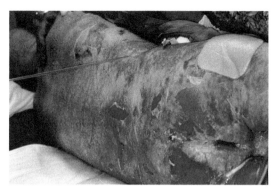

Fig. 4. Severe (grade 4) graft-versus-host disease, with erosion and desquamation.

confluent, poorly healing ulcers, sometimes persisting for months[32] (**Fig. 7**). Dissemination can occur, usually preceded by mucocutaneous involvement, highlighting the importance of prompt recognition and treatment of HSV in this population.[33] The incidence of acyclovir-resistant HSV in immunosuppressed patients is increasing, possibly owing to routine use of acyclovir prophylaxis.[34,35] Foscarnet or topical cidofovir may be required in such cases.[35] Mixed infections involving HSV and other pathogens (such as cytomegalovirus) also occur.[34] Although the most common presentation of varicella zoster virus infection in the immunosuppressed remains dermatomal vesicles and erosions, lesions can become bullous or necrotic, and disseminated disease can occur (**Fig. 8**). The primary morphology of the umbilicated vesicle is often identifiable, and can be a clue to diagnosis.[32,33]

Cutaneous Infections in the Immunosuppressed Patient: Opportunistic Fungal Infections

Prolonged neutropenia and/or altered T-cell function are risk factors for opportunistic fungal infections, and thus many occur in peri-SCT period or other chronically immunosuppressed patients. Cutaneous fungal infections in immunosuppressed patients can be divided broadly into primary cutaneous infections and secondary manifestations of hematogenous dissemination. *Aspergillus*, *Mucor*, *Rhizopus*, and *Fusarium* can present as primary cutaneous disease, often as scaly, crusted, or necrotic

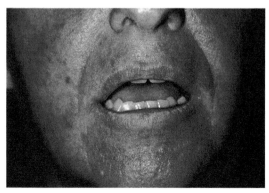

Fig. 5. Facial involvement in graft-versus-host disease, with involvement on the lips and chin with faint, pink to violet papules. This patient has early chronic graft-versus-host disease.

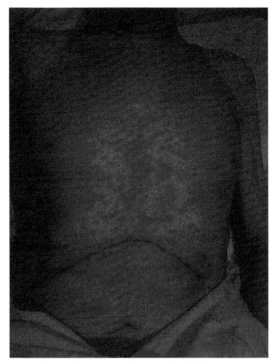

Fig. 6. Morbilliform eruption owing to graft-versus-host disease occurring in a patient who is recently post orthotopic liver transplant.

plaques at sites of broken skin, such as intravenous insertion sites or under occlusive dressings. The necrosis reflects the angioinvasive nature of these organisms (**Fig. 9**). Other presentations include acute paronychia (**Fig. 10**) or a cellulitic picture. Facial cellulitis, for example, can be a clue to underlying angioinvasive fungal sinusitis[36] (**Fig. 11**).

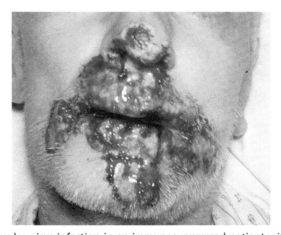

Fig. 7. Herpes simplex virus infection in an immunosuppressed patient with leukemia.

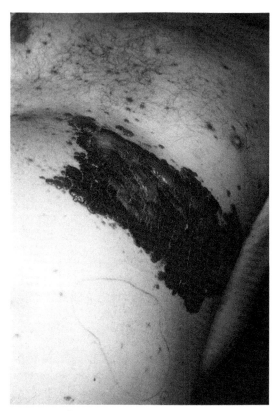

Fig. 8. Varicella zoster virus infection in an immunosuppressed patient, with hemorrhagic bullae and necrosis in the primary dermatomal lesion and disseminated erythematous papules and vesicles.

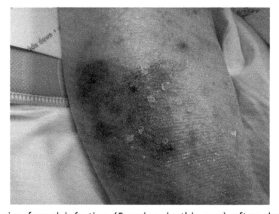

Fig. 9. Angioinvasive fungal infection (*Fusarium* in this case) often shows areas with a hemorrhagic or necrotic appearance.

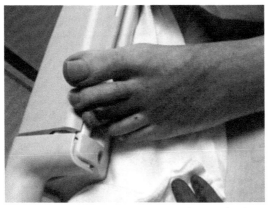

Fig. 10. *Fusarium* onychomycosis leading to paronychia and ultimately disseminated infection.

Skin lesions in disseminated fungal infections range from nonspecific pink papules or papulopustules (**Fig. 12**) to tender erythematous plaques with purpura or eschar.[36,37] Recognition of opportunistic fungal infections in immunosuppressed patients is an emergency, often requiring bedside biopsies to obtain tissue for rapid histologic evaluation and culture, because fungal blood cultures are negative in up to 75% of cases of disseminated disease.[36,38]

Sweet Syndrome

Sweet syndrome (SS), or acute febrile neutrophilic dermatosis, presents abruptly with tender, edematous plaques or nodules (**Fig. 13**), often accompanied by fever and peripheral neutrophilia.[39,40] Many cases of SS are malignancy-associated, particularly acute myelogenous leukemia.[39] SS can also be medication-induced, including granulocyte-colony stimulating factor or granulocyte macrophage-colony stimulating factor.[39,40] The main differential diagnosis includes cutaneous infection and leukemia cutis. Recognition of SS is important because SS responds rapidly to treatment with systemic corticosteroids, which are usually otherwise avoided in immunosuppressed, febrile patients.[40,41] Skin biopsy and culture can be helpful.[39,41]

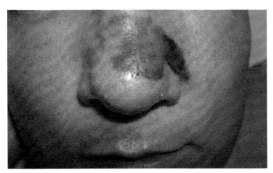

Fig. 11. Hemorrhagic, purpuric plaque on the face that is a clue to underlying fungal sinusitis with *Mucor*.

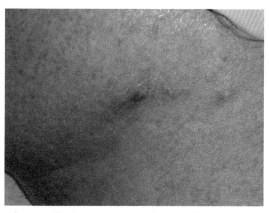

Fig. 12. Disseminated aspergillosis presenting with a nondescript pustule.

Contact Dermatitis

Contact dermatitis is commonly seen by dermatologists, and accounts for approximately 9% of inpatient or emergency room consultations.[42,43] Contact dermatitis can be irritant or allergic in nature. Frequent causes of contact dermatitis in inpatients include adhesives, topical antibiotics, and surgical scrubs. Adhesive contact dermatitis occurs from bandages or monitoring leads, presenting with geometric eczematous to vesicular plaques[44] (**Fig. 14**). Allergic contact dermatitis to substances used under dressings, such as liquid adhesive or topical antibiotics (particularly bacitracin and neomycin), may be more common than reactions to adhesives.[45] Contact dermatitis can occur to commonly used surgical scrubs, including chlorhexadine gluconate and povidone iodine. Povidone iodine also has a high rate of irritant reactions secondary to the oxidative effects of iodine in the skin.[44] Patients present with eczematous plaques around the surgical field, often with accentuation in skin folds or dependent areas where solutions accumulate or become occluded. Treatment of contact dermatitis involves avoidance of the inciting agent and use of moderate to high-potency topical steroids. Systemic corticosteroids may be required if the eruption is widespread, bullous, or progressive.

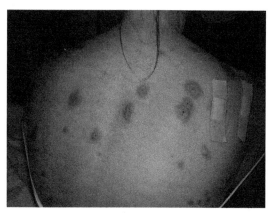

Fig. 13. Sweet syndrome, with edematous erythematous papules and plaques. These lesions often mimic cellulitis clinically and histologically.

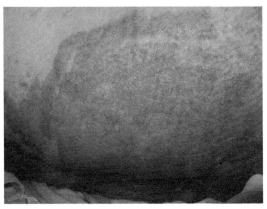

Fig. 14. Allergic contact dermatitis, presumably owing to surgical preparatory scrub; erythematous eczematous plaques often show edema and vesicles.

Red Legs in the Hospitalized Patient: Cellulitis and Mimickers

Cellulitis remains a frequent cause of inpatient hospitalization. Risk factors for lower leg cellulitis include age, obesity, previous cellulitis, previous deep venous thrombosis, edema/lymphedema, venous insufficiency, and disrupted skin barrier.[46,47] Practice guidelines by the Infectious Disease Society of America were recently updated[48]; because Streptococci is the most common organism implicated in uncomplicated lower limb cellulitis, antimicrobial treatment should cover Streptococci unless there are concerns for methicillin-resistant *S aureus* (penetrating trauma, intravenous drug use, known methicillin-resistant *S aureus*). In hospitalized patients, leg elevation should also be emphasized. A short course of oral corticosteroids (eg, prednisone 40 mg orally for 7 days) in those without contraindication added to antimicrobial therapy leads to faster resolution, shorter durations of hospital stay, and may reduce recurrence rates.[48,49]

Mimics of lower extremity cellulitis: venous stasis dermatitis and lipodermatosclerosis

Lower leg cellulitis is frequently overdiagnosed, particularly in the scenario of the patient with suspected "bilateral cellulitis," which is nearly always an alternative diagnosis.[50] One of the most frequent mimics is venous stasis disease, including stasis dermatitis (venous eczema).[8] Stasis dermatitis is an eczematous dermatitis occurring as a result of chronic venous insufficiency, frequently involves the lower leg, and presents with pruritic, fissured, and crusted eczematous papules and plaques (**Fig. 15**). The treatment of stasis dermatitis is 2-fold: midpotency topical steroids to treat the eczematous dermatitis, and compression or elevation to treat the edema.

Lipodermatosclerosis is an inflammatory panniculitis, presenting initially with deep-seated painful, erythematous, warm, cellulitic-appearing nodules and plaques, often on the ankles of women. With time, fibrosis occurs, leaving patients with sclerotic, hyperpigmented plaques and an overall "bound-down" appearance resembling an inverted champagne bottle.[50]

Skin Ulcers in the Hospitalized Patient

Dermatologists can aid in evaluating hospitalized patients with cutaneous ulcers. The differential diagnosis for a patient with a chronic ulcer is broad, and includes common causes such as venous stasis ulcers, pressure ulcers, and arterial ulcers, as well as

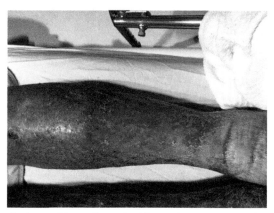

Fig. 15. Venous stasis dermatitis, with marked lower leg edema, erythema, and scale with areas of fissuring. This presentation is often confused with cellulitis; the bilateral nature argues against this.

less common entities, such as vasculitis and infectious processes, ranging from bacterial to deep fungal infections. A dermatology consultation can be particularly helpful in the case of unusual or recalcitrant ulcers, especially when primary dermatologic conditions are suspected. Some ulcerating conditions, such as calciphylaxis and pyoderma gangrenosum (PG), can arise during hospitalization, and are discussed elsewhere in this article.

Calciphylaxis

Calciphylaxis (calcific uremic arteriopathy) is an ulcerative condition of the skin owing to disordered calcium deposition in cutaneous vasculature. Calciphylaxis most frequently occurs in patients with chronic kidney disease on hemodialysis, occurring in 1% to 4% of hemodialysis patients. Calciphylaxis is increasingly reported in nonuremic patients, with risk factors including warfarin exposure, female sex, obesity, and protein C or S deficiency. Regardless of the etiology, calciphylaxis presents as exquisitely painful, retiform, purpuric to necrotic plaques, most frequently on the abdomen, thighs, and buttocks (**Fig. 16**). Diagnosis of calciphylaxis is made based on clinical

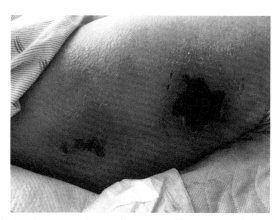

Fig. 16. Calciphylaxis, demonstrating stellate or retiform purpuric and necrotic plaques. Clinical clues are exquisite tenderness and a firm, deep plaque surrounding the eschar.

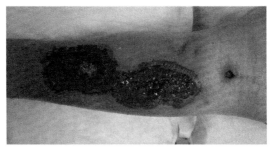

Fig. 17. Pyoderma gangrenosum, with a typical heaped up, violaceous border. Note pathergy at a long-standing surgical site just below the knee.

appearance and lesional biopsy showing medial calcification of arterioles. Calciphylaxis carries a poor prognosis, with mortality rates as high as 80% owing to wound sepsis. Treatment is with avoidance of triggering factors (especially anticoagulants, if implicated), infusion of sodium thiosulfate, and wound care.[51] Intralesional sodium thiosulfate may be an alternative for those who cannot tolerate intravenous infusions.[52]

Pyoderma gangrenosum

PG is a neutrophilic dermatosis that typically presents as painful ulcers with undermined edges and violaceous borders (**Fig. 17**). PG demonstrates pathergy, with the induction of new or worsening lesions at sites of skin trauma. The main differential diagnosis includes venous stasis ulceration, arterial ulceration, and infectious ulcers. Correct diagnosis is imperative because debridement of PG ulcers is usually counterproductive, and treatment may require immunosuppression. Approximately 70% of cases of PG occur in conjunction with other systemic diseases, including inflammatory bowel disease, rheumatoid arthritis, and hematologic malignancies.[53] PG also occurs postoperatively, particularly after operative procedures of the chest wall,[54] and can mimic wound infection. PG is a diagnosis of exclusion, and despite the risk of pathergy, skin biopsy is often performed by dermatologists to exclude atypical infections as treatment with systemic immunosuppression is often required.[53]

SUMMARY

Dermatology consultation can improve diagnostic accuracy in the hospitalized patient with cutaneous disease. Dermatology consultation can streamline and improve treatment plans, and potentially lead to cost savings. Dermatology consultants can be a valuable resource for education for trainees, patients, and families. Inpatient consultative dermatology spans a breadth of conditions, including inflammatory dermatoses, infectious processes, adverse medication reactions, and neoplastic disorders, many of which can be diagnosed based on dermatologic examination alone, but when necessary, bedside skin biopsies can contribute important diagnostic information.

REFERENCES

1. Nahass GT, Meyer AJ, Campbell SF, et al. Prevalence of cutaneous findings in hospitalized medical patients. J Am Acad Dermatol 1995;33:207–11.
2. Kirsner RS, Yang DG, Kerdel FA. Dermatologic disease accounts for a large number of hospital admissions annually. J Am Acad Dermatol 1999;41:970–3.

3. Falanga V, Schachner LA, Rae V, et al. Dermatologic consultations in the hospital setting. Arch Dermatol 1994;130:1022–5.
4. Ozyurt S, Kelekci KH, Seremet S, et al. Analysis of inpatient dermatologic consultations. Actas Dermosifiliogr 2014;105:799–800.
5. Hu L, Haynes H, Ferrazza D, et al. Impact of specialist consultations on inpatient admissions for dermatology-specific and related DRGs. J Gen Intern Med 2013; 28:1477–82.
6. Davila M, Christenson LJ, Sontheimer RD. Epidemiology and outcomes of dermatology in-patient consultations in a Midwestern U.S. University Hospital. Dermatol Online J 2010;16:12.
7. Arakaki RY, Strazzula L, Woo E, et al. The impact of dermatology consultation on diagnostic accuracy and antibiotic use among patients with suspected cellulitis seen at outpatient internal medicine offices: a randomized clinical trial. JAMA Dermatol 2014;150:1056–61.
8. Levell NJ, Wingfield CG, Garioch JJ. Severe lower limb cellulitis is best diagnosed by dermatologists and managed with shared care between primary and secondary care. Br J Dermatol 2011;164:1326–8.
9. Helms AE, Helms SE, Brodell RT. Hospital consultations: time to address an unmet need? J Am Acad Dermatol 2009;60:308–11.
10. McCleskey PE, Gilson RT, DeVillez RL. Medical Student Core Curriculum in Dermatology Survey. J Am Acad Dermatol 2009;61:30–5.e4.
11. Solomon BA, Collins R, Silverberg NB, et al. Quality of care: issue or oversight in health care reform? J Am Acad Dermatol 1996;34:601–7.
12. Cathcart SD, Theos A. Inpatient management of atopic dermatitis. Dermatol Ther 2011;24:249–55.
13. Kirsner RS, Yang DG, Kerdel FA. The changing status of inpatient dermatology at American academic dermatology programs. J Am Acad Dermatol 1999;40:755–7.
14. Barbieri JS, Nelson CA, James WD, et al. The reliability of teledermatology to triage inpatient dermatology consultations. JAMA Dermatol 2014;150:419–24.
15. Fox LP, Cotliar J, Hughey L, et al. Hospitalist dermatology. J Am Acad Dermatol 2009;61:153–4.
16. Bigby M, Jick S, Jick H, et al. Drug-induced cutaneous reactions. A report from the Boston Collaborative Drug Surveillance Program on 15,438 consecutive inpatients, 1975 to 1982. JAMA 1986;256:3358–63.
17. Bigby M. Rates of cutaneous reactions to drugs. Arch Dermatol 2001;137: 765–70.
18. Wintroub BU, Stern R. Cutaneous drug reactions: pathogenesis and clinical classification. J Am Acad Dermatol 1985;13:167–79.
19. Bircher AJ, Scherer Hofmeier K. Drug hypersensitivity reactions during hematopoietic stem cell transplantation. Curr Probl Dermatol 2012;43:150–64.
20. Gerson D, Sriganeshan V, Alexis JB. Cutaneous drug eruptions: a 5-year experience. J Am Acad Dermatol 2008;59:995–9.
21. James WD, Berger TG, Elston DM. Andrews' diseases of the skin. Philadelphia (PA): Saunders Elsevier; 2011.
22. Cotliar J. Approach to the patient with a suspected drug eruption. Semin Cutan Med Surg 2007;26:147–54.
23. Muir J, Storan ER. Response to 'experience with the dermatology inpatient hospital service for adults: Mayo Clinic, 2000-2010'. J Eur Acad Dermatol Venereol 2014;29(6):1236–7.
24. Wahie S, Lawrence CM. Wound complications following diagnostic skin biopsies in dermatology inpatients. Arch Dermatol 2007;143:1267–71.

25. Hu SW, Cotliar J. Acute graft-versus-host disease following hematopoietic stem-cell transplantation. Dermatol Ther 2011;24:411–23.
26. Sundram U. A review of important skin disorders occurring in the posttransplantation patient. Adv Anat Pathol 2014;21:321–9.
27. Lee T, Lee YS, Yoon SY, et al. Characteristics of liver injury in drug-induced systemic hypersensitivity reactions. J Am Acad Dermatol 2013;69:407–15.
28. Tong LX, Worswick SD. Viral infections in acute graft-versus-host disease: a review of diagnostic and therapeutic approaches. J Am Acad Dermatol 2015; 72(4):696–702.
29. Kuykendall TD, Smoller BR. Lack of specificity in skin biopsy specimens to assess for acute graft-versus-host disease in initial 3 weeks after bone-marrow transplantation. J Am Acad Dermatol 2003;49:1081–5.
30. Sharma A, Armstrong AE, Posner MP, et al. Graft-versus-host disease after solid organ transplantation: a single center experience and review of literature. Ann Transplant 2012;17:133–9.
31. Zhang Y, Ruiz P. Solid organ transplant-associated acute graft-versus-host disease. Arch Pathol Lab Med 2010;134:1220–4.
32. Tan HH, Goh CL. Viral infections affecting the skin in organ transplant recipients: epidemiology and current management strategies. Am J Clin Dermatol 2006;7: 13–29.
33. Shiley K, Blumberg E. Herpes viruses in transplant recipients: HSV, VZV, human herpes viruses, and EBV. Infect Dis Clin North Am 2010;24:373–93.
34. Saito K, Hatano Y, Okamoto T, et al. Severe cutaneous necrosis due to mixed infection with herpes simplex virus and fungi in an unrelated cord blood stem cell transplantation recipient. J Dermatol 2013;40:411–3.
35. Muluneh B, Dean A, Armistead P, et al. Successful clearance of cutaneous acyclovir-resistant, foscarnet-refractory herpes virus lesions with topical cidofovir in an allogeneic hematopoietic stem cell transplant patient. J Oncol Pharm Pract 2013;19:181–5.
36. Mays SR, Bogle MA, Bodey GP. Cutaneous fungal infections in the oncology patient: recognition and management. Am J Clin Dermatol 2006;7:31–43.
37. Chacon AH, Farooq U, Shiman MI, et al. Cutaneous aspergillosis masquerading as Sweet's syndrome in a patient with acute myelogenous leukemia. J Cutan Pathol 2013;40:66–8.
38. Grossman ME, Silvers DN, Walther RR. Cutaneous manifestations of disseminated candidiasis. J Am Acad Dermatol 1980;2:111–6.
39. Kazmi SM, Pemmaraju N, Patel KP, et al. Characteristics of Sweet syndrome in patients with acute myeloid leukemia. Clin Lymphoma Myeloma Leuk 2014; 15(6):358–63.
40. Raza S, Kirkland RS, Patel AA, et al. Insight into Sweet's syndrome and associated-malignancy: a review of the current literature. Int J Oncol 2013;42: 1516–22.
41. Anzalone CL, Cohen PR. Acute febrile neutrophilic dermatosis (Sweet's syndrome). Curr Opin Hematol 2013;20:26–35.
42. Penate Y, Guillermo N, Melwani P, et al. Dermatologists in hospital wards: an 8-year study of dermatology consultations. Dermatology 2009;219:225–31.
43. Jack AR, Spence AA, Nichols BJ, et al. Cutaneous conditions leading to dermatology consultations in the emergency department. West J Emerg Med 2011;12: 551–5.
44. Cheng CE, Kroshinsky D. Iatrogenic skin injury in hospitalized patients. Clin Dermatol 2011;29:622–32.

45. Widman TJ, Oostman H, Storrs FJ. Allergic contact dermatitis from medical adhesive bandages in patients who report having a reaction to medical bandages. Dermatitis 2008;19:32–7.
46. Hirschmann JV, Raugi GJ. Lower limb cellulitis and its mimics: part I. Lower limb cellulitis. J Am Acad Dermatol 2012;67:163.e1–12 [quiz: 175–6].
47. Tay EY, Fook-Chong S, Oh CC, et al. Cellulitis recurrence score: a tool for predicting recurrence of lower limb cellulitis. J Am Acad Dermatol 2015;72:140–5.
48. Stevens DL, Bisno AL, Chambers HF, et al. Practice guidelines for the diagnosis and management of skin and soft tissue infections: 2014 update by the Infectious Diseases Society of America. Clin Infect Dis 2014;59:e10–52.
49. Bergkvist PI, Sjobeck K. Antibiotic and prednisolone therapy of erysipelas: a randomized, double blind, placebo-controlled study. Scand J Infect Dis 1997;29:377–82.
50. Hirschmann JV, Raugi GJ. Lower limb cellulitis and its mimics: part II. Conditions that simulate lower limb cellulitis. J Am Acad Dermatol 2012;67:177.e1–9 [quiz: 185–6].
51. Vedvyas C, Winterfield LS, Vleugels RA. Calciphylaxis: a systematic review of existing and emerging therapies. J Am Acad Dermatol 2012;67:e253–60.
52. Strazzula L, Nigwekar SU, Steele D, et al. Intralesional sodium thiosulfate for the treatment of calciphylaxis. JAMA Dermatol 2013;149:946–9.
53. Su WP, Davis MD, Weenig RH, et al. Pyoderma gangrenosum: clinicopathologic correlation and proposed diagnostic criteria. Int J Dermatol 2004;43:790–800.
54. Liaqat M, Elsensohn AN, Hansen CD, et al. Acute postoperative pyoderma gangrenosum case and review of literature identifying chest wall predominance and no recurrence following skin grafts. J Am Acad Dermatol 2014;71:e145–6.

Teledermatology

John D. Whited, MD, MHS[a,b,*]

KEYWORDS

- Telemedicine • Teledermatology • Digital imaging • Diagnosis • Clinical outcomes
- User satisfaction

KEY POINTS

- Teledermatology can be performed using store and forward technology, real-time interactive technology, or a hybrid technique that combines both elements.
- Teledermatology has been found to be a diagnostically reliable means of diagnosing skin conditions. The evidence for diagnostic accuracy has been more equivocal.
- In-person dermatology visits decrease by an average of 45.5% to 61.5% for store and forward teledermatology and real-time interactive teledermatology, respectively.
- Clinical outcomes for patients being referred to or managed by teledermatology have been comparable with conventional care.
- Overall, patients are satisfied with teledermatology. Accessibility and averted travel are cited as positive features.

INTRODUCTION

Telemedicine has transitioned, albeit not completely, from an alternative method of health care delivery to simply a means of delivering health care. Teledermatology, one of the more common applications of telemedicine, is also one of the more mature disciplines in telemedicine. Primary care clinicians who are not current users

Funding source: This article contains a review of content from Department of Veterans Affairs, Office of Research and Development, Health Services Research and Development Awards IIR 95-045, IIR 98-159, and IIR-05-278 to the author.
Conflict of interest: Dr J.D. Whited: Coeditor and royalties for *Teledermatology: a user's guide* published by Cambridge University Press.
The views expressed in this article are those of the author and do not necessarily reflect the position or policy of the United States Department of Veterans Affairs or the United States Government.
[a] Research and Development, Durham Veterans Affairs Medical Center, Research and Development (151), 508 Fulton Street, Durham, NC 27705, USA; [b] Division of General Internal Medicine, Duke University School of Medicine, 411 West Chapel Hill Street, Suite 500, Durham, NC 27701, USA
* Durham Veterans Affairs Medical Center, Research (151), 508 Fulton Street, Durham, NC 27705.
E-mail address: john.whited@va.gov

of teledermatology will likely be exposed to teledermatology, or at least the opportunity to use teledermatology, in the future. Although increasingly ubiquitous, teledermatology does alter how care is delivered and affects the experience of the referring clinician, the patient, and the dermatologist. This article emphasizes how those features affect the referring clinician who, most often, is a primary care clinician. The evidence of most relevance to a primary care clinician, namely, diagnostic reliability, diagnostic accuracy, clinical outcomes, and user satisfaction, is the focus of this review.

TELEDERMATOLOGY MODALITIES

Teledermatology is performed by using either a store and forward technique or real-time interactive technology. A third method, a hybrid of these 2 methods, integrates aspects of both modalities. The key features of each modality are described in **Table 1**.

STORE AND FORWARD

The store and forward technique has emerged as the most commonly used modality in teledermatology. In general, it consists of high-resolution digital images bundled with standardized historical and clinical information. Questions such as the duration of presence of the referred condition, a change in size, or if the lesion is pruritic are typical components of a standardized history. Customarily, an imaging convention or protocol is followed to obtain the image set.[1] The consult requests are sent electronically from the site of the referring clinician and patient to the site of the consulting dermatologist, often via an electronic health record or any other electronic means that meets all applicable security and privacy requirements. The distinguishing feature of store and forward teledermatology is a separation of the referring clinician and patient from the dermatologist in both time and place. For example, a consult request placed on day 1 by a referring clinician from one geographic site is reviewed on day 2 by a

Table 1	
Key features of teledermatology modalities	
Modality	**Key Features**
Store and forward	• Uses still digital images • Includes historical information, often standardized • Patient and dermatologist are separated in space and time; asynchronous • No or minimal interaction between patient and dermatologist • Logistically straightforward
Real-time interactive	• Uses videoconferencing technology • Allows for verbal interaction between patient, referring clinician (if present), and dermatologist • Patient and dermatologist are separated by space but not time; synchronous • Logistically more complex
Hybrid	• Uses videoconferencing technology with higher-resolution still digital images as an adjunct • Allows for patient interaction • Patient and dermatologist are separated by space but not time; synchronous

dermatologist located at another geographic site. For the majority of store and forward consultations, there is no direct interaction between the dermatologist and the patient within the confines of the teledermatology consultation. The dermatologist's conclusions and recommendations are sent back to the referring clinician who conveys this information to the patient and implements the recommendations, if any.

Real-Time Interactive

The real-time interactive technique uses videoconferencing technology to perform the teledermatology consultation. The patient, dermatologist, and usually an individual at the referring site, facilitator, technician, or referring clinician, are present and interact via the videoconference. A functional difference of this modality compared with store and forward is that, although there is a separation of patient and dermatologist by space, there is not a separation in time. Therefore, a logistical consideration when using real-time interactive technology is scheduling both sites to be available at the same time. Consults performed across different time zones can add to the scheduling complexity. This technique does allow the dermatologist and patient to verbally interact in much the same manner as would occur in an in-person clinic visit.

Hybrid

As the name implies, hybrid modalities integrate features of both store and forward and real-time interactive technologies. High-resolution digital images are often reviewed in the context of the interactive features that videoconferencing allows. During the consult session, the dermatologist can direct the number and location of still digital images he or she feels is necessary to complete the evaluation. The higher-resolution still images augment the lower-resolution images that are typical of videoconferencing technology. Thus, this modality allows for the dermatologist to interact with the patient in real time and to review high-resolution still digital images of the affected skin before, during, and after the interaction.

DIAGNOSTIC RELIABILITY AND ACCURACY

A question relevant for referring clinicians to ask is how does teledermatology diagnosis compare with diagnosis that would be made if patients were evaluated via an in-person face to face evaluation? Likewise, this same question should be asked by patients and dermatologists. There are 2 salient features of the diagnostic process, interobserver diagnostic reliability and diagnostic accuracy.[2] Reliability refers to agreement or the repeatability or reproducibility of a diagnostic assessment. If 2 examiners independently evaluate the same skin lesion and both conclude that it is a basal cell carcinoma, then the diagnoses they provided are reliable. However, if one examiner believes the skin lesion to be a basal cell carcinoma and the other diagnoses it as sebaceous hyperplasia, then their diagnoses differ and are considered to be unreliable.

Accuracy reflects whether the diagnoses reached are correct or incorrect and is assessed by comparing the diagnosis with a reference standard test, also termed a gold standard test. If after a biopsy and histopathologic review of tissue (reference standard test) the above-mentioned lesion is determined to be a basal cell carcinoma, then in the first scenario both examiners provided an accurate diagnosis of basal cell carcinoma. In the second scenario, one examiner was accurate (basal cell carcinoma) and one was inaccurate (sebaceous hyperplasia). As a final alternative, if the biopsy reveals that the lesion is a squamous cell carcinoma, then, in both cases, the examiners provided inaccurate diagnoses.

Reliability of Teledermatology Modalities

Store and forward

Several studies have reported interobserver agreement between teledermatologists and dermatologists providing in-person evaluations. Simple percentage agreement has ranged from 41% to 100%.[3-25] As might be expected, greater agreement is noted when overlap between differential diagnoses is counted as agreement compared with agreement based only on a single most likely diagnosis (**Table 2**).

Two studies provided a context for teledermatologist versus in-person dermatologist agreement by assessing the level of agreement found among different in-person dermatologists. One of these studies found that 2 in-person dermatologists agreed on a diagnosis 54% of the time (95% confidence interval [CI], 46%–61%) for the single most likely diagnosis and 92% of the time (95% CI, 88%–96%) when agreement based on differential diagnoses was considered.[7] With the same patient sample, the range for agreement between teledermatologists and clinic-based dermatologists was 41% to 55% (95% CI, 34%–63%) for the single most likely diagnosis and 79% to 95% (95% CI, 72%–98%) when differential diagnoses were included. The overlapping confidence intervals provide no evidence to suggest a difference in reliability for the

Table 2
Interobserver reliability between teledermatologist and in-person dermatologist evaluations reported as simple percentage agreement: store and forward teledermatology

Reliability Assessment by Diagnostic Category		
Single Most Likely Diagnosis (%)	Differential Diagnoses Included (%)	Reference
61–64	67–70	Kvedar et al,[3] 1997
88	—	Zelickson & Homan,[4] 1997
90	—	Lyon & Harrison,[5] 1997
64–77	81–89	High et al,[6] 2000
41–55	79–95	Whited et al,[7] 1999
44–51	57–61	Taylor et al,[8] 2001
73–85	83–89	Lim et al,[9] 2001
41	51	Eminovic et al,[10] 2003
54	63	Du Moulin et al,[11] 2003
44–48	64–65	Mahendran et al,[12] 2005
53	64	Oakley et al,[13] 2006
56	68	Tucker & Lewis,[14] 2005
55	—	Bowns et al,[15] 2006
71–76	90–97	Ebner et al,[16] 2008
87–92	96–100	Silva et al,[17] 2009
69	—	Heffner et al,[18] 2009
78–84	92–98	Ribas et al,[19] 2010
88	—	Rubegni et al,[20] 2011
—	62	Lamel et al,[21] 2012
—	95	Kaliyadan et al,[22] 2013
72–73	88–92	Aguilera et al,[23] 2014
91	—	Nami et al,[24] 2015
46–76	79–91	Warshaw et al,[25] 2015

teledermatologist versus in-person dermatologist pairs when compared with diagnostic agreement found among different in-person dermatologists. Another study of similar design yielded similar results. Agreement between teledermatologists and in-person dermatologists was 78% to 84% (95% CI, 71%–89%) for the single most likely diagnosis and 92% to 98% (95% CI, 87%–100%) when differential diagnoses were included[19] this compared with 83% (95% CI, 77%–89%) agreement for in-person dermatologists for the single most likely diagnosis and 94% (95% CI, 90%–97%) agreement for differential diagnoses.

Real-time interactive
A smaller body of evidence has shown that interobserver diagnostic reliability values for real-time interactive consultations are fairly similar to store and forward interventions.[26–32] Between teledermatologists and in-person dermatologists, agreement on a single most likely diagnosis has ranged from 54% to 80% and agreement that includes differential diagnoses has ranged from 76% to 99% (**Table 3**). One study made simultaneous assessments of agreement among different in-person dermatologists compared with a teledermatologist versus in-person dermatologist pairing.[26] For the in-person dermatologists, agreement on the single most likely diagnosis was 94% (95% CI, 87%–100%) and 100% when differential diagnoses were included. For the teledermatologist versus in-person dermatologist pairing, agreement on the single most likely diagnosis was 78% (95% CI, 68%–88%) and 99% (95% CI, 97%–100%) for differential diagnoses. Thus, no evidence to suggest a difference in reliability was found.

Accuracy of Teledermatology Modalities

The assessment of accuracy in dermatology is difficult.[33] Accuracy evaluation requires the ability to apply a reference standard test. Histopathologic review of biopsied tissue can serve as a reference standard test, although its primary uses are to distinguish benign from malignant tumors and to support a clinicopathologic correlation. Because histopathologic assessment is often not definitively specific, applying this as a gold standard to the clinical diagnosis can be problematic.

Store and forward
With these limitations in mind, several studies have compared the accuracy of store and forward teledermatology with in-person dermatology with the use of reference standard tests.[7,13,34–41] The conclusions have varied, ranging from diagnostic superiority for teledermatology[36] and comparable accuracy rates[7,13,35,39–41] to inferiority of teledermatology (**Table 4**).[34,37,38]

Table 3
Interobserver reliability between teledermatologist and in-person dermatologist evaluations reported as simple percentage agreement: real-time interactive teledermatology

Reliability Assessment by Diagnostic Category		
Single Most Likely Diagnosis (%)	Differential Diagnoses Included (%)	Reference
78	99	Lesher et al,[26] 1998
54	80	Gilmour et al,[27] 1998
80	—	Lowitt et al,[28] 1998
60	76	Loane et al,[29] 1998
77	—	Phillips et al,[30] 1997
59	—	Phillips et al,[31] 1998
72	86	Nordal et al,[32] 2001

Table 4
Diagnostic accuracy rate comparing in-person evaluation: store and forward technology

| Modality | Accuracy Assessment by Diagnostic Category | | Reference |
	Single Most Likely Diagnosis (%) (95% CI)	Differential Diagnoses Included (%) (95% CI)	
In person	59–71 (48–81)	85 (77–93)	Whited et al,[7] 1999
Teledermatology	53–63 (42–74)	68–85 (58–93)	
In person	72 (53–87)	—	Oakley et al,[13] 2006
Teledermatology	71 (56–83)	—	
In person	—	80–97	Krupinksi et al,[34] 1999
Teledermatology	—	73–78	
In person	70–77	80–92	Whited et al,[35] 1998
Teledermatology	31–85	85	
In person	30–42 (15–53)	—	Lozzi et al,[36] 2007
Teledermatology	79 (72–93)	—	
In person	56 (53–60)	76 (73–79)	Warshaw et al,[37] 2009
Teledermatology	43 (39–47)	59 (56–63)	
In person	59	80	Warshaw et al,[38] 2009
Teledermatology	50	64	
In person	57 (39–74)	—	Rios-Yuil,[39] 2012
Teledermatology	67 (50–84)	—	
In person	84 (70–98)	—	Barnard & Goldyne,[40] 2000
Teledermatology	73 (56–90)	—	
In person	43 (35–51)	—	Jolliffe et al,[41] 2001
Teledermatology	47 (39–55)	—	

Real-time interactive

Only 1 study has evaluated the accuracy of real-time interactive technology.[28] Although the study primarily assessed diagnostic reliability, an accuracy assessment was performed from the 11 histopathologic findings that were available. For the in-person evaluation, 7 of 11 (64%) diagnoses were accurate and 8 of 11 (73%) diagnoses were accurate as made by a teledermatologist.

DERMATOLOGY CLINIC VISITS AVERTED

A feature relevant to both referring clinicians and dermatologists are the number of times teledermatology can avert a clinic-based visit with a dermatologist. Issues such as the feasibility of a particular patient or population to attend an in-person visit and geographic concerns, such as the distance or method of travel required to attend a dermatology clinic, can obviously influence these rates. Another factor is the ability of the referring clinician to perform any recommended interventions such as a skin biopsy or application of cryotherapy. The greater the number of interventions that the referring clinician can or is willing to perform based on the dermatologist's recommendations, the less likely the patient requires travel to the site of dermatology care for those interventions.

Store and Forward

Several studies have reported on the number of dermatology clinic visits averted with the use of store and forward teledermatology. The percentage of dermatology clinic visits averted has ranged widely from 13% to 81%.[8,10,12,15,16,42–54] The average rate of dermatology clinic visits that were avoided by store and forward teledermatology was 45.5%.

The store and forward teledermatology program initiated by the Veterans Affairs Puget Sound Health Care System warrants particular mention and description.[55] In what is perhaps the most sophisticated store and forward teledermatology program reported in the literature, the Veterans Affairs Puget Sound Health Care System Dermatology Service has implemented a curriculum for primary care clinicians that includes initial training, continuing education, development of patient care plans, and basic surgery skills training. Between baseline and year 1 of this program, a fairly dramatic change in clinical practice patterns was noted. At baseline, most dermatology care (61%) was referred to the remote dermatology clinics, whereas at year 1, only 15% of the patients were referred to remote dermatology clinics ($P<.01$). This result coincided with an increased number of procedures (eg, biopsies) being performed by the primary care clinicians through the training component of the teledermatology program.

Real-Time Interactive

For real-time interactive teledermatology, the rate of visit avoidance has ranged from 44.4% to 82%.[42,56–59] The average rate of clinic visit avoidance was 61.5% for real-time interactive technology. These values are higher than those reported for store and forward teledermatology as may be expected because the nature of real-time interactive teledermatology is more commonly meant to function as a substitute for an in-person evaluation, whereas store and forward teledermatology is more likely to be used, in part, as a triage mechanism to decide who does and does not need to be seen.[60]

CLINICAL OUTCOMES

Another referring clinician's question of relevance is how does teledermatology affect the clinical course of patients—would the patients be expected to fare better, worse, or the same if teledermatology is used? Similar to accuracy, assessments of clinical course can be difficult. If you are assessing a single disease and a disease-specific severity measure exists, then such a measure can be used. For example, if the target condition is psoriasis, then a measure such as the Psoriasis Area Severity Index can be used. However, the vast majority of skin conditions have no such instrument available.

Store and Forward

Three randomized trials have assessed clinical course with store and forward teledermatology.[61–63] Two of these studies were of similar design and used serial digital images as a means of assessing clinical course.[61,62] Serial digital images were used to assess the clinical course of a wide variety of referred ambulatory skin conditions. Both these studies yielded similar results. In the first study, between the time of referral and month 4, the percentage of conventionally referred patients rated as improved was 65% versus 64% for teledermatology; 32% were rated unchanged for conventional care compared with 33% for teledermatology; 3% were rated worse in the conventional care group versus 4% rated as worse for teledermatology.[61] The differences were not statistically significant ($P = .57$). For the second study, a larger number of categories were used to rate clinical course.[62] Between the time of referral and month 9, conventionally referred patients and teledermatology patients, respectively, were rated as resolved in 26% versus 25%; improved in 46% versus 47%; unchanged, not clinically relevant in 11% versus 10%; unchanged, clinically relevant in 13% versus 10%; worse in 4% versus 8%. There was no evidence to suggest a difference in ratings between the 2 referral groups (P = .88). A third study randomized patients to clinic-based follow-up or follow-up using smartphone technology to manage facial acne treated with isotretinoin.[63] A smartphone was used both to collect the images and to transmit clinical information between the patient and dermatologist. Clinical course was rated using the Global Acne Severity Scale and total lesion count. The severity of acne during 24 weeks of treatment improved in both groups with no evidence for a difference between the 2 management options (P = .38 as measured by the Global Acne Severity Scale and P = .95 as measured by the total lesion count).

Real-Time Interactive

Two studies conducted a retrospective medical record review of teledermatology consultations to assess clinical outcomes.[64,65] In one study, of 127 subjects reviewed, 58.3% were rated as showing clinical improvement, 16.5% were rated as no clinical improvement, 7.1% of the patients were rated noncompliant, and 18.1% were rated as not applicable to include chronic conditions that would not be expected to change.[64] In a second study, clinical improvement, as documented by a teledermatologist in a follow-up visit, was reported for 215 (68.7%) of the 313 patients managed by teledermatology with 2 or more teledermatology encounters.[65]

PATIENT AND REFERRING CLINICIAN SATISFACTION

Reliable and valid instruments have not been developed to assess satisfaction among users and participants of teledermatology. Reports in the literature are primarily composed of evaluations that have face validity. Face validity implies that the questions being asked seem to make a reasonable assessment of the relevant issues or address important features at face value.

Patient Satisfaction: Store and Forward

There are several studies that have assessed the satisfaction of patients who have used store and forward teledermatology.[15,22,63,66–73] Often, patients have not shown a clear preference for teledermatology or conventional care suggesting that they are satisfied with both modalities. With all things being equal, patients would likely prefer an in-person visit, but all things are not equal. For example, a patient may have no local access to dermatology care or travel may be associated with great difficulty. It is issues such as these, among others, that served as the genesis of telemedicine, including teledermatology. Nonetheless, patients have expressed a high level of overall satisfaction with store and forward teledermatology. This feature and other select comments about the patients' perspective on store and forward teledermatology appear in **Table 5**.

Referring Clinician Satisfaction: Store and Forward

Overall, referring clinicians have reported that store and forward teledermatology is a positive experience, with some exceptions.[15,66–69,71,72,74,75] The educational benefit is an oft-cited useful feature of the consult process. The feedback, often quicker than through traditional consult processes, lends itself at least to the perception that there is an educational benefit derived from the teledermatology consult content and dermatologist to referring clinician communication. In fact, the aforementioned Veteran Affairs Puget Sound Health Care System store and forward teledermatology program has demonstrated improved dermatology knowledge among primary care

Table 5
User satisfaction: store and forward teledermatology

Reported Positive Features	Reported Negative Features	Overall Satisfaction	Reference
Patient Satisfaction			
Would recommend teledermatology to others	Concern about the patient-provider relationship	42%	Weinstock et al,[66] 2002
Satisfied that concerns were addressed	—	4.56 on a 5-point scale	Kvedar et al,[68] 1999
Comfortable with use of digital images	Concern about incomplete information transmission	7.4 on a 10-point scale	van den Akker et al,[69] 2001
Teledermatology was convenient	Concern about not speaking with a dermatologist	93%	Williams et al,[70] 2001
Confidence in teledermatology	Concern about time required to learn about consult results	82%	Whited et al,[72] 2004
Preference for teledermatology over in-person care in 66% of respondents	Concern about proper treatment and follow-up	4.1 on a 5-point scale	Hsueh et al,[73] 2012
Referring Clinician Satisfaction			
Would recommend teledermatology	Consult process took too long	63%	Weinstock et al,[66] 2002
Found it convenient	Time requirements to generate the consult	—	Kvedar et al,[68] 1999
Improved access to specialists	Increased workload	21%	Collins et al,[71] 2004
Preference for teledermatology	—	92%	Whited et al,[72] 2004
Easy to use, would use system again	Uncertain that teledermatology would decrease consult time	—	Ou et al,[74] 2008
Educational benefit	Problems with information technology	71%	McFarland et al,[75] 2013

clinicians that used the teledermatology referral system.[55] A dermatology competency examination was administered to primary care providers at baseline and 1 year into the program. Scores on the examination improved from 63% correct to 74% correct at year 1 ($P = .01$).

Negative comments are voiced when the referring clinicians are responsible for generating and sending the teledermatology consults, which is understandable in busy primary care practices and suggests that teledermatology technicians or other staff dedicated to initiate and send teledermatology consults may be important, at least for clinics that would expect to generate a large volume of consults. This concept is analogous to the role that a phlebotomist plays when a blood test is ordered. This particular issue was reported in a study that assessed the perspectives of primary care clinicians who were users of teledermatology, primarily store and forward teledermatology.[76] A challenge reported by the primary care clinicians was the competing interest and deviation from their usual workflow processes imposed by the generation of the teledermatology consultation. Nonetheless, all surveyed primary care clinicians rated teledermatology as extremely valuable. A summary of other perceptions provided by referring clinicians appear in **Table 5**.

Patient Satisfaction: Real-Time Interactive

As with store and forward technology, patients generally express no strong preference for one modality over the other and generally perceive real-time interactive teledermatology favorably.[27,32,77–80] Representative findings from the literature appear in **Table 6**.

Referring Clinician Satisfaction: Real-Time Interactive

Only 2 studies have assessed referring clinician satisfaction with real-time interactive teledermatology.[27,81] As with store and forward teledermatology, a perceived educational benefit was a primary positive comment. Negative aspects, much like with store

Table 6			
User satisfaction: real-time interactive			
Reported Positive Features	**Reported Negative Features**	**Overall Satisfaction**	**Reference**
Patient Satisfaction			
Teledermatology was as good as or better than clinic-based care for contact with the dermatologist	Lack of hands-on examination	—	Nordal et al,[32] 2001
Teledermatology was as good as clinic-based care	Discomfort with the camera	—	Loane et al,[78] 1998
Teledermatology as good as clinic visits	—	88%	Hicks et al,[79] 2003
Less travel required	—	91%	Al Quran et al,[80] 2015
Referring Clinician Satisfaction			
Educational benefit	Problems with information technology	—	Gilmour et al,[27] 1998
Educational benefit	Consults were time consuming	—	Jones et al,[81] 1996

and forward consults, were reports that the consults were time consuming. In addition, problems with the quality of the visual and auditory features of the information technology were cited as a negative feature (see **Table 6**).

FUTURE CONSIDERATIONS/SUMMARY

Primary care clinicians who have not already encountered teledermatology are increasingly likely to do so in the future. Understanding the evidence that describes how teledermatology performs in areas that are relevant to the referring clinician and their patients should serve as a basis for informed decision making and planning regarding teledermatology implementation. The evidence to date indicates that teledermatology is comparable in diagnostic reliability with conventional consultations and there has been no evidence to suggest a difference in clinical outcomes with store and forward teledermatology. Any application of teledermatology would be expected to avert some proportion of dermatology clinic visits. The variability of this effect has been wide, in part, because of expectations of the consult process, geography, and the ability of referring clinicians to implement dermatologist's recommendations. Overall, teledermatology is well accepted by patients and referring clinicians; however, satisfaction is lower among referring clinicians who do not have support in place to generate teledermatology consultations. Diagnostic accuracy results have been less definitive, with some evidence indicating that teledermatology's accuracy is inferior to in-person assessments. This area may warrant future consideration as certain skin conditions or lesions may have different accuracy characteristics when reviewed by teledermatology modalities. The teledermatology literature is small, albeit growing, and as a maturing discipline these and other more refined research questions may be important topics for future consideration.

REFERENCES

1. McKoy K, Norton S, Lappan C. Quick guide for store-forward and live-interactive teledermatology for referring providers. American Telemedicine Association; 2012. Available at: http://www.americantelemed.org/resources/telemedicine-practice-guidelines/telemedicine-practice-guidelines/quick-guide-to-store-forward-live-interactive-teledermatology#.VcjiPzYw_cs. Accessed March 25, 2015.
2. Fletcher RH, Fletcher SW, Wagner EH. Clinical epidemiology – the essentials. 2nd edition. Baltimore (MD): Williams and Wilkins; 1988. p. 23–4.
3. Kvedar JC, Edwards RA, Menn ER, et al. The substitution of digital images for dermatologic physical examination. Arch Dermatol 1997;133(2):161–7.
4. Zelickson BD, Homan L. Teledermatology in the nursing home. Arch Dermatol 1997;133(2):171–4.
5. Lyon CC, Harrison PV. A portable digital imaging system in dermatology: diagnostic and educational applications. J Telemed Telecare 1997;3(S1):81–3.
6. High WA, Houston MS, Calobrisi SD, et al. Assessment of the accuracy of low-cost store-and-forward teledermatology consultation. J Am Acad Dermatol 2000;42(5):776–83.
7. Whited JD, Hall RP, Simel DL, et al. Reliability and accuracy of dermatologists' clinic-based and digital image consultations. J Am Acad Dermatol 1999;41(5):693–702.
8. Taylor P, Goldsmith P, Murray K, et al. Evaluating a telemedicine system to assist in the management of teledermatology referrals. Br J Dermatol 2001;144(2):328–33.
9. Lim AC, Egerton IB, See A, et al. Accuracy and reliability of store-and-forward teledermatology: preliminary results from the St. George Teledermatology Project. Australas J Dermatol 2001;42(4):247–51.

10. Eminovic N, Witkamp L, Ravelli AC, et al. Potential effect of patient-assisted tele-dermatology on outpatient referral rates. J Telemed Telecare 2003;9(6):321–7.

11. Du Moulin MF, Bullens-Goessens YI, Henquet CJ, et al. The reliability of diag-nosis using store-and-forward teledermatology. J Telemed Telecare 2003;9(5):249–52.

12. Mahendran R, Goodfield MJ, Sheehan-Dare RA. An evaluation of the role of a store-and-forward teledermatology system in skin cancer diagnosis and manage-ment. Clin Exp Dermatol 2005;30(3):209–14.

13. Oakley AM, Reeves F, Bennett J, et al. Diagnostic value of written referral and/or images for skin lesions. J Telemed Telecare 2006;12(3):151–8.

14. Tucker WF, Lewis FM. Digital imaging: a diagnostic screening tool? Int J Dermatol 2005;44(6):479–81.

15. Bowns IR, Collins K, Walters SJ, et al. Telemedicine in dermatology: a randomized controlled trial. Health Technol Assess 2006;10(43):1–39.

16. Ebner C, Wurm EM, Binder B, et al. Mobile teledermatology: a feasibility study of 58 subjects using mobile phones. J Telemed Telecare 2008;14(1):2–7.

17. Silva CS, Souza MB, Duque IA, et al. Teledermatology: diagnostic correlation in a primary care service. An Bras Dermatol 2009;84(5):489–93.

18. Heffner VA, Lyon VB, Brousseau DC, et al. Store-and-forward teledermatology versus in-person visits: a comparison in pediatric dermatology clinic. J Am Acad Dermatol 2009;60(6):956–61.

19. Ribas J, Cunha Mda G, Schettini AP, et al. Agreement between dermatological diagnoses made by live examination compared to analysis of digital images. An Bras Dermatol 2010;85(4):441–7.

20. Rubegni P, Nami N, Cevenini G, et al. Geriatric teledermatology: store-and-forward vs.face-to-face examination. J Eur Acad Dermatol Venereol 2011;25(11):1334–9.

21. Lamel SA, Haldeman KM, Ely H, et al. Application of mobile teledermatology for skin cancer screening. J Am Acad Dermatol 2012;67(4):576–81.

22. Kaliyadan F, Amin TT, Kuruvilla J, et al. Mobile teledermatology – patient satisfac-tion, diagnostic and management concordance, and factors affecting patient refusal to participate in Saudi Arabia. J Telemed Telecare 2013;19(6):315–9.

23. Aguilera GR, del Calle PC, Iglesias EV, et al. Interobserver reliability of store-and-forward teledermatology in a clinical practice setting. Actas Dermosifiliogr 2014;105(6):605–13.

24. Nami N, Massone C, Rubegni P, et al. Concordance and time estimation of store-and-forward mobile teledermatology compared to classical face-to-face consul-tation. Acta Derm Venereol 2015;95(1):35–9.

25. Warshaw EM, Gravely AA, Nelson DB. Reliability of store and forward telederma-tology for skin neoplasms. J Am Acad Dermatol 2015;72(3):426–35.

26. Lesher JL, Davis LS, Gourdin FW, et al. Telemedicine evaluation of cutaneous dis-eases: a blinded comparative study. J Am Acad Dermatol 1998;38(1):27–31.

27. Gilmour E, Campbell SM, Loane MA, et al. Comparison of teleconsultations and face-to-face consultations: preliminary results of a United Kingdom multicentre teledermatology study. Br J Dermatol 1998;139(1):81–7.

28. Lowitt MH, Kessler II, Kauffman CL, et al. Teledermatology and in-person exam-inations: a comparison of patient and physician perceptions and diagnostic agreement. Arch Dermatol 1998;134(4):471–6.

29. Loane MA, Corbett R, Bloomer SE, et al. Diagnostic accuracy and clinical man-agement by realtime teledermatology. Results from the Northern Ireland arms of the UK multicentre teledermatology trial. J Telemed Telecare 1998;4(2):95–100.

30. Phillips CM, Burke WA, Shechter A, et al. Reliability of dermatology teleconsultations with the use of teleconferencing technology. J Am Acad Dermatol 1997; 37(3):398–402.

31. Phillips CM, Burke WA, Allen MH, et al. Reliability of telemedicine in evaluating skin tumors. Telemed J E Health 1998;4(1):5–7.

32. Nordal EJ, Moseng D, Kvammen B, et al. A comparative study of teleconsultations versus face-to-face consultations. J Telemed Telecare 2001;7(5):257–65.

33. Whited JD. Teledermatology: current status and future directions. Am J Clin Dermatol 2001;2(2):59–64.

34. Krupinski EA, LeSueur B, Ellsworth L, et al. Diagnostic accuracy and image quality using a digital camera for teledermatology. Telemed J E Health 1999;5(3):257–63.

35. Whited JD, Mills BJ, Hall RP, et al. A pilot trial of digital imaging in skin cancer. J Telemed Telecare 1998;4(2):108–12.

36. Lozzi GP, Soyer HP, Massone C, et al. The additive value of second opinion teleconsulting in the management of patients with challenging inflammatory, neoplastic skin diseases: a best practice model in dermatology? J Eur Acad Dermatol Venereol 2007;21(1):30–4.

37. Warshaw EM, Lederle FA, Grill JP, et al. Accuracy of teledermatology for nonpigmented neoplasms. J Am Acad Dermatol 2009;60(4):579–88.

38. Warshaw EM, Lederle FA, Grill JP, et al. Accuracy of teledermatology for pigmented lesions. J Am Acad Dermatol 2009;61(5):753–65.

39. Rios-Yuil JM. Correlation between face-to-face assessment and telemedicine for the diagnosis of skin disease in case conferences. Actas Dermosifiliogr 2012; 103(2):138–43.

40. Barnard CM, Goldyne ME. Evaluation of an asynchronous teleconsultation system for diagnosis of skin cancer and other skin diseases. Telemed J E Health 2000;6(4):379–84.

41. Jolliffe VM, Harris DW, Whittaker SJ. Can we safely diagnose pigmented lesions from stored video images? A diagnostic comparison between clinical examination and stored video images of pigmented lesions removed for histology. Clin Exp Dermatol 2001;26(1):84–7.

42. Loane MA, Bloomer SE, Corbett R, et al. A comparison of real-time and store-and-forward teledermatology: a cost-benefit study. Br J Dermatol 2000;143(6): 1241–7.

43. White H, Gould D, Mills W, et al. The Cornwall dermatology electronic referral and image-transfer project. J Telemed Telecare 1999;5(S1):85–6.

44. Whited JD, Hall RP, Foy ME, et al. Teledermatology's impact on time to intervention among referrals to a dermatology consult service. Telemed J E Health 2002; 8(3):313–21.

45. Moreno-Ramirez D, Ferrandiz L, Bernal AP, et al. Teledermatology as a filtering system in pigmented lesion clinics. J Telemed Telecare 2005;11(6):298–303.

46. Moreno-Ramirez D, Ferrandiz L, Nieto-Garcia A, et al. Store and forward teledermatology in skin cancer triage: experience and evaluation of 2009 teleconsultations. Arch Dermatol 2007;143(7):479–84.

47. Knol A, van den Akker TW, Damstra RJ, et al. Teledermatology reduces the number of patient referrals to a dermatologist. J Telemed Telecare 2006;12(2):75–8.

48. Martinez-Garcia S, del Boz-Gonzalez J, Martin-Gonzalez T, et al. Teledermatology: review of 917 teleconsults. Actas Dermosifiliogr 2007;98(5):318–24.

49. Eminovic N, de Keizer NF, Wyatt JC, et al. Teledermatologic consultations and reduction in referrals to dermatologists: a cluster randomized controlled trial. Arch Dermatol 2009;145(5):558–64.

50. van der Heijden JP, de Keizer NF, Voorbaak FP, et al. A pilot study of tertiary dermatology: feasibility and acceptance of telecommunication among dermatologists. J Telemed Telecare 2010;16(8):447–53.

51. van der Heijden JP, de Keizer NF, Bos JD, et al. Teledermatology applied by following patient selection by general practitioners in daily practice improves efficiency and quality of care at lower costs. Br J Dermatol 2011;165(5):1058–65.

52. van der Heijden JP, de Keizer NF, Witkamp L, et al. Evaluation of a tertiary teledermatology service between peripheral and academic dermatologists in the Netherlands. Telemed J E Health 2013;20(4):332–7.

53. Lester J, Weinstock MA. Teletriage for provision of dermatologic care: a pilot program in the Department of Veterans Affairs. J Cutan Med Surg 2014;18(3):170–3.

54. Tandjung R, Badertscher N, Kleiner N, et al. Feasibility and diagnostic accuracy of teledermatology in Swiss primary care: process analysis of a randomized controlled trial. J Eval Clin Pract 2015;21(2):326–31.

55. McFarland LV, Raugi GJ, Taylor LL, et al. Implementation of an education and skills programme in a teledermatology project for rural veterans. J Telemed Telecare 2012;18(2):66–71.

56. Loane MA, Bloomer SE, Corbett R, et al. A randomized controlled trial assessing the health economics of realtime teledermatology compared with conventional care: an urban versus rural perspective. J Telemed Telecare 2001;7(2):108–18.

57. Wootton R, Bloomer SE, Corbett R, et al. Multicentre randomized control trial comparing real time teledermatology with conventional outpatient dermatological care: a societal cost-benefit analysis. BMJ 2000;320:1252–6.

58. Lamminen H, Tuomi ML, Lamminen J, et al. A feasibility study of realtime teledermatology in Finland. J Telemed Telecare 2000;6(2):102–7.

59. Granlund H, Thoden CJ, Carlson C, et al. Realtime teleconsultations versus face-to-face consultations in dermatology: immediate and six-month outcome. J Telemed Telecare 2003;9(4):204–9.

60. Pathipati AS, Lee L, Armstrong AW. Tailpiece – Health care delivery methods in teledermatology: consultative, triage, and direct-care models. J Telemed Telecare 2011;17(4):214–6.

61. Pak H, Triplett CA, Lindquist JH, et al. Store-and-forward teledermatology results in similar clinical outcomes to conventional clinic-based care. J Telemed Telecare 2007;13(1):26–30.

62. Whited JD, Warshaw EM, Kapur K, et al. Clinical course outcomes for store and forward teledermatology versus conventional consultation: a randomized trial. J Telemed Telecare 2013;19(4):197–204.

63. Fruhauf J, Krock S, Quehenberger F, et al. Mobile teledermatology helping patients control high-need acne: a randomized controlled trial. J Eur Acad Dermatol Venereol 2015;29(5):919–24.

64. Marcin JP, Nesbitt TS, Cole SL, et al. Changes in diagnosis, treatment, and clinical improvement among patients receiving telemedicine consultations. Telemed J E Health 2005;11(1):36–43.

65. Lamel S, Chambers CJ, Ratnararthorn M, et al. Impact of live interactive teledermatology on diagnosis, disease management, and clinical outcomes. Arch Dermatol 2012;148(1):61–5.

66. Weinstock MA, Nguyen FQ, Risica PM. Patient and provider satisfaction with teledermatology. J Am Acad Dermatol 2002;47(1):68–72.

67. Pak HS, Welch M, Poropatich R. Web-based teledermatology consult system: preliminary results from the first 100 cases. Stud Health Technol Inform 1999;64:179–84.

68. Kvedar JC, Menn ER, Baradagunta S, et al. Teledermatology in a capitated delivery system using distributed information architecture: design and development. Telemed J E Health 1999;5(4):357–66.
69. van den Akker TW, Reker CH, Knol A, et al. Teledermatology as a tool for communication between general practitioners and dermatologists. J Telemed Telecare 2001;7(4):193–8.
70. Williams TL, May CR, Esmail A, et al. Patient satisfaction with teledermatology is related to perceived quality of life. Br J Dermatol 2001;145(6):911–7.
71. Collins K, Walters S, Bowns I. Patient satisfaction with teledermatology: quantitative and qualitative results from a randomized controlled trial. J Telemed Telecare 2004;10(1):29–33.
72. Whited JD, Hall RP, Foy ME, et al. Patient and clinician satisfaction with a store-and-forward teledermatology consult system. Telemed J E Health 2004;10(4): 422–31.
73. Hsueh MT, Eastman K, McFarland LV, et al. Teledermatology patient satisfaction in the Pacific Northwest. Telemed J E Health 2012;18(5):377–81.
74. Ou MH, West GA, Lazarescu M, et al. Evaluation of TELEDERM for dermatological services in rural and remote areas. Artif Intell Med 2008;44(1):27–40.
75. McFarland LV, Raugi GJ, Reiber GE. Primary care provider and imaging technician satisfaction with a teledermatology project in rural Veterans Health Administration clinics. Telemed J E Health 2013;19(11):815–25.
76. Armstrong AW, Kwong MW, Chase EP, et al. Teledermatology operational considerations, challenges, and benefits: the referring providers' perspective. Telemed J E Health 2012;18(8):580–4.
77. Reid DS, Weaver LE, Sargeant JM, et al. Telemedicine in Nova Scotia: a report of a pilot study. Telemed J E Health 1998;4(3):249–58.
78. Loane MA, Bloomer SE, Corbett R, et al. Patient satisfaction with realtime teledermatology in Northern Ireland. J Telemed Telecare 1998;4(1):36–40.
79. Hicks LL, Boles KE, Hudson S, et al. Patient satisfaction with teledermatology services. J Telemed Telecare 2003;9(1):42–5.
80. Al Quran HA, Khader YS, Ellauzi ZM, et al. Effect of real-time teledermatology on diagnosis, treatment, and clinical improvement. J Telemed Telecare 2015;21(2): 93–9.
81. Jones DH, Crichton C, Macdonald A, et al. Teledermatology in the Highlands of Scotland. J Telemed Telecare 1996;2(S1):7–9.

Index

Note: Page numbers of article titles are in **boldface.**

A

ABCDEs, of melanoma, 1329–1330
Absorbable sutures, 1311
Accuracy, of teledermatology, 1367–1370
Acitretin, for lupus, 1292
Acne, 1179, 1181, 1200–1204
    topical medications for, 1168–1169, 1174
Actinic keratoses, 1169, 1175, 1327
Acute cutaneous lupus, 1287–1289
Acute generalized exanthematous pustulosis, 1260, 1341–1342
Adalimumab, 1184–1187, 1189
Adapalene, 1174, 1202
Adverse drug reactions, cutaneous, **1337–1348**
Alclometasone, for atopic dermatitis, 1278
Allergens
    in atopic dermatitis, 1282–1283
    top ten, 1247
Allergic contact dermatitis, 1246–1247
Allergic rhinitis, with atopic dermatitis, 1270
Alopecia, 1204–1210
    androgenic, 1207–1209
    classification of, 1205–1206
    diagnosis of, 1204–1205
    female pattern, 1207–1209
    in morphea, 1297
    telogen effluvium and, 1209–1210
Alopecia areata, 1205–1207, 1221
Aluminum chloride antiperspirants, for hyperhidrosis, 1198
American Academy of Dermatology Consensus group criteria, for atopic dermatitis, 1271, 1273–1274
American Board of Internal Medicine, "Choosing Wisely" program of, 1214
American Society of Dermatology, "Choosing Wisely" program of, 1214
Aminoglycosides, for pseudomonal nail infection, 1217
Amlodpine, for chilblains, 1256
Ammonium lactate, 1174
Androgenic alopecia, 1207–1209
Androgens, as targets, for acne treatment, 1203–1204
Anesthesia, for procedures, 1306
Angiosarcoma, 1332
Anthralin, for alopecia, 1207
Antifungal medications, 1173, 1213–1217
Antihistamines

Med Clin N Am 99 (2015) 1381–1399
http://dx.doi.org/10.1016/S0025-7125(15)00174-1
0025-7125/15/$ – see front matter © 2015 Elsevier Inc. All rights reserved.

Antihistamines (*continued*)
    for arthropod bites, 1250
    for atopic dermatitis, 1280, 1282
Antimicrobials, 1168, 1172–1173
Antinflammatories, for atopic dermatitis, 1276–1284
Antinuclear antibodies
    in dermatomyositis, 1295
    in lupus, 1289
Antiparasitic medications, 1173
Antiperspirants, for hyperhidrosis, 1198
Antiseptics, for procedures, 1306
Apocrine glands, physiology of, 1196
Arthralgia, in morphea, 1297
Arthropod bites, bullous reactions to, 1249–1250
Asteatotic eczema, 1169, 1176
Asthma, with atopic dermatitis, 1270
Atherosclerosis, in psoriasis, 1231–1232
Atopic dermatitis, **1269–1285**
    areas involved in, 1270–1271
    differential diagnosis of, 1273–1274
    incidence of, 1269
    laboratory tests for, 1271, 1273–1276
    pathophysiology of, 1270
    patient history for, 1269–1270
    physical examination for, 1270–1274
    symptoms of, 1269–1270
    treatment of, 1276–1284
Atopic march, 1270
Atrial fibrillation, in psoriasis, 1230–1231
Atrophy, after intralesional injection, 1315
Autoimmune diseases
    alopecia in, 1207
    blistering, 1250–1255
Avoidance, in allergic contact dermatitis, 1247
Avulsion technique, for onychomycosis, 1217
Axillary hyperhidrosis, 1197–1199
Azathioprine
    for atopic dermatitis, 1280–1281
    for dermatomyositis, 1296
    for lichen planus, 1220
    for lupus, 1292
Azelaic acid, 1174, 1202
Azithromycin, for acne, 1203

B

Bacterial impetigination, 1175–1177
Baker-Gordon formula peel, 1319
Barbiturate bullae (coma bullae), 1256–1257
Basal cell carcinoma, 1324–1326
Bathing, for atopic dermatitis, 1284

Bed bug bites, bullous reactions to, 1249–1250
Belimumab, for lupus, 1292
Benzoyl peroxide, 1172, 1179, 1202
Betamethasone, 1170
    for atopic dermatitis, 1278
    for eczema, 1177
Biologic therapies, **1183–1194**
    for psoriasis, 1233
    interleukin-17 inhibitors, 1185, 1188–1189
    interleukin-12/interleukin-23 inhibitors, 1185, 1187–1189
    intravenous immunoglobulin, 1185, 1189–1191
    rituximab, 1185, 1188–1189, 1292.1296
    tumor necrosis factor inhibitors, 1184–1187, 1189, 1233
Biopsies, 1306–1312. *See also individual diseases.*
    complications of, 1311–1312
    excisional, 1310, 1312
    for atopic dermatitis, 1273, 1276
    for blistering diseases, 1246
    for cutaneous adverse drug reactions, 1340
    for melanoma, 1331, 1333
    for pigmented lesions, 1310
    in immunosuppressed patient, 1352
    indications for, 1306
    postoperative care for, 1311
    punch, 1309–1310
    shave, 1306–1309
Bites, arthropod, bullous reactions to, 1249–1250
Blackheads, 1200
Bleach bath, for atopic dermatitis, 1283
Bleeding, after biopsy, 1311–1312
Bleomycin, for verrucae, 1218–1219
Blistering diseases, **1243–1267**
    autoimmune, 1250–1255
    diagnostic approach to, 1244
    drugs causing, 1254–1261, 1266
    external triggers causing, 1246–1250
    in infections, 1262–1266
    internal diseases causing, 1250, 1256–1262
    laboratory tests for, 1246
    patient history of, 1245
    physical examination for, 1244–1246
    rituximab for, 1190
Botulinum toxin
    for hyperhidrosis, 1199
    procedure for, 1317
Bowen disease, of nail, 1222
Briakinumab, for psoriasis, 1233
Brimonidine, 1174
Brodalumab, 1188
Budesonide, for atopic dermatitis, 1278
Bullae, definition of, 1245

Bullous cellulitis, 1265
Bullous diabeticorum, 1250, 1252, 1256
Bullous diseases. *See* Blistering diseases.
Bullous impetigo, 1264, 1266
Bullous lupus, 1252–1253
Bullous morphea, 1299
Bullous neutrophilic dermatoses, 1258, 1262
Bullous pemphigoid, 1252, 1261
Bullous pyoderma gangrenosum, 1258, 1262
Bullous tinea, 1265
Burow solution, for paronychia, 1218
Butterfly rash, in lupus, 1288–1289

C

Calcineurin inhibitors, for atopic dermatitis, 1279
Calciphylaxis, 1360–1361
Calcipotriene, 1174
Cancer. *See also* Melanoma; Skin cancer.
    due to tumor necrosis factor inhibitors, 1186
    in dermatomyositis, 1296
Candida infections, of nail, 1215–1217
Carcinoma
    basal cell, 1324–1326
    Merkel cell, 1332
    microcystic adnexal, 1332
    sebaceous, 1332
    squamous cell, 1326–1328
Cardiomyopathy, in psoriasis, 1230
Cardiovascular disease, psoriasis and, **1227–1242**
    pathophysiology of, 1231–1232
    prevalence of, 1228–1231
    risk factors for, 1233–1234
    screening for, 1233–1234
    therapies effects on, 1232–1233
Celiac disease, dermatitis herpetiformis in, 1255
Cellulitis, 1265, 1359
Cerebrovascular disease, in psoriasis, 1230–1231
Chemical denervation, 1317
Chemical peels, 1318–1319
Chemotherapy, for melanoma, 1333
Chickenpox, 1264
Chilblains, 1256
Chlorhexidine, for procedures, 1306
Chloroqine, for dermatomyositis, 1296
Chloroquine, for lupus, 1292
"Choosing Wisely" program, 1214
Chronic cutaneous lupus, 1287
Ciclopirox, 1178–1179, 1217
Clindamycin, 1172, 1202
Clobetasol, 1170, 1278

Clocortolone, for atopic dermatitis, 1278
Clonidine, for hyperhidrosis, 1199
Clotrimazole, 1173
Colchicine, for small vessel vasculitis, 1262
Cold exposure, chilblains in, 1256
Coma bullae, 1256–1257
Comedolytics, 1201–1203
Comedones, 1200–1204
Compensatory hyperhidrosis, 1197–1199
Consultation, inpatient, **1349–1364**
    barriers to, 1350
    cost savings and, 1350
    reasons for, 1349–1350
    teaching role in, 1350
Contact dermatitis
    allergic, 1246–1247
    consultation on, 1358
    irritant, 1247–1248
    of nail, 1221
Coronary artery disease, in psoriasis, 1230
Corticosteroids
    for allergic contact dermatitis, 1247
    for alopecia, 1207
    for arthropod bites, 1250
    for atopic dermatitis, 1277–1280
    for bullous neutrophilic dermatoses, 1262
    for dermatomyositis, 1249, 1296
    for irritant contact dermatitis, 1248
    for lichen planus, 1220
    for lupus, 1292
    for morphea, 1299–1300
    for paronychia, 1221
    for small vessel vasculitis, 1262
    intralesional injections of, 1314–1315
    topical, 1167–1168, 1170–1171
Cosmetic procedures, 1316–1317
Coup de sabre, in morphea, 1299
Creams, for atopic dermatitis, 1277–1278
Cryosurgery, 1313–1314
    for basal cell carcinoma, 1326
    for verrucae, 1218
Curettage, 1312–1313
    for basal cell carcinoma, 1326
    for hyperhidrosis, 1199
Cutaneous adverse drug reactions, **1337–1348**
    acute generalized exanthematous pustulosis, 1341–1342
    complicated versus uncomplicated, 1338–1340
    definition of, 1337
    diagnosis of, 1338–1340
    DRESS/DIHS (drug reaction with eosinophilia and systemic symptoms/drug-induced
        hypersensitivity syndrome, 1344–1346

Cutaneous (*continued*)
    epidemiology of, 1337
    morbilliform, 1351–1352
    spectrum of, 1337
    Stevens-Johnson syndrome, 1342–1344
    toxic epidermal necrolysis, 1342–1344
Cutaneous lupus. *See* Lupus.
Cutaneous lymphoma, 1333
Cyclosporine, for atopic dermatitis, 1280–1281
Cyst(s), digital mucous, 1223
Cytokines, in psoriasis, 1231–1232

D

Dandruff, 1179–1180
Dapsone, 1172
    for acne, 1202
    for lupus, 1292
    for small vessel vasculitis, 1262
Deep vein thrombosis, in psoriasis, 1229–1230
Denervation, chemical, 1317
Dermatitis
    allergic contact, 1246–1247
    atopic. *See* Atopic dermatitis.
    contact. *See* Contact dermatitis.
    irritant contact, 1247–1248
    seborrheic, 1179–1180, 1273, 1275
    stasis, 1359
    topical medications for, 1167–1168
Dermatitis herpetiformis, 1255
Dermatofibrosarcoma protuberans, 1332
Dermatology
    adverse drug reactions, **1337–1348**
    atopic dermatitis, **1269–1285**
    biologic therapies, **1183–1194**
    dermatomyositis, 1292–1297
    diffuse blisters, **1243–1267**
    inpatient consultation, **1349–1364**
    lupus, 1287–1303
    morphea, 1297–1300
    nail disease, **1213–1226**
    procedures, **1305–1321**
    psoriasis. *See* Psoriasis and psoriatic arthritis.
    rheumatologic disorders, **1287–1303**
    skin appendage disorders, **1195–1211**
    skin cancer. *See* Melanoma; Skin cancer.
    teledermatology, **1365–1379**
    topical therapy, **1167–1182**
Dermatomyositis, 1292–1297
Dermatophyte infections, of nail, 1214–1217
Desonide, 1171, 1179, 1278

Desoximetasone, 1170, 1278
Dexamethasone, for atopic dermatitis, 1278
Diabetes mellitus
    blistering in, 1250, 1252, 1256
    in psoriasis, 1229
Diagnosis, teledermatology for, **1365–1379**
Diclofenac, 1175
Diffuse blisters. *See* Blistering diseases.
Diflorasone, for atopic dermatitis, 1278
Digital images, for teledermatology, 1365–1379
Digital mucous cysts, 1223
Diphenylcyclopropenone
    for alopecia, 1207
    for verrucae, 1218–1219
Direct immunofluorescence test, for blistering diseases, 1246
Discoid cutaneous lupus, 1290
Distal-lateral subungual onychomycosis, 1216
DMARDs, 1186
Double-stranded DNA, antibodies to, in lupus, 1289
Doxycycline, for acne, 1202–1203
DRESS/DIHS (drug reaction with eosinophilia and systemic symptoms/drug-induced
    hypersensitivity syndrome, 1344–1346
Drug(s), adverse reactions to, **1337–1348**
    bullous eruptions, 1259, 1265–1266
    lupus, 1288
Drug chart, 1352
Dyslipidemia, in psoriasis, 1228–1229, 1234

E

Eccrine glands, physiology of, 1195–1196
Econazole, 1173
Eczema, 1177. *See also* Atopic dermatitis.
    asteatotic, 1169, 1176
Eczema herpeticum, 1283–1284
Edema bullae, 1257
Efinaconazole, 1173, 1179, 1217
Eikenella infections, of nail fold, 1217–1218
Electrodessication, for basal cell carcinoma, 1326
Emollients, for atopic dermatitis, 1177, 1275–1277, 1284
Environmental factors
    in atopic dermatitis, 1282–1283
    in psoriasis, 1228
Epidermolysis bullosa aquisita, 1253
Epidermophyton infections, of nails, 1214
Epinephrine, added to anesthesia, 1306
Erythema multiforme, 1260, 1290–1291
Erythromycin, for acne, 1202
Erythronychia, longitudinal, 1222
Erythropoetin, for porphyria, 1258
Esthetic procedures, 1316–1317

Etanercept, 1184–1189, 1233
Excessive (hyperhidrosis) sweating, 1197–1199
Excision, for basal cell carcinoma, 1326
Exercise, for dermatomyositis, 1296
Exostosis, subungual, 1222

F

Fatigue, in morphea, 1297
Female pattern alopecia, 1207–1209
Fibroxanthoma, atypical, 1332
Filaggrin defects, in atopic dermatitis, 1270
Fillers, injectable, 1317
Finasteride
    for acne, 1204
    for alopecia, 1209
Fixed drug eruption, 1259
Flaccid bullae, definition of, 1245
Flea bites, bullous reactions to, 1249–1250
Fluconazole, for onychomycosis, 1217
Fluocinonide, 1170–1171, 1278
Fluoroquinolone, for pseudomonal nail infection, 1217
5-Fluorouracil, 1175
Flurandrenolide, for atopic dermatitis, 1278
Fluticasone, for atopic dermatitis, 1278
Fungal infections
    in immunosuppressed patient, 1354–1356
    of nail, 1213–1217
Furocoumarins, toxicity of, 1248–1249

G

Gels, for atopic dermatitis, 1277
Generalized cutaneous lupus, 1290
Generalized plaque morphea, 1297
Genetic factors
    in adverse drug reactions, 1342
    in DRESS/DIHS, 1344
    in psoriasis, 1231–1232
Glomus tumor, of nail, 1222
Glycolic acid, for chemical peel, 1319
Glycopyrrolate, for hyperhidrosis, 1198–1199
Goeckerman therapy, for atopic dermatitis, 1280
Graft-versus-host disease, acute, 1353
Grotton pappules, in dermatomyositis, 1293
Gustatory hyperhidrosis, 1197–1199
Guttate morphea, 1299

H

Hair follicles, physiology of, 1195–1196
Hair loss, 1204–1210, 1297

Hair pull test, 1204–1205
Halcinonide, for atopic dermatitis, 1278
Halobetasol, 1170, 1278
Hand, dermatitis of, 1177
Heart, disorders of, in dermatomyositis, 1294
Heart failure, in psoriasis, 1230
Heliotrope rash, in dermatomyositis, 1293
Hematomas, after biopsy, 1311–1312
Hemorrhage, after biopsy, 1311–1312
Hemostasis, for biopsies, 1308–1309
Hepatitis, in DRESS/DIHS, 1345
Hepatitis B
    reactivation of, in rituximab therapy, 1190
    screening for, before medication prescription, 1184–1185
Hepatitis C, screening for, before medication prescription, 1184–1186
Herpes group infections, in immunosuppressed patient, 1352–1353
Herpes simplex virus infections, blisters in, 1263
HIV infection, screening for, before medication prescription, 1186
Hormones, for acne, 1203–1204
Human papillomavirus infections, warts in, 1218–1219
Hybrid technique, in teledermatology, 1366–1367
Hydrocortisone, 1171, 1179
    for atopic dermatitis, 1278
    for hyperhidrosis, 1198
Hydroxychloroquine, 1258
    for chilblains, 1256
    for dermatomyositis, 1296
    for lupus, 1291–1292
Hygiene hypothesis, 1270
Hyperhidrosis, 1197–1199
Hyperpigmentation
    after chemical peels, 1318–1319
    in morphea, 1297
    in phytophotodermatitis, 1248–1249
Hypertension, in psoriasis, 1229
Hypopigmentation, after intralesional injection, 1315
Hypothalamus, hyperhidrosis and, 1197
Hypothalamus-pituitary axis dysfunction, 1279

I

Id reaction, 1246
Imiquimod, 1175
Immunosuppressed patient
    herpes group infections in, 1352–1353
    opportunistic fungal infections in, 1353–1354
    rash in, 1352
    varicella zoster infection in, 1356
Immunotherapy
    for melanoma, 1333
    intralesional, for verrucae, 1218–1219

Impetigination, bacterial, 1175–1177
Impetigo, bullous, 1264, 1266
Infections
    after biopsy, 1311–1312
    bullous dermatoses in, 1262–1266
    in atopic dermatitis, 1283–1284
    of nail unit, 1213–1219
    topical medications for, 1168
Inflammation, topical medications for, 1167–1168
Inflammatory acne, 1202–1203
Inflammatory dermatoses, of nail unit, 1219–1221
Infliximab, 1184–1187, 1189
Ingenol mebutate, 1175
Injectable fillers, 1317
Injections, intralesional, of corticosteroids, 1314–1315
Interleukin-12/23 inhibitors, 1185, 1187–1189, 1233, 1273
Interleukin-17 inhibitors, 1185, 1188–1189, 1233
Internal diseases, blistering diseases in, 1250, 1256–1262
Intraepidermal split, in autoimmune disorders, 1266
Intralesional injections, of corticosteroids, 1314–1315
Intravenous immunoglobulin, 1185, 1189–1191
Iontophoresis, for hyperhidrosis, 1199
iPledge program, 1203
Irritant contact dermatitis, 1247–1248
Isopropyl alcohol, for procedures, 1306
Isotretinoin
    for acne, 1203
    for lupus, 1292
Itraconazole, for onychomycosis, 1216–1217
Ivermectin, 1173
Ixekizumab, 1188

J

Jessner solution, for chemical peel, 1319
Jo-1 antigen, antibodies to, in dermatomyositis, 1295

K

Kaposi sarcoma, 1332
Keloidal morphea, 1299
Keloids, after biopsy, 1312
Keratinocytes
    apoptosis of, 1342–1344
    atypical proliferation of, 1326–1328
Keratolytics, for verrucae, 1218–1219
Ketoconazole, 1173, 1179
Kidney disease
    calciphylaxis in, 1360–1361
    in psoriasis, 1229

L

Laser therapy
    for onychomycosis, 1217
    for verrucae, 1219
    procedure for, 1317
Leiomyosarcoma, 1333
Lenalidomide, for lupus, 1292
Lichen planus
    lupus overlap with, 1290
    of nail unit, 1220
Lichen sclerosis, morphea and, 1297
Lichenification, in atopic dermatitis, 1271
Lidocaine, for procedures, 1306
Linear IgA bullous dermatosis, drug-induced, 1261, 1266
Linear morphea, 1298–1299
Lipodermatosclerosis, 1359
Liposuction technique, for hyperhidrosis, 1199
Liquid nitrogen, for cryotherapy, 1218, 1313–1314
Liver involvement, in DRESS/DIHS, 1345
Local anesthesia, for procedures, 1306
Longitudinal erythronychia, 1222
Longitudinal melanonychia, 1221–1222
Lotions, for atopic dermatitis, 1277–1278
Lung, interstitial disease of, dermatomyositis, 1295–1296
Lupus, 1287–1303
    blistering in, 1252–1253
    classification of, 1287
    clinical findings in, 1288–1291
    dermatomyositis overlaps with, 1296
    disorders overlapping with, 1290–1291
    history of, 1287–1288
    natural history of, 1288
    treatment of, 1291–1292
Lupus profundus, 1291
Lymphoma
    cutaneous, 1333
    due to tumor necrosis factor inhibitors, 1186

M

Malar erythema, in lupus, 1288–1289
Malignancy. *See* Cancer; Melanoma; Skin cancer.
Malignant fibrous histiocytoma, 1332
MDAS antibodies, in dermatomyositis, 1295
Mechanic's hands, in dermatomyositis, 1293, 1295
Melanoma, 1328–1333
    biopsy for, 1311–1312
    detection of, 1329–1331
    epidemiology of, 1328–1329
    treatment of, 1331, 1333

Melanonychia, longitudinal, 1221–1222
Merkel cell carcinoma, 1332
Metabolic syndrome, in psoriasis, 1228–1229
Metastasis, from squamous cell carcinoma, 1328
Methotrexate
    for atopic dermatitis, 1280–1281
    for dermatomyositis, 1296
    for lupus, 1292
    for morphea, 1300
    for psoriasis, 1232–1233
Metronidazole, 1172
Mi-2 antibodies, in dermatomyositis, 1295
Microcomedones, 1200–1204
Microcystic adnexal carcinoma, 1332
Microscopy, for onychomycosis, 1214
Microsporum infections, of nails, 1214
Microvascular disease, in psoriasis, 1229–1230
Minocycline, for acne, 1202–1203
Minoxidil, for alopecia, 1209
Mohs micrographic surgery, 1316
    for basal cell carcinoma, 1324–1326
    for melanoma, 1333
    for squamous cell carcinoma, 1328
Moisturizers, for atopic dermatitis, 1275–1276
Mometasone, for atopic dermatitis, 1278
Morbilliform drug eruptions, 1351–1352
Morphea, 1297–1300
Morpheaform basal cell carcinoma, 1324–1325
Mosquito bites, bullous reactions to, 1249–1250
Mucosa, lupus affecting, 1291
Multifocal basal cell carcinoma, 1324–1325
Mupirocin, 1172
Muscle disorders, in dermatomyositis, 1292–1297
Myalgia, in morphea, 1297
Mycophenolate mofetil
    for atopic dermatitis, 1280, 1282
    for dermatomyositis, 1296
    for lupus, 1292
    for morphea, 1300
Mycosis fungoides, 1333
Myocardial infarction, in psoriasis, 1230
Myositis, in dermatomyositis, 1292–1297

N

Nail(s), physiology of, 1195–1196
Nail disease, **1213–1226**
    infections, 1213–1219
    inflammatory dermatoses, 1219–1221
    neoplasms, 1221–1223
National Comprehensive Cancer Network criteria, 1324

National Psoriasis Foundation, 1233–1234
Neoplasms. *See also* Melanoma; Skin cancer.
   list of, 1332–1333
   of nail unit, 1221–1223
Nevi, melanoma risk and, 1329
Nifedipine, for chilblains, 1256
Nikolsky sign, 1245, 1339
Nodular basal cell carcinoma, 1324–1325
Nodulocystic acne, 1203
Nonabsorbable sutures, 1311
Nonsteroidal anti-inflammatory drugs, cutaneous reactions to, 1339
North American Contact Dermatitis Group, top ten allergen list of, 1247

O

Obesity, in psoriasis, 1228, 1234
Ocular involvement, in Stevens-Johnson syndrome, 1342–1343
Oil formulations, for atopic dermatitis, 1277–1278
Ointments, for atopic dermatitis, 1277–1278
Onycholysis, 1178–1179
Onychomycosis, 1213–1217
Open-spray cryotherapy, 1313–1314
Oral contraceptives, for acne, 1204
Oral involvement, in Stevens-Johnson syndrome, 1342–1343
Outcomes, in teledermatology, 1371–1372
Oxybutynin, for hyperhidrosis, 1199

P

P-155/140 antibodies, in dermatomyositis, 1295
Paget disease, 1332
Pain, after biopsy, 1311–1312
Palmar hyperhidrosis, 1197–1199
Panniculitis, lupus, 1291
Pansclerotic morphea, 1297–1298
Papilloma, nail bed, 1222
Papules
   basal cell carcinoma, 1324–1325
   in atopic dermatitis, 1270
Paronychia
   acute, 1217–1218
   chronic, 1221
Patch test, for irritant contact dermatitis, 1248
Peels, chemical, 1318–1319
Pemphigoid gestationis, 1254
Pemphigus foliaceus, 1251
Pemphigus vulgaris, 1251, 1261
Periodic acid-Schiff test, for onychomycosis, 1214
Peripheral arterial disease, in psoriasis, 1230
Periungual verrucae, 1218–1219
Permethrin, 1173

Petrolatum, 1168
Photodynamic therapy
    for basal cell carcinoma, 1326
    for onychomycosis, 1217
Photoprotection, for porphyria, 1258
Photosensitivity, in lupus, 1289
Phototherapy
    for atopic dermatitis, 1280
    for morphea, 1299–1300
    for psoriasis, 1233
Phototoxic bullous eruption, 1248–1249
Phototoxic drug eruption, 1260
Phytophotodermatitis, 1248–1249
Pigmented lesions
    basal cell carcinoma, 1324–1325
    biopsy for, 1311
Pimecrolimus, 1174, 1279
Pioglitazone, for psoriasis, 1234
Plantar hyperhidrosis, 1197–1199
Plants, furocoumarins in, toxicity of, 1248–1249
Plaque(s)
    in atopic dermatitis, 1270
    in morphea, 1297–1299
Poison ivy dermatitis, 1246
Polymerase chain reaction, for blistering diseases, 1246
Porphyria cutanea tarda, 1257–1258
Potassium hydroxide test, for onychomycosis, 1214
Povidone-iodine, for procedures, 1306
Prednisone
    for alopecia, 1207
    for dermatomyositis, 1296
Pregnancy, pemphigoid gestationis in, 1254
Pressure, coma bullae due to, 1256–1257
Primary hyperhidrosis, 1197–1199
Procedures, **1305–1321**
    advanced, 1315–1319
    antiseptics for, 1306
    biopsies. *See* Biopsies.
    cryosurgery, 1218, 1313–1314
    curettage, 1199, 1312–1313
    local anesthesia for, 1306
    patient preparation for, 1305–1306
    saucerization, 1308
Proximal subungual onychomycosis, 1215
Prurigo, in atopic dermatitis, 1271
Pruritus
    in allergic contact dermatitis, 1246–1247
    in arthropod bites, 1249–1250
    in atopic dermatitis, 1269–1285
Pseudomonal nail infection, 1217
Pseudoporphyria, drug-induced, 1261

Psoralen with phototherapy, for atopic dermatitis, 1280
Psoriasis and psoriatic arthritis
    biologic therapy for, 1184–1185, 1188–1189
    cardiovascular disease and, **1227–1242**
    of nail unit, 1219–1220
    topical medications for, 1168–1169, 1174
    versus atopic dermatitis, 1273
Psoriasis Area and Severity Index, 1187
Psoriasis Longitudinal Assessment and Registry, 1187
Pulmonary embolism, in psoriasis, 1229–1230
Punch biopsies, 1309–1310
Pustulosis, acute generalized exanthematous, 1341–1342
Pyoderma gangrenosum, 1361

Q

Quinacrine, for lupus, 1292

R

Radiotherapy, for basal cell carcinoma, 1326
Rash. *See also* Blistering diseases.
    in allergic contact dermatitis, 1246–1247
    in atopic dermatitis, 1269–1285
    in dermatomyositis, 1292–1297
    in immunosuppressed patient, 1352
    in lupus, 1287–1303
    in morphea, 1297–1300
Raynaud phenomenon, in morphea, 1299
Real-time interactive technique, in teledermatology, 1366–1375
Red legs, 1359
Reliability, of teledermatology, 1368–1369
Retinoids
    for acne, 1202–1203
    for lichen planus, 1220
    for lupus, 1292
    for psoriasis, 1232–1233
Rheumatologic skin diseases, **1287–1303**
    dermatomyositis, 1292–1297
    lupus, 1252–1253, 1287–1292
    morphea, 1297–1300
Rituximab, 1185, 1188–1189
    for dermatomyositis, 1296
    for lupus, 1292
Rodent-ulcer, in basal cell carcinoma, 1324–1325
Rosacea, topical medications for, 1168–1169, 1174
Rowell syndrome, 1290–1291
Ruxolitinib, for alopecia, 1207

S

Salicylic acid, 1174
    for acne, 1202

Salicylic (*continued*)
    for chemical peel, 1319
    for verrucae, 1218–1219
Sarcoma, Kaposi, 1332
Satisfaction, with teledermatology, 1372–1375
Saucerization, 1308
Scabies
    bullous reactions in, 1249–1250
    versus atopic dermatitis, 1273
Scalp
    hair loss in, 1204–1210
    morphea in, 1297
Scarring
    after biopsy, 1311–1312
    after chemical peels, 1318–1319
Scissor biopsies, 1308
Sclerosing variant, of basal call carcinoma, 1324–1325
Sebaceous carcinoma, 1332
Sebaceous glands
    acne development in, 1200–1204
    physiology of, 1195–1196
Seborrheic dermatitis, 1179–1180, 1273, 1275
Secondary hyperhidrosis, 1197–1199
Seconkinumab, 1188
Secukinumab, 1185
Severity of Illness Score for Toxic Epidermal Necrolysis, 1344
Shave biopsies, 1306–1309
Shawl sign, in dermatomyositis, 1293
Skin appendages, disorders of, **1195–1211**
    acne, 1179, 1181, 1200–1204
    alopecia, 1204–1210
    hyperhidrosis, 1197–1199
    pathophysiology of, 1195–1196
Skin barrier
    dysfunction of, in atopic dermatitis, 1270
    restoration of, for atopic dermatitis, 1275–1276
Skin cancer, **1323–1335**. *See also* Melanoma.
    basal cell carcinoma, 1324–1326
    epidemiology of, 1323–1324
    potential of, 1332–1333
    squamous cell carcinoma, 1326–1328
    topical medications for, 1169, 1175
Small vessel vasculitis, 1262
Smith antigen, antibodies to, in lupus, 1289
Snip biopsies, 1308
Society for Rheumatology Biologics Registry, 1186
Sodium hypochlorite, for atopic dermatitis, 1283
Soft tissue augmentation, 1317
Specimen processing, 1309
Spironolactone
    for acne, 1204

for alopecia, 1209
Squamous cell carcinoma, 1326–1328
Squaric acid butyl ester
    for alopecia, 1207
    for verrucae, 1218–1219
SSA antibodies, in lupus, 1289
Staphylococcus aureus infections
    in atopic dermatitis, 1283–1284
    of nail fold, 1217
Stasis dermatitis, 1359
Stevens-Johnson syndrome, 1259, 1266, 1342–1344, 1351–1352
Streptococcal infections
    of nail fold, 1217–1218
    red legs in, 1359
Stroke, in psoriasis, 1230–1231
Subacute cutaneous lupus, 1287, 1289–1290
Subungual exostosis, 1222
Subungual onychomycosis, 1214–1215
Sulfacetamide-sulfur, 1172, 1202
Sunscreen
    for dermatomyositis, 1296
    for lupus, 1292
Superficial basal cell carcinoma, 1324–1325
Superficial morphea, 1299
Superficial white onychomycosis, 1214–1215
Supportive care, for Stevens-Johnson syndrome, 1343–1344
Sutures, for biopsies, 1309–1312
Swallowing difficulty, in dermatomyositis, 1293
Sweating, excessive (hyperhidrosis), 1197–1199
Sweet syndrome, 1258, 1262, 1356
Sympathectomy, for hyperhidrosis, 1199
Synthetase, antibodies to, in dermatomyositis, 1295
Systemic sclerosis
    dermatomyositis overlaps with, 1296
    versus morphea, 1297, 1299

T

Tacrolimus, 1174
    for atopic dermatitis, 1279
    for paronychia, 1221
Tanning, as melanoma risk, 1329
Tavaborole, for onychomycosis, 1217
Tazarotene, 1174, 1202
Tea tree oil, for acne, 1202
Teacher, dermatologist as, 1350
Telangiectasia, in dermatomyositis, 1293
Teledermatology, **1365–1379**
    averting clinic visits with, 1370–1371
    clinical outcomes of, 1371–1372
    diagnostic reliability and accuracy of, 1367–1370

Teledermatology (*continued*)
    modalities of, 1366–1367
    satisfaction with, 1372–1375
Telogen effluvium, 1209–1210
Tense bullae, definition of, 1245
Terbinafine, 1173, 1216–1217
Thalidomide, for lupus, 1292
Tinea, bullous, 1265
Tinea pedis, 1266
Tinea unguium, 1178–1179, 1214
Topical therapy
    case studies using, 1169, 1175–1180
    for acne, 1200–1204
    for basal cell carcinoma, 1326
    for hyperhidrosis, 1198–1199
    for onychomycosis, 1217
    for pseudomonal nail infection, 1217
    medications for, 1167–1175
Toxic epidermis necrolysis, 1259, 1266, 1351–1352
Transplantation
    as squamous cell carcinoma risk, 1327
    graft-versus-host disease in, 1353
Travel, to clinics, teledermatology and, 1370–1371
Tretinoin, 1174, 1179
Triamcinolone, 1169–1170
    for atopic dermatitis, 1278
    for lupus, 1292
Trichloroacetic acid, for chemical peel, 1319
Trichophyton infections, 1178–1179, 1214
Tuberculosis screening, before medication prescription, 1184–1185
Tumid lupus, 1291
Tumor(s)
    list of, 1332–1333
    malignant. *See* Melanoma; Skin cancer.
Tumor necrosis factor inhibitors, 1184–1187, 1189, 1233

U

Ulcers, 1359–1360
    in calciphylaxis, 1360–1361
    in pyoderma gangrenosum, 1361
    in squamous cell carcinoma, 1328
Ultraviolet light
    as basal cell carcinoma risk factor, 1324
    as melanoma risk, 1329
    as squamous cell carcinoma risk, 1326–1327
    for atopic dermatitis, 1280
    for morphea, 1299–1300
    furocoumarin reaction with, 1248–1249
Urea, 1174
Uremia, calciphylaxis in, 1360–1361

Usetkinumab, for psoriasis, 1233
Ustekinumab, 1185, 1189

V

Varicella infections, 1264, 1356
Vasculitis, small vessel, 1262
Vehicles, for topical medications, 1169
Venous thromboembolism, in psoriasis, 1229–1230
Verrucae, periungual, 1218–1219
Vesicles, definition of, 1245
Veterans Affairs Puget Sound Health Care System Dermatology Service, 1371–1372, 1374
Vibrio vulnificus infections, blisters in, 1265–1266
Videoconferencing, for teledermatology, 1365–1379
Vitamin D deficiency, in lupus, 1292
Voice, difficulty with, in dermatomyositis, 1293

W

Warts, periungual, 1218–1219
Wet wraps, for atopic dermatitis, 1284
Whiteheads, 1200
Wound dehiscence, after biopsy, 1312

United States Postal Service

Statement of Ownership, Management, and Circulation
(All Periodicals Publications Except Requestor Publications)

1. Publication Title	2. Publication Number	3. Filing Date
Medical Clinics of North America	3 3 7 - 3 4 0	9/18/15

4. Issue Frequency	5. Number of Issues Published Annually	6. Annual Subscription Price
Jan, Mar, May, Jul, Sep, Nov	6	$255.00

7. Complete Mailing Address of Known Office of Publication (Not printer) (Street, city, county, state, and ZIP+4®)

Elsevier Inc.
360 Park Avenue South
New York, NY 10010-1710

Contact Person
Stephen R. Bushing
Telephone (Include area code)
215-239-3688

8. Complete Mailing Address of Headquarters or General Business Office of Publisher (Not printer)

Elsevier Inc. 360 Park Avenue South, New York, NY 10010-1710

9. Full Names and Complete Mailing Addresses of Publisher, Editor, and Managing Editor (Do not leave blank)

Publisher (Name and complete mailing address)

Linda Belfus, Elsevier Inc. 1600 John F. Kennedy Blvd., Suite 1800, Philadelphia, PA 19103

Editor (Name and complete mailing address)

Jessica McCool, Elsevier Inc. 1600 John F. Kennedy Blvd., Suite 1800, Philadelphia, PA 19103-2899

Managing Editor (Name and complete mailing address)

Adrianne Brigido, Elsevier Inc. 1600 John F. Kennedy Blvd., Suite 1800, Philadelphia, PA 19103-2899

10. Owner (Do not leave blank. If the publication is owned by a corporation, give the name and address of the corporation immediately followed by the names and addresses of all stockholders owning or holding 1 percent or more of the total amount of stock. If not owned by a corporation, give the names and addresses of the individual owners. If owned by a partnership or other unincorporated firm, give its name and address as well as those of each individual owner. If the publication is published by a nonprofit organization, give its name and address.)

Full Name	Complete Mailing Address
Wholly owned subsidiary of	1600 John F. Kennedy Blvd, Ste. 1800
Reed/Elsevier, US holdings	Philadelphia, PA 19103-2899

11. Known Bondholders, Mortgagees, and Other Security Holders Owning or Holding 1 Percent or More of Total Amount of Bonds, Mortgages, or Other Securities. If none, check box ☐ None

Full Name	Complete Mailing Address
N/A	

12. Tax Status (For completion by nonprofit organizations authorized to mail at nonprofit rates) (Check one)
The purpose, function, and nonprofit status of this organization and the exempt status for federal income tax purposes:
☐ Has Not Changed During Preceding 12 Months
☐ Has Changed During Preceding 12 Months (Publisher must submit explanation of change with this statement)

13. Publication Title	14. Issue Date for Circulation Data Below
Medical Clinics of North America	July 2015

PS Form 3526, July 2014 (Page 1 of 3 (Instructions Page 3)) PSN 7530-01-000-9931 PRIVACY NOTICE: See our Privacy policy in www.usps.com

---

15. Extent and Nature of Circulation			Average No. Copies Each Issue During Preceding 12 Months	No. Copies of Single Issue Published Nearest to Filing Date
a. Total Number of Copies (Net press run)			1605	1279
b. Legitimate Paid and/or Requested Distribution (By Mail and Outside the Mail)	(1)	Mailed Outside-County Paid/Requested Mail Subscriptions stated on PS Form 3541. (Include paid distribution above nominal rate, advertiser's proof copies and exchange copies)	714	549
	(2)	Mailed In-County Paid/Requested Mail Subscriptions stated on PS Form 3541. (Include paid distribution above nominal rate, advertiser's proof copies and exchange copies)		
	(3)	Paid Distribution Outside the Mails Including Sales Through Dealers And Carriers, Street Vendors, Counter Sales, and Other Paid Distribution Outside USPS®	286	280
	(4)	Paid Distribution by Other Classes of Mail Through the USPS (e.g. First-Class Mail®)		
c. Total Paid and or Requested Circulation (Sum of 15b (1), (2), (3), and (4))			1000	829
d. Free or Nominal Rate Distribution (By Mail and Outside the Mail)	(1)	Free or Nominal Rate Outside-County Copies included on PS Form 3541	123	110
	(2)	Free or Nominal Rate In-County Copies included on PS Form 3541		
	(3)	Free or Nominal Rate Copies mailed at Other classes Through the USPS (e.g. First-Class Mail®)		
	(4)	Free or Nominal Rate Distribution Outside the Mail (Carriers or other means)		
e. Total Nonrequested Distribution (Sum of 15d (1), (2), (3) and (4))			123	110
f. Total Distribution (Sum of 15c and 15e)			1123	939
g. Copies not Distributed (See Instructions to publishers #4 (page #3))			482	340
h. Total (Sum of 15f and g)			1605	1279
i. Percent Paid and/or Requested Circulation (15c divided by 15f times 100)			89.05%	88.29%

* If you are claiming electronic copies go to line 16 on page 3. If you are not claiming Electronic copies skip to line 17 on page 3.

16. Electronic Copy Circulation	Average No. Copies Each Issue During Preceding 12 Months	No. Copies of Single Issue Published Nearest to Filing Date
a. Paid Electronic Copies		
b. Total paid Print Copies (Line 15c) + Paid Electronic copies (Line 16a)		
c. Total Print Distribution (Line 15f) + Paid Electronic Copies (Line 16a)		
d. Percent Paid (Both Print & Electronic copies) (16b divided by 16c X 100)		

☐ I certify that 50% of all my distributed copies (electronic and print) are paid above a nominal price

17. Publication of Statement of Ownership
If the publication is a general publication, publication of this statement is required. Will be printed in the **November 2015** issue of this publication.

18. Signature and Title of Editor, Publisher, Business Manager, or Owner	Date
Stephen R. Bushing	September 18, 2015
Stephen R. Bushing – Inventory Distribution Coordinator	

I certify that all information furnished on this form is true and complete. I understand that anyone who furnishes false or misleading information on this form or who omits material or information requested on the form may be subject to criminal sanctions (including fines and imprisonment) and/or civil sanctions (including civil penalties).

PS Form 3526, July 2014 (Page 3 of 3)

Moving?

Make sure your subscription moves with you!

To notify us of your new address, find your **Clinics Account Number** (located on your mailing label above your name), and contact customer service at:

Email: journalscustomerservice-usa@elsevier.com

800-654-2452 (subscribers in the U.S. & Canada)
314-447-8871 (subscribers outside of the U.S. & Canada)

Fax number: 314-447-8029

Elsevier Health Sciences Division
Subscription Customer Service
3251 Riverport Lane
Maryland Heights, MO 63043

ELSEVIER

Printed and bound by CPI Group (UK) Ltd, Croydon, CR0 4YY

03/10/2024

01040487-0010